PROBLEM-ORIENTATED
CLINICAL MICROBIOLOGY
AND INFECTION

CHURCHILL LIVINGSTONE
Medical Division of Pearson Professional Limited

Distributed in the United States of America by Churchill Livingstone
Inc., 650 Avenue of the Americas, New York, N.Y. 10011, and by
associated companies, branches and representatives throughout the
world.

First published 1996

ISBN 0 443 04914 9

British Library Cataloguing in Publication Data
A catalogue record for this book is available from the British Library

Library of Congress Cataloging in Publication Data
A catalog record for this book is available from the Library of
Congress

Medical knowledge is constantly changing. As new information
becomes available, changes in treatment, procedures, equipment
and the use of drugs becomes necessary. The authors and the
publishers have, as far as it is possible, taken care to ensure that the
information given in the text is accurate and up to date. However,
readers are strongly advised to confirm that the information,
especially with regard to drug usage, complies with current legislation
and standards of practice.

Printed in Hong Kong
WW/01

For Churchill Livingstone
Publisher: Timothy Horne
Project Editors: James Killgore, Janice Urquhart
Copy Editor: Jennifer Bew
Indexer: John Sampson
Project Controller: Nancy Arnott
Design Direction: Erik Bigland

PROBLEM-ORIENTATED CLINICAL MICROBIOLOGY AND INFECTION

HILARY HUMPHREYS

MD BCh BAO FRCPI MRCPath
Senior Lecturer in Microbiology, University of Nottingham, Nottingham;
Honorary Consultant, University Hospital, Nottingham;
Honorary Consultant, Public Health Laboratory Service

WILLIAM L. IRVING

MA MB BChir MRCP PhD MRCPath
Senior Lecturer in Clinical Virology, University of Nottingham, Nottingham;
Honorary Consultant, University Hospital, Nottingham;
Honorary Consultant, Public Health Laboratory Service

Foreword by
DAVID C. E. SPELLER

MA BM BCh FRCP FRCPath
Head of the Antibiotic Reference Unit, Central Public Health Laboratory, Colindale, London;
Emeritus Professor of Clinical Microbiology, University of Bristol, Bristol, UK

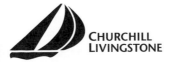

CHURCHILL LIVINGSTONE

NEW YORK EDINBURGH LONDON MADRID MELBOURNE SAN FRANCISCO TOKYO 1996

CONTENTS

Foreword   *vii*
How to use this book   *vii*
Acknowledgements   *viii*
Abbreviations   *ix*

1. CENTRAL NERVOUS SYSTEM

Case 1	Nigel, a 3-year-old boy with lethargy and a skin rash	*1*
Case 2	Mr Aldridge, a 45-year-old accountant with odd behaviour and a fever	*3*
Case 3	Jim, a 72-year-old man with progressive headache	*6*
Case 4	John, a 75-year-old with muscle weakness	*9*
Case 5	Andrew, a 20-year-old student with fever, nausea and headache	*10*
Case 6	Mr Grundy, a 62-year-old histopathology technician who has become forgetful and disorientated	*12*

2. RESPIRATORY SYSTEM

Case 7	Darren, a hot and irritable 12-month-old infant	*15*
Case 8	Susan, a 21-year-old student with a runny nose and imminent exams	*17*
Case 9	Peter, a 19-year-old student with a sore throat	*19*
Case 10	Respiratory distress and fever in Catriona, a 1-year-old infant	*21*
Case 11	Mrs Smith, 32-year-old, with a cough and generalized muscle aches and pains	*22*
Case 12	Sarah, a 55-year-old woman with rigors, cough and chest pain	*26*
Case 13	Dermot, a 57-year-old smoker with increasing dyspnoea and confusion	*28*
Case 14	Dyspnoea, wheeze and a productive cough in Tony, a 55-year-old smoker	*30*
Case 15	Shula, 5 months old, off colour and feeding poorly	*32*
Case 16	Productive cough in Benjamin, a 14-year-old with cystic fibrosis	*35*

3. GASTROINTESTINAL SYSTEM

Case 17	Bertrand, a 35-year-old Frenchman with nausea, abdominal pain and diarrhoea	*38*
Case 18	Damien, a 13-month-old baby, with vomiting and diarrhoea	*41*
Case 19	Fraser, a 37-year-old business executive with abdominal pain, diarrhoea and flatulence	*43*
Case 20	Bob, a 55-year-old retired coal miner with abdominal pain	*45*
Case 21	Belinda, a 25-year-old non-Caucasian with malaise, myalgia and fever	*47*

Case 22   Anorexia, malaise and nausea in Eddie, 25 years old   *50*

Case 23   Upper abdominal pain in Gareth, a 46-year-old sheep farmer   *55*

Case 24   Continuous non-bloody diarrhoea in Paul, a 35-year-old aid worker   *57*

Case 25   Colicky abdominal pain and diarrhoea in Winston, a 68-year-old man with chronic leukaemia   *58*

4. GENITOURINARY SYSTEM

Case 26   Gillian, a 23-year-old receptionist with frequency, dysuria and haematuria   *60*

Case 27   Joan's cloudy bag   *62*

Case 28   Elizabeth, a 28-year-old prostitute, attends the clinic for a check-up   *64*

Case 29   Sharon, a 24-year-old personnel manager with a blistering genital rash   *67*

Case 30   Jane, 27, requests an AIDS test   *70*

Case 31   Suprapubic pain and haematuria in Gavin, a 35-year-old sales executive   *72*

Case 32   Mark, a 42-year-old solicitor, has a lump on his penis   *73*

5. SKIN AND MUCOUS MEMBRANES

Case 33   Howard, a 10-year-old boy with scaly skin lesions   *75*

Case 34   Hannah, a 67-year-old widow with a leg ulcer   *77*

Case 35   Victoria, 4 years old, with painful mouth ulcers   *79*

Case 36   Jamie, a 5-year-old with a troublesome graze   *81*

Case 37   Simon, a 4 year old, develops a rash   *84*

Case 38   Emma, 8 years old, also develops a rash   *86*

Case 39   Steven, a 42-year-old accountant with a red painful eye   *89*

Case 40   Extensive rash, headache, fever and myalgia in Avril, a 20-year-old woman   *91*

Case 41   Wiliam and Mary, both aged 30, with blisters on their hands   *93*

Case 42   Skin rash and arthralgia in Eammon, a 25-year-old man   *95*

Case 43   Father Pat, a 45-year-old priest with a skin rash   *96*

6. SYSTEMIC INFECTIONS

Case 44   Mary, a 35-year-old engineer with nausea, weakness and rigors   *98*

Case 45   Tony, a 65-year-old man with vomiting, abdominal pain and fever   *101*

Case 46   Eric, a pyrexial 76-year-old war veteran with a heart murmur   *104*

Case 47   Margaret returns from Africa with a fever and headache   *107*

Case 48   Thomas, a 35-year-old schoolteacher, who is anti-HIV positive   *110*

Case 49 Karim, a 65-year-old cachectic man with fever 113

Case 50 Gordon, a 35-year-old Scottish vet with fever 116

Case 51 Complications of a road traffic accident in Brian, a retired 63-year-old barrister 119

Case 52 Fever, sweating and weight loss in Richard, recently returned from east Africa 122

Case 53 Dilip, a 45-year-old motor mechanic with diabetes and renal failure 124

7. PREGNANCY AND THE NEONATE

Case 54 Irritability, feeding difficulties and hypoxia in Sarah just after birth 128

Case 55 Deborah, 23 years old and 12 weeks pregnant, develops a rash 130

Case 56 A sticky eye, in Daniel, 5 days old 133

Case 57 A pregnant woman, whose son has developed chicken-pox 134

Case 58 Mrs Fisher, 25 years old, pregnant, and a history of genital herpes 136

Case 59 An unexpected blood count from Mrs Archer, 16 weeks pregnant 137

8. MISCELLANEOUS

Case 60 David, a 22-year-old student with a swollen testis 141

Case 61 Lenny, a 38-year-old Jamaican, with a palpable skin rash 142

Case 62 Richard, a young man with lethargy and breathlessness 144

Case 63 Michael, a medical student recently returned from Africa with a fever 146

Case 64 Polyarthralgia in Susan, a 25-year-old 148

Case 65 Problems on a Friday afternoon for Virginia, a junior house officer 149

APPENDICES

1. Rational use of the microbiology laboratory 152

2. Immunisation against infectious diseases (UK recommendations) 153

3. Some of the more commonly used antimicrobial agents 155

4. AIDS defining illnesses 160

INDEX

161

FOREWORD

All infection specialists can remember vivid teaching, with lasting impact, based on patients with individual clinical problems. Those of us who teach trainees or medical students know that the use of clinical material, at best at the bedside, but failing this in the lecture theatre or tutorial room, is an effective alerting system. Dr Hilary Humphreys and Dr Will Irving have seized this approach and used it ingeniously to cover the most important information and skills in clinical microbiology and infectious diseases.

This design has many advantages. The case presentations provide interest and pose problems, for self-questioning, before answers are given. These answers and the additional information are represented in a practically useful manner, and are readily assimilable by the stimulated reader. In the text, the boxes summarize and highlight significant material, and give a framework for learning or revision. At the same time, the table of contents and the extensive index allow the book to be used for reference, and the appendices tabulate the minimum systematic information needed, on microbiology, antibiotics, etc.

This book is particularly welcome at a time when we are more than ever conscious of information overload in medicine. This problem is being faced while Continuing Medical Education is developed formally and the undergraduate curriculum and learning methods undergo reform. The format of this book makes it suitable for self-conducted learning, and by concentrating on an assembly of patients with relevant clinical problems it defines the essential syllabus in the study of infection.

David C. E. Speller

HOW TO USE THIS BOOK

Medical education is undergoing something of a revolution. The General Medical Council in the United Kingdom is encouraging more 'student-centred learning' and has raised the concept of a core curriculum with options, rather than complete mastery of all the myriad specialities that comprise modern-day medicine. We have been guided by these principles when compiling this book. The book is designed to be a microbiological text for clinical medical students, presented in a novel and enjoyable format.

There are essentially two components: the body of the book consists of 65 Case Presentations, each describing the patient's presentation. The reader is asked to assess this information and answer an appropriate question. The case unfolds as more information is provided (e.g. the results of investigations) and further questions are raised. Our aims in this aspect of the book are to inculcate the basic principles involved in the investigation and management of patients with infection, and to encourage the student to formulate his/her own thoughts in a logical fashion.

The cases are clustered together according to the principal organ systems involved. If additional information related to particular organisms is required, reference must be made to the index.

However, the book is intended to be more than just a collection of clinical cases. We hope to equip the clinical medical student with the relevant microbiological information he or she will need to deal effectively with clinical problems of an infectious nature in most fields of medicine. Thus, in addition to the linear evolution of each particular case there are digressions in the text that allow us to discuss and enlarge upon material which, although not directly concerned with the case in question, is nevertheless important. This is the way in which we have attempted to solve the problem of not realistically being able to present clinical cases exhibiting every possible variation and manifestation of every possible infectious disease. These diversions are distinguished from the main text by being enclosed within appropriately labelled Tables and Boxes. These also serve as useful revision summaries prior to examinations.

Although we firmly believe that an understanding of the principles of clinical microbiology and infection is essential for doctors in almost all branches of medicine, we acknowledge that not everyone will be as fascinated by the vagaries of parasites, fungi, bacteria and viruses as we are! In deciding what to include and exclude from this book, we hope that our own views on what constitutes an essential core of microbiology is realistic. Above all, we hope you enjoy and benefit from the format adopted herein.

H.H
W.L.I.

ACKNOWLEDGEMENTS

We are indebted to Professor Speller, for his encouragement, enthusiasm and perspicacious comments. We wish to thank the following for their helpful comments and suggestions during the writing of this book: Dr Daniel Peckham, Dr Frank E. Murray, Mrs Dee Deardon, Mrs Ann Calrow, Dr Gerry Dolan, Professor Nick Rutter, Dr Christine Bowman, Professor David Greenwood, Dr Graham Lennox, Dr S. Vernon and Dr Bob Winter.

We acknowledge the following for the use of illustrations: Dr I. Ahmed-Jousef (Fig. 32.1), Dr B. R. Allen (Figs 33.1 and 33.2), Dr A. P. Ball (Figs 37.1 and 55.1), Dr Erwin Brown (Fig. 40.1), Dr K. L. Dalziel (Fig. 34.1), Dr R. T. D. Emond (Fig. 37.2), Dr M. Everard (Figs. 15.3), Ms A. Feldon and Ms N. Jackson (Fig. 46.2), Professor Roger Finch (Figs 27.1 and 43.1), Professor David Greenwood (Figs 19.1 and 47.1), Dr A. Haynes (Fig. 61.1), Dr M. Hewitt (Fig. 2.1), Dr Henry Irving (Figs 16.1, 20.1, 23.1 and 49.1), Professor David Isaacs (Figs 9.1, 35.1 and 35.2), Dr John Kurtz (Fig. 11.1), Dr John V. Lee (Fig. 13.1), Dr James Lowe (Figs 6.1 and 6.2), Dr Michael McKendrick (Figs 22.1, 38.1 and 38.2), Dr Colm O. Mahoney (Fig. 60.1), Professor N. Rutter (Figs 7.1 and 56.1), Mr Andrew Shelton (Figs 18.1 and 18.2), Dr Alan Stevens (Fig. 49.3), Mr S. Vernon (Fig. 39.1), the Radiology Department, Queen's Medical Centre (Figs 12.1B, 48.1 and 51.1).

Finally, we wish to thank Mr George Sharp and Mr Malcolm Baker for photographing laboratory material and all our colleagues, friends and families for their support and encouragement.

ABBREVIATIONS

AIDS	Acquired Immune Deficiency Syndrome
Alk Phos	Alkaline Phosphatase (liver function test)
ALT	Alanine Aminotransferase
ARDS	Adult Respiratory Distress Syndrome
ATLL	Adult T cell Leukaemia Lymphoma
AZT	Azidothymidine
BCG	Bacillus Calmette-Guérin (TB vaccine)
BMT	Bone Marrow Transplant
BSE	Bovine Spongiform Encephalopathy
CAPD	Continuous Ambulatory Peritoneal Dialysis
CDC	Centre for Disease Control (Atlanta, Georgia, USA)
CDSC	Communicable Disease Surveillance Centre (London, UK)
CFT	Complement Fixation Test (antibody detection technique)
CFU	Colony Forming Units (number of bacteria)
CJD	Creutzfeldt-Jakob Disease
CMV	Cytomegalovirus
CNS	Central Nervous System
CPE	Cytopathic Effect
CRP	C-Reactive Protein (acute phase protein)
CSF	Cerebrospinal Fluid
CT	Computerised Tomography (scan)
CXR	Chest X-Ray
CFU	Colony Forming Units (bacterial counts)
CIE	Counter Immuno-Electrophoresis (antigen detection technique)
DEAFF	Detection of Early Antigen Fluorescent Foci
DPT	Diphtheria-Pertussis-Tetanus (vaccine)
EBV	Epstein-Barr Virus
ECG	Electrocardiograph
EEG	Electroencephalogram
ELISA	Enzyme-Linked Immunoassay (serological technique)
EM	Electron Microscopy
ESR	Erythrocyte Sedimentation Rate (acute phase protein)
EV	Enterovirus
FEV_1 & FVC	Forced Expiratory Volume in 1 second & Forced Vital Capacity (lung function tests)
FTA	Fluorescent Treponemal Antigen (serological test for syphilis)
FUO	Fever of Unknown Origin
H	Haemagglutinin (antigen of influenza virus)
HAV	Hepatitis A Virus
HAM	HTLV-1 Associated Myelopathy (see also TSP)
Hb	Haemoglobin
HBcAg	Hepatitis B core Antigen
HBeAg	Hepatitis B extractable Antigen

HBsAg	Hepatitis B surface Antigen
HBV	Hepatitis B Virus
HCV	Hepatitis C Virus
HDV	Hepatitis D Virus (formerly known as Delta agent)
HEV	Hepatitis E Virus
HHV6,7	Human Herpesvirus 6,7
HiB	*Haemophilus influenzae* type b (capsulate)
HIV	Human Immunodeficiency Virus
HPV	Human Papillomavirus
HSE	Herpes Simplex Encephalitis
HSV	Herpes Simplex Virus
HTLV	Human T cell Lymphotropic Virus (two types, I & II)
IFN	Interferon
IgG, IgM	Immunoglobulin of the G or M class
im	intramuscular
ITU	Intensive Therapy Unit
iv	intravenous
IVP	Intravenous Pyelogram (kidney X-ray)
kD	Kilodaltons
LRTI	Lower Respiratory Tract Infection
MBC & MIC	Minimum Bactericidal Concentration & Minimum Inhibitory Concentration (quantification of antibacterial activity)
MMR	Measles-Mumps-Rubella (vaccine)
MRI	Magnetic Resonance Imaging
MRSA	Methicillin-Resistant *Staphylococcus aureus*
MSU	Mid-Stream Urine
N	Neuraminidase (antigen of influenza virus)
NANBH	Non-A Non-B Hepatitis
NPA	Nasopharyngeal Aspirate
NSU	Non-Specific Urethritis
PB	Paul Bunnell (test for infectious mononucleosis)
PCP	*Pneumocystis carinii* Pneumonia
PCR	Polymerase Chain Reaction (molecular technique)
PGL	Progressive Generalised Lymphadenopathy
PID	Pelvic Inflammatory Disease
Plts	Platelets
PML	Progressive Multifocal Leucoencephalopathy
PMNL	Polymorphonuclear Leucocyte
PrP^{c,Sc}	Protease-resistant Protein (cellular and scrapie isoforms)
PUO	Pyrexia of Unknown Origin
RPR	Rapid Plasma Reagin (serological test for syphilis)
RSV	Respiratory Syncytial Virus
SBE	Subacute Bacterial Endocarditis
SCBU	Special Care Baby Unit
SGOT	Serum Glutamic-Oxaloacetic Transaminase (liver function test)

SPAG	Small Particle Aerosol Generator
SRSV	Small Round Structured Virus
SRV	Small Round Virus
SSPE	Subacute Sclerosing Panencephalopathy
TB	Tuberculosis
TPHA	Treponemal Particle Haemagglutination (serological test for syphilis)
TSP	Tropical Spastic Paraparesis
TSS	Toxic Shock Syndrome
TSST-1	Toxic Shock Syndrome Toxin
URTI	Upper Respiratory Tract Infection
US	Ultrasound
UTI	Urinary Tract Infection
VDRL	Venereal Disease Reference Laboratory (indicates serological test for syphilis)
VHF	Viral Haemorrhagic Fever
VZIg	Varicella-Zoster Immunoglobulin
VZV	Varicella-Zoster Virus
WCC	White Cell Count
WHO	World Health Organization
WR	Wassermann Reaction (serological test for syphilis)
ZN	Ziehl-Neelsen (special stain for mycobacteria)

CASE 1
Nigel, a 3-year-old boy with lethargy and a skin rash

Nigel, a 3-year-old boy, is referred to hospital with a 2-day history of lethargy, irritability and poor feeding. On examination he is pyrexial, drowsy, and has 2–3 purplish-red lesions on the trunk and extremities (Fig. 1.1) which, according to his parents, were not present when he was seen earlier by the family practitioner. There is no neck stiffness.

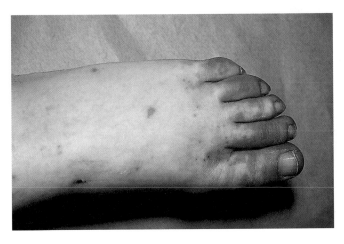

Fig. 1.1 Purplish-red lesions on foot.

Q What is the most likely diagnosis? What investigations should be carried out to confirm it?

A Acute bacterial meningitis must be excluded in a sick infant as described here, even in the absence of neck stiffness. Cerebrospinal fluid (CSF) should be obtained by lumbar puncture (LP) for biochemical and microbiological analysis. An LP is contraindicated if there is clinical evidence of raised intracranial pressure, such as rapid changes in pulse, blood pressure and level of consciousness, papilloedema or focal neurological signs. Blood cultures are also essential, as septicaemia often accompanies bacterial meningitis.

Q What is the significance of the age of the patient in predicting the likely aetiology of meningitis:

1. in this case?
2. in a 3-day-old neonate?
3. in a 25-year-old pregnant woman with a prodromal flu-like illness?
4. in a 75-year-old comatose man?

A Certain organisms are more likely to be involved at specific times in life, especially during the neonatal period. Bacterial meningitis is more common during childhood and early adulthood, and the most common cause is *Neisseria meningitidis* (the meningococcus). Capsulated *Haemophilus influenzae* type B (see Case 7) is usually confined to nonvaccinated children less than 5 years of age, as after this age they have acquired antibodies to capsular antigens. *Streptococcus pneumoniae* (the pneumococcus) can cause meningitis throughout life (Box 1.1).

1. The age of the patient and the presence of a purpuric rash are very suggestive of meningococcal meningitis.

2. *Escherichia coli* and β-haemolytic streptococcus group B, which are part of the normal vaginal flora, are the most likely causes but are rare outside the neonatal period (>1 month old).

3. Viral meningitis is much more common than that due to bacteria. Likely viral causes include enteroviruses (Coxsackieviruses, echoviruses and polioviruses; see

Case 35), mumps and occasionally Herpes simplex. *Listeria monocytogenes* must be considered as a possible cause during pregnancy or postpartum, and in the neonate (see Case 54). This opportunist pathogen may be acquired from the ingestion of certain foods, e.g. soft cheeses, pâté or cook–chill foods that have been inadequately prepared. Consequently, pregnant women should be advised to avoid these for the duration of pregnancy.

4. *S. pneumoniae* is relatively more common in the elderly, and this organism, together with the presence of coma, heralds a poor prognosis.

B1.1 Aetiology of acute meningitis
Bacteria

N. meningitidis
H. influenzae type B (<5 years old)
S. pneumoniae
E. coli (neonatal)
Group B streptococcus (neonatal)
L. monocytogenes (pregnant
    women, neonates – see Case 54)
Staphylococci (often trauma or
    surgery-associated)
Treponema pallidum
Leptospira species

Viruses
Enteroviruses (see Case 35) Mumps (see Case 60)

Nigel's CSF, obtained from lumbar puncture, is cloudy and contains 540 white cells/mm³ (90% polymorphs) and 5 red blood cells/mm³. CSF protein is 8 g/l and glucose 0.3 mmol/l (blood glucose 5.7 mmol/l). The Gram stain reveals Gram-negative intracellular diplococci.

Q Which of the above values are abnormal? What type of meningitis is this and what is the likely pathogen?

A A cloudy or turbid CSF, together with raised white cells (normal <5/mm³) with neutrophils predominant, a raised protein (normal 1.5–4.0 g/l) and a glucose concentration less than 60% of the blood level is highly suggestive of bacterial rather than viral meningitis. The organisms seen on the Gram film are almost certainly *N. meningitidis*. The following day small grey colonies were growing on chocolate and blood agar which were oxidase positive and biochemically confirmed as *N. meningitidis*.

Causes of meningitis which present with an 'aseptic' CSF pattern, i.e. raised white cells with lymphocytes predominant, slightly raised protein but normal glucose, include viruses (e.g. enteroviruses, mumps), *Treponema pallidum* (syphilis), leptospirosis and tuberculosis (high CSF protein, glucose usually low, presentation not so acute). Occasionally the predominant cells may be lymphocytes rather than polymorphs in the very early stages of meningitis caused by bacteria.

Q What is the antibiotic of choice here?

A Intravenous penicillin for 10–14 days is the treatment of choice for meningococcal meningitis. Penicillin is also indicated to treat pneumococcal meningitis, although resistance to penicillin is being increas-

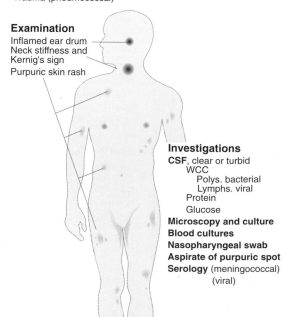

History
Duration of symptoms (>1 week suggests viral aetiology or TB)
Otitis media (*H.influenzae* possible)
Contact with a case recently (meningococcal)
Trauma (pneumococcal)

Examination
Inflamed ear drum
Neck stiffness and
Kernig's sign
Purpuric skin rash

Investigations
CSF, clear or turbid
    WCC
        Polys. bacterial
        Lymphs. viral
    Protein
    Glucose
Microscopy and culture
Blood cultures
Nasopharyngeal swab
Aspirate of purpuric spot
Serology (meningococcal)
                (viral)

Fig. 1.2 Diagnosis of meningitis.

ingly reported and is a particular problem in Spain and South Africa. Blind therapy, where the aetiology is either unknown or *H. influenzae* (up to 20% β-lactamase positive) is possible, i.e. <5 years of age and unvaccinated, is a third-generation cephalosporin such as cefotaxime or, alternatively, chloramphenicol.

Q Was it preferable in this instance to delay starting treatment pending investigations?

A The rapid development of a purpuric rash indicates meningococcal septicaemia, which is a medical emergency as death may occur within minutes. Intravenous penicillin should be administered *before* a lumbar puncture is carried out, even if this means that an organism will not be recovered from blood or CSF. This is one of the rare instances where treatment should precede microbiological investigations.

Nigel was started on high-dose intravenous penicillin and gradually improved over the next 48–72 hours. Pamela, his mother, expressed some concern as to the risk to his brother Lenny, aged 2, and sister Cynthia, aged 7.

Q What measures, if any, can be taken to minimize the risk to Nigel's close contacts?

A Chemoprophylaxis should be administered to all close contacts and vaccination may be indicated depending upon aetiology or type of organism (see Box 1.2).

Summary: Meningitis
Presentation
Headache, vomiting, fever, irritability, drowsiness (especially children), rash (meningococcal)
Diagnosis (See Fig. 1.2)
CSF for microscopy, biochemical analysis and culture, plus blood cultures, serology
Management
i.v. penicillin (meningococcal + pneumococcal) or cefotaxime (aetiology unknown or if haemophilus likely) Rifampicin to index case and contacts Prevention by vaccination (haemophilus and some strains of meningococcus)

B1.2 Prevention of meningitis
Chemoprophylaxis
Meningococcal – for all close contacts that is, family members, those sharing accommodation with the index case, 'kissing partners' and the index patient. This prevents acquisition by contacts and spread if already acquired. Treatment of the index case with penicillin does not always eradicate nasopharyngeal carriage. Not usually indicated for medical or nursing staff caring for the patient. Rifampicin: ×2 days Ciprofloxacin: alternative *Haemophilus* – close contacts if there is an unvaccinated child under 5 in the household. Rifampicin: ×4 days
Vaccination
Most cases in temperate climates are due to *N. meningitidis* group B, for which there is as yet no effective vaccine. Close contacts or fellow class members of schoolchildren should be vaccinated if there are two or more cases due to group A or group C, for which there are effective vaccines. Conjugated polysaccharide *Haemophilus influenzae* type b is now recommended for all infants from 2 months of age.

CASE 2
Mr Aldridge, a 45-year-old accountant with odd behaviour and a fever

Mr Aldridge, a 45-year-old accountant, is brought to the Casualty Department by his wife. Earlier in the day he was found wandering in his local park, muttering unintelligibly to himself. His wife feels that as the day has passed he has become more and more detached from what is going on around him, although he has been able to answer direct questions. When talking to Mr Aldridge it is difficult to elicit sensible answers, and in between his reponses he appears very drowsy. His past medical history, taken from his wife, reveals no serious illnesses and he is on no regular medication. However, he has been complaining over the past few days of feeling off colour, and yesterday he returned home early from work with a headache and a fever, for which he took some paracetamol. On examination he has a temperature of 37.9°C, but apart from his decreased level of consciousness and dysphasia there are no other abnormal physical signs.

Q What is the differential diagnosis?

A The most striking features about Mr Aldridge are his recent behavioural changes and his impaired level of consciousness. In the absence of any localizing signs the most likely diagnosis is encephalitis, of which there is a multitude of possible causes. The prodromal illness and fever are suggestive of an infectious aetiology, of which viral encephalitis is the most common, but other diagnoses, including tuberculous meningoencephalitis, cerebral abscesses, tumours or strokes, cannot be ruled out at this stage.

Q What are the viral causes of encephalitis?

A Viral causes of encephalitis are listed below:

Herpes simplex virus types 1 and 2
- the commonest cause of sporadic viral encephalitis
- any age, including newborn (neonatal herpes)

Mumps virus (see Case 60)
- meningoencephalitis

Measles virus (see Case 37)
- postinfectious encephalitis
- subacute sclerosing panencephalitis

Varicella-zoster virus (see Case 38)
- postinfectious encephalitis (after chicken pox).
- zoster encephalitis as a complication of herpes zoster

Enteroviruses (see Case 35)
- direct viral invasion of brain substance

Influenza virus (see Case 11)
- postinfectious encephalitis
- (possibly) encephalitis lethargica

Rubella virus (see Case 55)
- panencephalitis as part of congenital rubella syndrome

Rabies virus (see Case 5)

Arthropod-borne viruses (geographically localized, the following examples do not exist in the UK)
- e.g. tick-borne encephalitis (Eastern Europe), Japanese B encephalitis (SE Asia, China), St Louis encephalitis (USA).

Q Does herpes simplex encephalitis (HSE) always arise from primary infection with HSV?

A No. HSV types 1 and 2 are two of the seven herpesviruses known to infect humans (see Box 2.1). All

---

B2.1 Human herpesviruses
Herpes simplex type 1
Herpes simplex type 2
Varicella-zoster virus
Epstein–Barr virus
Cytomegalovirus
Human herpes virus type 6
Human herpes virus type 7

---

herpesviruses are capable of undergoing latency. This means that infection with one of these viruses is followed by lifelong carriage, with the virus establishing a latent infection at some site within the body. This latent virus can be reactivated at any stage in later life, thus giving rise to a secondary, or reactivated, infection. Individuals can also be re-exposed to the virus and become reinfected. It is therefore possible to undergo the following types of infection with a herpes virus:

Primary – i.e. the very first exposure to the virus

Secondary – which can be either reactivation of endogenous latent virus or reinfection with exogenous virus.

HSE may be a manifestation of either primary or, more commonly, secondary (reactivated) HSV infection.

Q As herpes simplex virus is the commonest infectious cause of encephalitis, would it be useful to know whether Mr Aldridge has any past or recent history of herpetic disease, i.e. recurrent cold sores or genital herpes?

A No. A history of past or current external herpetic infection is of no discriminatory value in assessing the diagnosis of HSE. Patients with HSE give a past history of herpetic disease no more frequently than the general population. The presence or absence of a recurrent herpetic lesion at the time of presentation similarly gives no useful information about whether the virus has spread to the brain. Cold sores in particular can be misleading, as a recurrence may arise as a consequence of any intercurrent illness.

Q What is the pathogenesis of the damage to the brain in HSE?

A There are many important unanswered questions in relation to the pathogenesis of HSE, not the least being how does the virus

spread to the brain? However, it is clear that virus *is* present at the site of the affected tissue. The histological picture is one of acute haemorrhagic necrosis, which arises either as a direct result of virus-induced cell death, or possibly because of the host immune response to virus-infected cells.

Q How can a diagnosis of HSE be proven?

A Diagnosis is difficult, and until recently has relied upon the following approaches (in decreasing order of sensitivity):

1. Brain biopsy. Virus can be detected at the affected site by immunofluorescence with appropriate monoclonal antibodies, by electron microscopy, or by isolation in tissue culture. However, most clinicians feel that this invasive procedure cannot be justified. Viable virus is *not* usually present in CSF obtained by lumbar puncture.

2. Clinical and neurological investigations – the mainstay of acute diagnosis if a brain biopsy is not performed. The most commonly affected area of the brain is the temporal lobe: this underlies the bizarre behavioural changes which may be present in the history. The CSF is rarely, if ever, normal, but the changes are not specific – the presence of red cells arises from the haemorrhagic nature of the pathology (see above); the white cell pleocytosis is not necessarily severe. The lesions in the brain are almost always focal – neurological diagnostic techniques such as EEG and CT or MRI scan should reveal this. The presence of a focal lesion seen by brain imaging is the most sensitive indicator of a diagnosis of HSE, other than brain biopsy.

3. Microbiological investigation – the demonstration of a rise in serum anti-HSV antibody titres and of intrathecal synthesis of such anti-

bodies. The latter requires both assay of anti-HSV in the CSF and a contemporaneous measure of blood–brain barrier function, which is usually provided by comparing blood and CSF anti-HSV titres with blood and CSF albumin concentrations. The major drawback to this diagnostic approach is that it may take several days, if not weeks, for positive results to develop.

Q How, therefore, should Mr Aldridge be investigated?

A Investigations should include:

- a full blood count
- urea and electrolytes
- blood glucose
- a serum sample for viral serology. This can be paired with a later sample if need be, and various antibody titres assayed
- a throat swab in virus transport medium and a faecal sample for viral culture; these may provide the only clue to a diagnosis of enteroviral encephalitis
- cerebral imaging, as Mr Aldridge's pathology is most likely to be cerebral, e.g. EEG, CT or MRI scan
- lumbar puncture, provided raised intracranial pressure has been excluded.

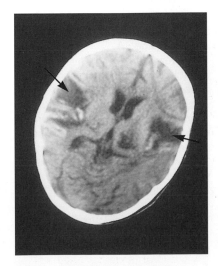

Fig. 2.1 Mr Aldridge's CT scan.

Mr Aldridge is admitted to hospital and a CT scan ordered, the results of which are shown in Figure 2.1. A full blood count is normal, as are urea and electrolytes and blood sugar. A lumbar puncture is performed, yielding the following information:

Slightly bloodstained fluid
700 red blood cells ×10⁶/l
43 white cells ×10⁹/l, 60% lymphocytes
No organisms seen. Culture results to follow
CSF sugar 3.6 mmol/l (blood sugar 5.0)
Protein 1.6 g/l

Q How are these results interpreted?

A CSF is almost always abnormal in HSE, but the changes are not specific. The lumbar puncture results are compatible with a diagnosis of HSE (see above). The commonest CSF abnormality in HSE is the presence of red cells, reflecting the haemorrhagic necrosis within the brain substance caused by the virus.

The CT scan shows focal areas of low attenuation in both temporal lobes containing flecks of haemorrhage and exerting a mass effect (arrows). The commonest site of involvement of HSE is the temporal lobe, and bilateral involvement is not unusual, therefore this also supports the diagnosis of HSE.

Q What is the treatment of herpes simplex encephalitis?

A Acyclovir. This antiviral agent is phosphorylated to an active form by a virally encoded enzyme (thymidine kinase). Thus, in uninfected cells the drug remains inactive and therefore non-toxic. Acyclovir triphosphate inhibits viral DNA polymerase, thereby preventing viral replication.

On the basis of the CSF findings and the CT scan a provisional diagnosis of herpes simplex encephalitis is made, and Mr Aldridge is started on intravenous acyclovir 10 mg/kg three times a day.

Q Should laboratory confirmation of the diagnosis have been awaited before therapy was started?

A No. It is vital that specific antiviral therapy be started as soon as the diagnosis is suspected, as any delay may have dire consequences in terms of residual morbidity on recovery.

Five days later the laboratory results show that the serum sample taken on the day of admission contained no anti-HSV as determined by a complement fixation test, and that the cultures inoculated with the CSF are not showing any cytopathic effect (CPE).

Q In the light of this new information, should the diagnosis be revised?

A No. The initial diagnosis of HSE was eminently correct. Mr Aldridge gave a classical history, the CSF findings were compatible with the diagnosis, and the CT scan revealed focal haemorrhagic lesions in the temporal lobes. In reality, most cases of HSE will in fact be much harder to diagnose than this one.

The absence of anti-HSV in the acute serum sample is irrelevant. The value of procuring this sample is that it may be possible to demonstrate a rise in CFT titre when a second, later, sample is taken.

Failure to isolate HSV from the CSF is the norm, not the exception, in HSE. This result therefore has no bearing on the diagnosis.

Mr Aldridge improves considerably following his admission to hospital and the initiation of acyclovir therapy. By day 5 his

temperature has settled, his speech has improved and he shows no further episodes of bizarre behaviour.

Q Should his acyclovir now be stopped?

A No. There are reports of relapses of HSE following cessation of anti-viral therapy, and there is also evidence from repeated lumbar punctures that HSE may be a more chronic disease than hitherto suspected. Hence it is advisable to continue therapy for a minimum of 10 days, even in the presence of the excellent response shown by Mr Aldridge.

Q Is there any recent advance which may make the diagnosis of HSE at the acute stage less problematic, without requiring a brain biopsy to be performed?

A The polymerase chain reaction (PCR) assay for the detection of specific sequences of DNA may revolutionize HSE diagnosis. This assay is exquisitely sensitive and can identify very low numbers of copies of the DNA of interest. HSV DNA is present in acute CSF, even

though viable virus cannot be grown from CSF. However, there are limitations: the extreme sensitivity of the assay makes it prone to the generation of false positive results because of cross-contamination of samples. The assay is not yet sufficiently robust that it can be adopted widely by laboratories that have no previous experience of the assay, so at the time of writing PCR diagnosis remains the prerogative of specialized research laboratories.

Summary: Herpes simplex encephalitis
Presentation
Variable. May include fever, decreasing conscious level, focal neurological signs, speech and behavioural changes.
Diagnosis
Clinical, with evidence of a focal lesion by any brain imaging technique. Rapid virological diagnosis by PCR may be possible
Treatment
Immediate high-dose intravenous acyclovir for at least 10 days unless diagnosis is revised

CASE 3
Jim, a 72-year-old man with progressive headache

Jim, a 72-year-old man, complains of a severe progressive headache over 1 month. There is no accompanying vomiting or photophobia, and he has otherwise been in good health until now. He does not smoke and drinks only occasionally. His close family have noticed that he is more lethargic of late, and he has also been observed having short-term memory lapses. On examination Jim has a temperature of 37.5°C and a pulse rate of 80/min. There is no neck stiffness, papilloedema, focal neurological signs or abnormalities of any of the other organ systems. Following referral to hospital, he is admitted for further investigations.

Q What is the likely differential diagnosis?

A The recent onset of severe and progressive headache is ominous and suggestive of intracranial pathology. This includes:

- a cerebral neoplasm (primary or secondary)
- cerebrovascular accident, cerebral infarction
- meningitis, encephalitis
- chronic subdural haematoma
- subdural empyema
- brain abscess.

Sinusitis, arthritis of the spine or jaw and temporal arteritis might present with some of the features described above, but exclusion of intracranial pathology is essential first.

Q What initial investigations are indicated?

A A full blood count, serum urea and electrolytes and erythrocyte sedimentation rate (ESR) or plasma viscosity, although non-specific, should exclude a connective tissue disorder (e.g. temporal arteritis) and may indicate systemic disease or point to an infective process. A lumbar puncture is required to exclude meningitis and is not contra-indicated here (see Case 1). A heavily bloodstained cerebrospinal fluid (CSF) which persists during the procedure, or xanthochromia, may indicate a recent intracranial haemorrhage. A CT or MRI scan, however, is likely to be the most useful investigation in confirming intracranial pathology, and many would prefer to carry this out in advance of a lumbar puncture in case of raised intracranial pressure not evident clinically. Other investigations, such as skull X-rays, arteriography, isotope brain scans and electroencephalograms (EEG), have largely been superseded by the sensitivity of CT and MRI scans.

The initial results of investigations are: haemoglobin 12.5 g/l; white cell count 9.5 ×10⁹/l (60% polymorph neutrophils); platelet count 250/mm³; and an ESR of 40 mm/h. Serum urea and electrolytes are normal. Lumbar puncture results in clear CSF under normal pressure with 3 red blood cells/mm³, 85 white cells/mm³ (50% polymorphs), a protein of 11 g/l (normal 1.5–4 g/l) and a CSF glucose of 3.2 mmol/l (serum, 4.5 mmol/l). Gram and Ziehl–Neelsen stains are negative and there is no growth from bacterial, including mycobacterial, and viral cultures. The CT scan is shown in Figure 3.1.

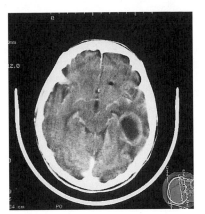

Fig. 3.1 CT scan at presentation.

Q Comment on the results of these investigations. What is the likely diagnosis?

A The ESR is unremarkable for a 72-year-old man and precludes the diagnosis of temporal arteritis. The CSF is abnormal (pleocytosis, elevated protein) but does not indicate specific pathology. In the absence of recent antibacterial agents bacterial meningitis is unlikely, and despite the failure to isolate a virus from CSF culture viral encephalitis is still possible, with herpes simplex the most likely (see Case 2). The CT scan suggests a mass in the temporal lobe which is circumscribed by ring enhancement and surrounded by cerebral oedema, all highly suggestive of a brain abscess. MRI is said to be more sensitive than CT, and may in addition detect satellite lesions, but it is not always available. Figure 3.2 highlights important features in the pathogenesis of cerebral abscess.

Jim is taken to the operating theatre and undergoes a craniotomy: 3 ml of purulent fluid are removed from the right temporal lobe. Gram's stain of this reveals numerous pus cells and Gram-positive cocci in chains.

Q What is the likely microbiological aetiology?

A Gram-positive cocci in chains are very indicative of streptococci, and here *Streptococcus milleri* is the most likely pathogen. This bacterium is part of the normal respir-

atory and gastrointestinal flora, grows best under microaerophilic conditions (sufficient CO₂), is characteristically associated with brain and liver abscesses, and on artificial media such as blood agar has a sweet caramel-like aroma. Other possibilities include anaerobic streptococci, viridans streptococci such as *S. mitis*, and *S. pneumoniae* (see Table 3.1).

Q What antimicrobial agents should be started pending the results of culture and sensitivity testing?

A Often where an abscess can be drained antibiotics may not be required, provided all the infected material has been removed and the patient has no systemic evidence of

infection. This does not strictly apply here, because of the inaccessibility of the infected site and the consequences of relapse requiring further surgery or drainage with considerable associated morbidity. The choice of agent is governed by the likely pathogen, the antimicrobial sensitivity pattern and the ability of the agent to cross the blood–brain barrier and achieve adequate concentrations in brain

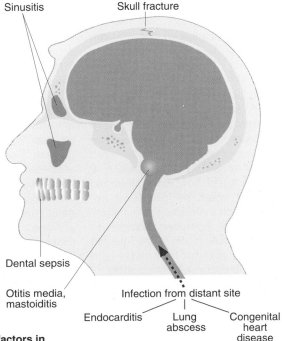

Fig. 3.2 Predisposing factors in cerebral abscess.

Sinusitis

Skull fracture

Dental sepsis

Otitis media, mastoiditis

Endocarditis

Infection from distant site

Lung abscess

Congenital heart disease

tissue. Certain antimicrobial agents, such as the aminoglycosides, do not cross the blood–brain barrier in appreciable concentrations, even in the presence of inflammation or meningitis. Chloramphenicol and the third-generation cephalosporins reach relatively high concentrations in the CSF and brain, as does metronidazole, which will cover most anaerobes. Whilst awaiting the results of culture, a combination of intravenous cefotaxime and metronidazole would be a sensible choice. Cefotaxime is preferred to penicillin G or ampicillin to cover Gram-negative bacilli which may not be visible on the Gram's stain.

Table 3.1 Aetiology of brain abscess according to anatomical location

Site	Predisposing factors	Organisms
Frontal	Sinusitis Dental sepsis	Streptococci, Bacteroides, *Staphylococcus aureus*, *Haemophilus* spp.
Temporal	Otitis media Mastoiditis	Streptococci, Bacteroides, Enterobacteriaceae
Frontal, temporal, parietal etc.	Trauma Penetrating wound	*S. aureus*, Clostridia
Multiple	Infective endocarditis Congenital heart disease Lung abscess	*S. aureus*, viridans streptococci Fusobacteria Nocardia

A pure growth of *S. milleri*, sensitive to penicillin and the cephalosporins, is isolated from the material aspirated during surgery. Jim makes a slow but gradual recovery, and on discharge from hospital 3 weeks later is much less lethargic and fully orientated. The CT scan at 4 weeks shows considerable resolution of the initial abnormality but with residual ring enhancement, but at 6 months is reported as normal.

Q How long should Jim remain on antibiotics?

A There are no hard data indicating how long treatment should be continued in this case. As the isolate is sensitive to penicillin the cefotaxime should be replaced by high-dose intravenous penicillin, which will reduce the cost of treatment and is less likely to result in superinfections arising from a broad-spectrum cephalosporin. Intravenous treatment should be continued for 2–3 weeks and should be followed by oral amoxicillin. The duration of treatment and how long parenteral therapy should be continued depends upon the organism, its sensitivity pattern, operative findings – in particular how much of the infected material could be removed – and the initial response to antibiotics.

Q What is the prognosis from brain abscess?

A Since the arrival of antibacterial agents mortality has fallen from about 50% to approximately 10%. An adverse outcome is dictated by a number of factors (see Box 3.1). The incidence of seizures following diagnosis and treatment ranges from 30 to 70% and there may be a role in many cases for prophylactic anticonvulsant therapy. Prognosis is also influenced by underlying disease and aetiology: fungal abscesses, e.g. *Candida albicans*, *Aspergillus* spp., often reflect severe immunosuppression and neutropenia, and antifungal agents do not achieve high concentrations in brain tissue.

B3.1 Risk factors predicting an unfavourable outcome from brain abscess

- Delayed diagnosis
- Posterior fossa location
- Multiple, deep or multiloculated lesions
- Rupture into the ventricles
- Coma (>50% mortality)
- Fungal aetiology

Summary: Brain abscess

Presentation

Headache, drowsiness, change in personality which may come on over weeks or months

Diagnosis

Exclusion of other causes of intracranial pathology, e.g. tumour. Definitive diagnosis now is by CT or MRI scan

Management

Aspiration of pus by craniotomy or by burr hole, and i.v. antibiotics for 2–3 weeks

CASE 4
John, a 75-year-old man with muscle weakness

John, a 75-year-old man, is referred to the medical outpatients department with a 4-day history of muscle weakness and cramps, especially of the lower limbs, and difficulty in swallowing solids. He smokes 5–10 cigarettes a day and drinks occasionally at weekends. He is on hydrochlorthiazide for mild hypertension and temazepam for difficulty in sleeping. On examination he is apyrexial, his blood pressure is 160/90 mmHg and his pulse rate is 90/min. There is generalized abdominal rigidity but with normal bowel sounds and increased muscle tone, which is most marked in the adductor muscles of the upper limbs. Sensation is normal.

Following admission to hospital for investigation and management his symptoms worsen over the next 2 days. There is increased clenching of the fists, extension of the lower limbs and, later, difficulty in swallowing liquids. On the third day following admission John has a respiratory arrest, is resuscitated and immediately transferred to the intensive therapy unit (ITU). There he is ventilated and a chest X-ray shows patchy consolidation of the superior segments of the right upper lobe, suggestive of aspiration pneumonia.

Q What conditions might explain this combination of signs and symptoms?

A The above clinical picture describes abnormalities of the peripheral and bulbar motor systems. A number of possibilities arise:

- Oculogyric crisis due to phenothiazines; temazepam is unlikely to cause this
- Hypocalcaemic or alkalotic tetany, excluded by serum calcium and blood pH
- Intracranial mass or haemorrhage; exclusively motor presentation makes this less likely
- Strychnine poisoning; excluded by history or toxic screen
- Meningitis; absence of fever and nuchal rigidity make this less likely
- Tetanus; possible.

Q What is the most likely diagnosis, therefore?

A A combination of increased muscle tone and rigidity, difficulty swallowing and respiratory muscle paralysis of fairly recent origin suggests tetanus, which is caused by a toxin, tetanospasmin, released by *Clostridium tetani*. The diagnosis of tetanus is usually made on

clinical grounds' other possible causes having been excluded by lumbar puncture (normal CSF) and a negative CT scan. The classic features, including lockjaw and *risus sardonicus* (sardonic smile), however, may often be absent. A history of trauma with isolation of the bacterium from the infected site may help in diagnosis, but in many cases this is absent. A history of immunization in a child or a booster dose of the vaccine within the last 5 years makes the diagnosis unlikely.

Q What other conditions resulting in neuroparalytic disease may be caused by *Clostridium* spp?

A Botulism, an unusual form of food poisoning caused by toxins released by *C. botulinum*, also causes muscle weakness. There are important autonomic abnormalities, more prominent than in tetanus, such as reduced salivation, ileus and urinary retention. The main features of botulism are shown in Box 4.1.

Q What are the principles of management for a patient with tetanus?

A Patients require immediate referral to hospital and usually admission to ITU for ventilation. As

B4.1 Botulism

- Food-borne disease caused by a neurotoxin released by *Clostridium botulinum*
- Most potent toxin known. Prevents release of acetylcholine at peripheral cholinergic synapses
- Incubation period of 12–36 hours followed by muscle weakness, dizziness, dry mouth, urinary retention, double vision and symmetrical muscle weakness
- Diagnosis confirmed by detection of toxin in blood, food or faeces, or by the isolation of *C. botulinum* from incriminated food
- Treatment involves admission to intensive care, ventilation and antitoxin

this condition is toxin mediated and it is difficult to counteract the effects of tetanospasmin once it is within the neuronal axons (see Figure 4.1), the primary objective of management is to avoid the complications of paralysis until the toxin levels fall. Benzodiazepines such as diazepam reduce anxiety, sedate and act as a central anticonvulsant. Antiarrhythmic agents may be required to treat unstable cardiac rhythm and antibiotics are indicated to treat complicating infections such as pneumonia. Wound debridement and penicillin are indicated early on if there is a history of trauma, but often patients present some time after this. Human tetanus immunoglobulin, administered intramuscularly, will oppose the action of any tetanospasmin that has not entered the nervous system, but there is little evidence to support the injection of this antitoxin around the site of the initial wound or injury, as by the time of diagnosis there will be no toxin remaining locally. Finally, parenteral or enteral feeding and good nursing care to prevent decubitus ulcers, venous thrombosis and pulmonary embolism, are essential features of overall management.

Q What is the prognosis for this patient?

A Mortality is highest at the extremes of life. The majority of children with neonatal tetanus die, but this probably reflects more their poor social and nutritional background. Approximately 40% of those over 50 years of age die, and this is largely influenced by the presence of pre-existing disease such as ischaemic heart disease, and the quality of intensive care in preventing complications following prolonged ventilation. Muscle spasms usually persist for 10 days or so, but in the absence of the complications referred to above recovery is usually complete.

John requires prolonged ventilation owing to aspiration pneumonia and adult respiratory distress syndrome (ARDS). He subsequently develops renal failure and requires dopamine to maintain blood pressure. Two weeks following admission John dies of multiple organ failure.

Q How is tetanus prevented?

A There is an effective vaccine available for use in the prevention of tetanus – this is not the case in botulism. This is usually administered in childhood as part of a triple vaccine with diphtheria toxoid and bordetella (killed vaccine) at 2, 3 and 4 months, with boosters at 4–5 and 15 years of age. Adequate

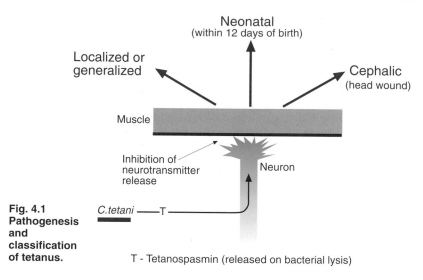

Fig. 4.1
Pathogenesis and classification of tetanus.

T - Tetanospasmin (released on bacterial lysis)

Table 4.1 Guidelines for the use of toxoid and tetanus immunoglobulin				
Previous effective vaccination or booster	Clean wounds		Other wounds	
<5 years ago	TV–	TIG–	TV–	TIG–
5–10 years ago	TV–	TIG–	TV+	TIG–
>10 years or unknown	TV+	TIG–	TV+	TIG+
TV, tetanus vaccine; TIG, tetanus immunoglobulin; –, not required; +, required				

immunity is believed to persist for approximately 10 years. In the light of the age of the patient described above, it is probable that he was never vaccinated or had not received a booster in the last 10 years. Alternatively, antibody levels may have declined with advancing age. Wound debridement and the aspiration of pus are also important measures in prevention, and penicillin is indicated if the wound is likely to be infected with anaerobic bacteria. A patient presenting to the Accident and Emergency department may also require tetanus immunoglobulin at the time of wound debridement (see Table 4.1).

Summary: Tetanus
Diagnosis
Largely clinical from motor signs present in the limbs and bulbar muscle groups, other possible causes having been excluded. History of wound not always present and isolation of *C. tetani* rare.
Management
Supportive, e.g. ventilation, artificial feeding etc. Also intramuscular tetanus immunoglobulin and penicillin if bacterium likely to be still present; toxoid vaccine with boosters every 5–10 years is protective

CASE 5
Andrew, a 20-year-old student with fever, nausea and headache

Andrew, a 20-year-old student, presents with a 5-day history of fever, malaise, anorexia, nausea and headache. He also reports difficulty in sleeping, and when he does sleep he is disturbed by vivid nightmares. Over the same period he has noticed a tingling sensation in a patch of skin on his left arm. He has no significant past medical history, and is on no regular medication. On examination he is febrile but there is little else of note, apart from a ragged healed scar on his left arm, which Andrew confirms is the site of abnormal sensation.

Q What are the initial impressions of Andrew's presentation?

A Most of the symptoms and signs described here are very non-specific and not suggestive of any particular pathology, but the history of abnormal sensation arising in a scar is of interest.

On further enquiry, it transpires that Andrew was bitten by a dog 3 months ago while backpacking in South America. Apart from thoroughly washing the area of the bite, he took no further action.

Q What diagnosis should now be considered?

A The obvious worry now is that Andrew may be suffering from rabies. Clinical rabies presents with a non-specific prodrome, lasting 2–7 days, which may include all of the symptoms mentioned as well as vomiting, diarrhoea, sore throat, cough and myalgia. Many patients also report behaviour disturbances, including hyperactivity, insomnia, hallucinations, anxiety and aggression. Abnormal sensation at the site of a previous bite occurs in about 50%. The history of a bite is therefore critical, but a bite some 3–6 months previously may easily be forgotten by the patient and the telltale scar may be missed by the physician.

Andrew is admitted to hospital for observation. Over the next 3 days he becomes increasingly restless and agitated, exhibiting purposeless movements of his limbs in response to tactile and auditory stimuli. He suffers intense spasms of the muscles involved in swallowing and the accessory muscles of respiration, lasting 10 seconds or so, accompanied by frothing at the mouth. The frequency and severity of these spasms initially increase, but begin to decrease after 2 days, when Andrew's conscious level declines into coma; he dies 24 hours later.

Q Why is rabies sometimes referred to as 'hydrophobia'?

A Hydrophobia is manifested by uncontrollable violent jerking movements as fluid is brought to the mouth, leading to the onset of a spasm which may be accompanied by retching, vomiting and generalized convulsions. It is evident in about 50% of cases of rabies. Spasms may also be precipitated by other stimuli, such as eating or a draught of air (aerophobia).

Q How may rabies be classified clinically?

A 'Furious' rabies, the more common form, as suffered by Andrew, is characterized by hyperexcitability, spasms and hydrophobia.

'Dumb' rabies presents with an ascending paralysis, which may be clnically indistinguishable from the Guillain–Barré syndrome.

However, these syndromes may overlap. Dumb rabies poses the greatest diagnostic problems. There may be a typical prodrome, with paralysis often involving the bitten limb first before spreading rapidly and symetrically.

Q What is the pathogenesis of rabies infection?

A 1. *Entry of virus.* Intact skin is impermeable to the virus, but infection may occur across undamaged mucous membranes. Rabid animals have virus in the saliva and so can spread infection by inoculating virus at the site of a bite, or by licking abraded skin.
2. *Viral replication.* This occurs initially in muscle cells at the site of the bite.
3. *Ascent to the central nervous system (CNS).* Following release from muscle cells, virus enters peripheral nerves and is translocated in their axoplasm to the spinal cord, and thence rapidly to the brain.
4. *Spread within the CNS.* There is extensive viral replication

within the brain, although curiously this results in very little gross structural damage.
5. *Descent from the CNS.* Virus travels back down axoplasmic routes to sites throughout the body, including salivary glands, myocardium, lung, liver, skin, retina and cornea. Involvement of the salivary gland mucosal epithelium results in virus being shed in salivary secretions, from where it may be transmitted to others. Patients with infectious virus in their bodily secretions thus pose an infection risk to those involved in their care. Human-to-human transmission is, however, a rare occurrence.

The incubation period prior to the development of disease is highly variable (up to a year, but on average 30–90 days). The shortest periods are seen in children and in bites close to the central nervous system, i.e. the head rather than foot wounds.

Q What factors influence the transmission of rabies from animal to man?

A Bites from rabid animals do not always cause disease. Factors which may influence this process include:

- the severity of the bite (may determine viral dose)
- the site of the bite: head and neck bites carry the greatest risk
- mortality is almost certainly higher for wounds inflicted through bare, rather than clothed, skin.

Q What is the likely outcome of a patient suspected of rabies?

A Despite the best efforts of modern intensive care and experimental treatment with antiviral and immunomodulatory drugs, the prognosis of a patient presenting with rabies is bleak. The disease is almost invariably fatal within a short time period.

Q How can the diagnosis be confirmed?

A There are a number of possible approaches:

Ante mortem:

- Demonstration of the virus by specific immunofluorescence in corneal impressions (taken by gently abrading the cornea with a microscope slide), or skin biopsy (best taken from the neck or face)
- Culture of the virus from saliva or other bodily secretions. This requires access to a laboratory that has the necessary containment facilities to allow safe culture of rabies virus
- Detection of antibodies to rabies virus in an individual who has not received vaccine.

Post mortem

- Histological examination of brain tissue for the presence of Negri bodies, i.e. intracytoplasmic eosinophilic inclusions in nerve cells
- Immunofluorescent detection of rabies antigen in the brain
- Transmission of virus to laboratory animals
- Electron microscopic detection of virus particles (which have a bullet-shaped morphology).

Q Where, and in which animals, is rabies endemic?

A Rabies is enzootic in all continents except Australasia and Antarctica. There are other disease-free areas (e.g. the United Kingdom, Japan), mostly islands where stringent quarantine regulations are enforced.

All warm-blooded animals are susceptible to the virus, including bats and birds. Urban rabies is prevalent mostly in feral and domestic dogs. Sylvatic rabies involves a wide range of species (e.g. foxes, skunks, racoons), the predominant animal varying in different geographical areas.

Q Could Andrew's fatal attack of rabies have been prevented?

A Yes. Both active (rabies vaccines) and passive (human rabies immunoglobulin) immunization against rabies is available, safe and effective. Rabies vaccination has a long and chequered history. Vaccines derived from virus grown in nervous tissue are poorly immunogenic and give rise to post-vaccination encephalitis in almost 1 in 1000 vaccinees. These are being replaced by safer vaccines grown in tissue culture (see below), but the latter are more expensive.

Q What is the correct management of a patient exposed to a possibly rabid animal?

A
1. Immediate thorough cleansing of the wound
2. Initiation of a course of post-exposure vaccination as soon as possible (see Box 5.1)
3. Individuals with high-risk exposures, e.g. deep or multiple bites, bites on the face, neck or hands, should also be given a stat dose of human rabies immunoglobulin, one half infiltrated around the wound itself and the remainder by intramuscular injection. This provides antibodies during the early critical period, before the development of active immunity.

The above regimen, when properly administered, is highly successful in preventing the transmission of rabies.

B5.1 Post-exposure rabies vaccination

- Vaccine consists of virus grown in human diploid cells and inactivated by β-propiolactone
- WHO recommendations are for a course of six intramuscular injections (deltoid muscle) on days 0, 3, 7, 14, 28 and 90, where day 0 is the day of the first dose
- Injection should *not* be into the gluteal region, as vaccine failure may arise owing to the poorer immunogenicity of vaccine injected into fat.

Summary: Rabies

Presentation
Non-specific prodrome (malaise, headache, tingling at site of bite) followed by either 'furious' rabies (hyperexcitability, spasms, hydrophobia) or 'dumb' rabies (ascending paralysis)

Prognosis
Universally fatal once clinically evident

Prevention
Pre-exposure: vaccination. Postexposure: vaccination following *any* possible exposure, plus passive immunization if risk of infection is high

---

CASE 6
Mr Grundy, a 62-year-old histopathology technician who has become forgetful and disorientated

Mr Grundy is brought to the surgery by his wife. He is 62 years old and works in the local hospital as a histopathology technician. He had been well until 6 weeks ago, since when he has become increasingly anxious and forgetful, with difficulty in speaking and walking. On direct questioning Mr Grundy appears somewhat confused and disorientated. He exhibits a number of multifocal myoclonic jerks on

examination, and has evidence of both receptive and expressive dysphasia. Mr Grundy is admitted to hospital for further investigation. Routine investigations, including urea and electrolytes, liver function tests and blood gases, are normal. During the next 2 weeks he becomes unsteady on his feet, with a number of falls, and his mental state deteriorates to one of dementia, with memory loss, impaired judgement and a decline in virtually all aspects of mental function. There is no family history of dementing illnesses. CT scan and CSF examination are normal. His EEG reveals repetitive high-voltage polyphasic discharges. A clinical diagnosis is made (see below). No treatment is offered and Mr Grundy's condition continues to deteriorate. He dies 2 months after admission to hospital. Postmortem studies of his brain reveal the abnormalities shown in Figure 6.1. (Fig. 6.2 shows a normal brain.)

Q What is the diagnosis?

A The striking features of Mr Grundy's illness were his relentlessly progressive dementia and ataxia. Routine investigations ruled out a metabolic cause (e.g. liver, renal or respiratory failure). There are a large number of dementing illnesses (e.g. Alzheimer's disease, Lewy body dementia), but the history of myoclonic jerks plus the abnormal EEG is suggestive of Creutzfeldt–Jakob disease (CJD). The majority of patients with CJD present with deficits in higher cortical function, which progress to a state of profound dementia. A minority may present with cerebellar or visual defects, which are usually rapidly followed by the onset of dementia. Over 85% of patients exhibit myoclonus, which persists in sleep and may be elicited by

sudden stimuli such as loud noises or bright lights.

Mr Grundy's brain histology confirms the diagnosis by showing the spongiform changes characteristic of this disease. Higher-power studies of the brain would confirm that these changes were due to vacuolation *within* the nerve cells rather than *between* them (as might occur in Alzheimer's disease, owing to the rapid loss of neurons from the brain).

Q Is CJD caused by an infectious agent?

A Inoculation of CJD brain into an experimental animal results in transmission of the disease, hence the classification of CJD as infectious. CJD is one of a group of human and animal diseases sharing a number of distinctive features and known by a variety of names:

- *Transmissible dementias* (transmissible to experimental animals, dementia is the pre-eminent feature of the disease in humans)
- *Spongiform encephalopathies* (neuronal vacuolation in the brain produces a spongy appearance)
- *Prion diseases* (prions believed to be the causative agents, see below)
- *Slow infections* (prolonged incubation period, infectious).

These diseases and the animals in which they occur include:

- scrapie: *Sheep, goats*
- transmissible mink encephalopathy: *Mink*
- chronic wasting disease: *Mule, deer and elk*
- bovine spongiform encephalopathy ('mad-cow disease'): *Cows*
- kuru: *Humans (cannibals)*
- Creutzfeldt–Jakob disease: *Humans*
- Gerstmann–Straussler–Sheinker syndrome (very rare): *Humans*.

The salient features of these diseases are:

- central nervous system pathology only
- prolonged incubation period
- progressive and fatal clinical course
- reactive astrocytosis and vacuolation of neurons on histology

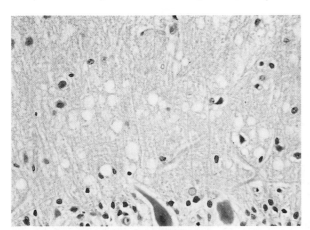

Fig. 6.1 Cerebral tissue from Mr Grundy.

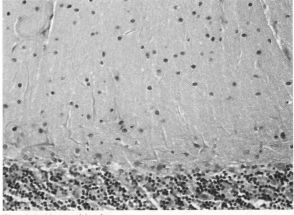

Fig. 6.2 Normal brain.

- transmissible to experimental animals by intracerebral inoculation of diseased tissue.

Q What is unusual about the causative agents of these diseases?

A The infectious agent is believed to consist entirely of protein. The term 'prion' was coined to describe this novel agent, being originally derived from the phrase 'proteinaceous infectious particle'. This radical hypothesis is based on the following lines of evidence:

- Infectivity of scrapie brain in experimental animals is resistant to a wide range of physical and chemical treatments which destroy nucleic acids, but is, however, affected by treatments that destroy or alter protein molecules.
- Despite intensive efforts by many research groups, no-one has succeeded in identifying any nucleic acid in the scrapie agent.
- A protein of molecular weight 27–30 kD has been identified in scrapie brain, whose concentration parallels the infectivity of experimental inocula.

The concept that a protein molecule has the wherewithal to direct its own replication challenges the very foundations of molecular biology. The gene encoding the prion protein (PrP) is in fact a normal cellular gene, the product of which appears to exist in two versions, known as isoforms. The scrapie isoform is able to induce its own production in a cell by catalysing the conversion of the normal isoform into itself. The cell then synthesizes more normal product, which in turn is altered to the scrapie isoform, which thus accumulates (see Fig. 6.3).

Thus experimental inoculation of material containing the scrapie isoform will result in transmission of the disease, as the abnormal isoform of PrP is generated in the recipient brain.

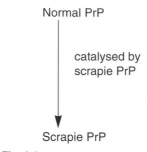

Normal PrP

catalysed by
scrapie PrP

Scrapie PrP

Fig. 6.3

Q How may accidental human-to-human transmission of CJD occur?

A CJD brain is infectious and prions are unusually resistant to inactivation by conventional means (e.g. autoclaving at 121°C). Thus any article contaminated by CJD brain can inadvertently transmit the disease if it is subsequently inoculated into another patient. Such transmission may occur via:

- contaminated intracerebral EEG electrodes and other neuro-surgical instruments
- corneal grafts
- dura mater grafts
- human pituitary-derived growth hormone (usually given to children as replacement therapy), and follicle-stimulating hormone (given to women to treat infertility). Such human-derived hormones are no longer used.

Iatrogenic transmission of CJD accounts for a tiny minority of cases. The route of transmission in the majority of cases of sporadic CJD is unknown.

Of cases of CJD, 10–15% are hereditary. Analysis of the PrP gene in families thus afflicted shows that the gene is mutated in affected individuals, which presumably increases the likelihood of spontaneous conversion of PrP from the normal to the scrapie isoform.

Q Was Mr Grundy's occupation significant?

A Certain health-care professionals are more likely than the general population to be exposed to CJD brain, e.g. neurosurgeons, pathologists, laboratory technicians. Cases of CJD have been described in such individuals, although at present there is no evidence that these occupational groups are over-represented. However, it is clear that appropriate guidelines to reduce the risk of occupational exposure to these agents should be instigated.

Q Are 'mad cows' safe to eat?

A Bovine spongiform encephalopathy (BSE), or 'mad-cow disease' arose in the UK owing to the practice (now banned) of feeding ruminant offal to cows. Whether BSE is due to transmission of scrapie from sheep to cows, or whether there has always been an endogenous bovine agent which has become amplified through the feeding cycle, is not clear. Several expert governmental committees have assessed the risk of transmission of BSE to humans via the oral route, and have concluded that such a risk is miniscule. Others disagree. Time will tell!

Summary: CJD
Presentation
Progressive dementia, ataxia, myoclonus
Diagnosis
Spongiform pathology and presence of PrP 27–30 seen at postmortem
Causative agent
Prion; may consist entirely of protein. Product of normal gene, with post-translational modification. May catalyse its own formation
Iatrogenic infection
May arise from contaminated neurosurgical instruments, human pituitary-derived hormones, dura mater grafts

CASE 7
Darren, a hot and irritable 12-month-old infant

A 12-month-old male child, Darren, is off form for 24–36 hours and is noticed by his parents to be hot and irritable. The illness fails to settle with paracetamol and he is therefore brought to his GP for assessment.

Q What should be looked for on examination?

A General examination should include vital signs such as temperature, heart rate and degree of irritability. Following on from that specific signs should be sought. The absence of a purpuric rash and neck stiffness makes meningitis, especially meningococcal meningitis, less likely, but this could only be excluded following a lumbar puncture; lower respiratory tract infection may be excluded by the absence of tachypnoea, difficulty with breathing, increased respiratory secretions or abnormal signs on auscultation. Tenderness over the ear (easier to assess in the older child, who may complain of earache) might suggest an ear infection, but whether this sign is present or absent auroscopy should be performed.

Examination reveals a bulging, opaque eardrum (Fig. 7.1). A presumptive diagnosis of otitis media (to be distinguished from otitis externa – see Box 7.1) is made, ampicillin to be given by mouth is prescribed, and Darren's parents are instructed to bring him back if he does not settle.

B7.1 Otitis externa

- Skin condition of the external auditory meatus, in any age group, characterized more by inflammation than infection, i.e. a form of local dermatitis
- Often chronic or relapsing
- Gram-negative bacilli (including *Proteus* and *Pseudomonas* spp.) and fungi such as *Candida* or even *Aspergillus* may be isolated from swabs
- Local toilet with or without topical antibiotics such as polymyxin is the first approach to management
- Infection with *Pseudomonas aeruginosa* in the elderly diabetic patient may lead to deep infection of the bone and meningitis (malignant otitis externa)

Q Should the GP have taken any specimens for microbiological confirmation?

A The management of uncomplicated otitis media does not usually warrant investigations. A Gram stain of pus or drainage fluid and culture is possible and to be recommended if the eardrum has perforated, or if a myringotomy is carried out. Blood cultures should be done if the child is toxic or to exclude another

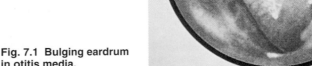

Fig. 7.1 Bulging eardrum in otitis media.

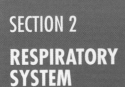

SECTION 2

RESPIRATORY SYSTEM

possible focus of infection, especially if admission to hospital is required.

Q What are the most common causes of otitis media?

A The commonest causes in order of frequency are:

- *Streptococcus pneumoniae*
- *Haemophilus influenzae*
- β-haemolytic streptococcus groups A (*S. pyogenes*), C and G
- *Staphylococcus aureus*
- Less commonly, *Moraxella catarrhalis*, coliforms such as *Escherichia coli*, viruses and *Mycoplasma pneumoniae*.

Q Is oral ampicillin a good choice here?

A Ampicillin, or preferably amoxycillin (better absorbed), is most commonly prescribed in this setting or while awaiting the results of culture and sensitivity tests. Penicillin V (oral penicillin) is poorly absorbed and inactive against Gram-negative bacilli.

Two days later Darren is only marginally better, and as the swelling of the eardrum has worsened the child is referred to hospital, where fluid from the middle ear is aspirated and sent to the microbiology laboratory for culture. *Haemophilus influenzae* **(see Box 7.2), resistant to ampicillin/amoxycillin, is isolated and following a 7-day course of co-amoxyclar (amoxycillin/ clavulanic) acid the child makes an uneventful recovery.**

Q What is clavulanic acid?

A This is a β-lactam antibiotic which has a broad spectrum of activity but low potency. It inhibits the destruction of β-lactamases produced by some bacteria, a common mechanism of resistance. It is used in a fixed ratio with amoxycillin or ticarcillin.

Q How common is ampicillin-resistant *H. influenzae*?

A The majority of isolates are ampicillin sensitive but approxi-

Table 7.1 *Haemophilus influenzae type B*	Non-capsulated *Haemophilus influenzae*
Meningitis (see Case 1)	Otitis media
Epiglottitis	Sinusitis
Bacteraemia (see Case 44)	Bronchitis (see Case 14)
Pneumonia (see Case 12)	Conjunctivitis
Septic arthritis and osteomyelitis (see Case 51)	
Cellulitis (see Case 36)	

B7.2 Haemophilus influenzae

- Small Gram-negative bacillus
- Human pathogen only
- Requires X (iron-containing pigment) and V (coenzyme) factors for growth in vitro
- 50% of healthy people are carriers, 5% carry capsulated strains
- Recent viral infection facilitates colonization and infection

mately 15–20% are resistant, usually owing to the production of β-lactamase, which can be counteracted by the addition of clavulanic acid as discussed above. A smaller proportion of isolates are resistant by a different mechanism, such as alteration in cell permeability or binding proteins. This form of resistance may be accompanied by resistance to other agents, such as trimethoprim and chloramphenicol (less frequently used now). Apart from ampicillin and ampicillin/ clavulanic acid, other agents useful in the blind therapy of otitis media include oral cephalosporins (cefaclor, cefixime), trimethoprim and erythromycin (poor activity against *Haemophilus*, however). Tetracyclines are contraindicated in the growing child because of deposition in teeth (resulting in staining) and bone.

Q Should Darren have been vaccinated against *Haemophilus influenzae*?

A Yes. The vaccine protects against infection with capsulated type B strains. This is a non-live conjugate vaccine in which the haemophilus capsular polysaccharides are linked to proteins which enhance immunogenicity, especially in children less than 1 year of age. It should be

offered to all infants from the age of 2 months and is administered by deep subcutaneous or intramuscular injection in three doses, with an interval of 1 month between doses. It will reduce the incidence of invasive disease due to type B (see Table 7.1), which occurs more frequently in children under 5 years but will not affect the incidence of otitis media caused by non-capsulate strains.

Q What complications may ensue from otitis media?

A Most cases resolve spontaneously, but a delayed diagnosis or inadequate treatment may result in:

- chronic suppurative otitis media – chronic discharge of pus with hearing loss
- glue ear – mucinous effusion in the middle ear, with fluctuating hearing loss and delayed childhood development
- mastoiditis – may proceed to meningitis and brain abscess (see Case 3).

Summary: Otitis media
Presentation
Fever, irritability, painful ear, inflamed eardrum
Diagnosis
Bulging tympanic membrane on auroscopy (fluid + blood for culture if severe)
Management
Antipyretics, antibiotics (amoxycillin, co-amoxyclar, trimethoprim, oral cephalosporin), occasionally myringotomy. Hearing tests on follow-up if severe or complicated

CASE 8

Susan, a 21-year-old student with a runny nose and imminent exams

Susan, a 21-year-old university student, complains of a runny nose and headache. She was well until yesterday, when she began sneezing and felt some irritation at the back of her throat, which has now progressed to a cough and sore throat. She is anxious as she has heard that there is a lot of 'flu' about, and she has an important examination to sit in 1 week's time. There are no abnormal physical signs; she is apyrexial and has no lymphadenopathy.

Q What is your diagnosis?

A Rhinitis (runny nose), headache, sore throat and cough are all features of the common cold (coryza). The absence of systemic symptoms and signs (e.g. fever, myalgia) distinguishes this syndrome from classical influenza (see Case 11).

Q What can Susan be told about the likely course of her illness?

A Headache, sneezing and sore throat usually disappear after 2–3 days. A clear and watery nasal discharge usually becomes mucopurulent and tenacious after a few days. These nasal symptoms tend to be more persistent and severe than other symptoms. Cough also peaks after 4–5 days and may persist. This is a composite view of the common cold syndrome, and it should be noted that individuals may vary in their perception of the relative severity of their different symptoms. There is little or no fever, and systemic manifestations are rare. Overall, patients are most miserable after 3–5 days but have recovered completely by 7–10 days.

Q How may respiratory tract infections be classified?

A There are a number of ways, e.g. by aetiological agent or by anatomical site affected. Clinically, the most important distinction is between *upper* and *lower* respiratory tract infections (URTI and LRTI). In general, the former are considerably more common but are associated with less morbidity than the latter, which may be life-threatening. URTI include the syndromes of otitis media, rhinitis or common cold, sinusitis, conjunctivitis, pharyngitis, laryngitis, croup and laryngotracheobronchitis. The relative frequencies of these syndromes differ with age. Whereas some syndromes are distinctive (e.g. otitis media), there is considerable clinical and aetiological overlap between many others, e.g. a patient with a sore throat may be classified as having a cold, a pharyngitis or a glandular fever-like illness, depending on the presence of other symptoms or signs and the degree to which the sore throat is the dominant symptom.

Q What is the aetiology of the common cold?

A Rhinoviruses and coronaviruses are the two most common causative agents, accounting for well over 50% of illnesses, although the syndrome may arise from infection with a wide range of other viruses, including respiratory syncytial virus (RSV (see Case 15)), parainfluenza, enteroviruses, adenoviruses, and even on occasions influenza viruses.

Q Why is the common cold so common?

A Quite simply because there are so many causative agents. There are over 100 serotypes of rhinovirus: different serotypes circulate in different years, and infection with one serotype does not induce protective immunity against others. On average, in the UK, common colds occur at the rate of almost one per person per year, although this varies with age, being higher in the first few years of life.

Q Should antibiotics be prescribed for Susan?

A No. Antibacterials are not indicated as her illness is viral in aetiology and indiscriminate antibiotic use in this setting may result in increased resistance and super-infections, e.g. oral candidiasis. Despite intensive efforts, no successful specific antiviral agent has been developed. However, it should be possible to achieve at least some symptomatic relief with appropriate analgesics, sympathomimetic nasal decongestants, antitussives and antihistamines. A range of over-the-counter medicines are available, although hot whisky or other home-brewed cocktails may be just as comforting!

Q What complications may arise from an acute rhinovirus infection?

A

- Sinusitis. Radiological evidence of involvement of the epithelium of the sinuses is common. Rhinoviruses have been isolated from sinus fluid, but of greater clinical importance is secondary bacterial sinusitis, the key features of which are shown in Box 8.1.
- Otitis media (see Case 7). The role of rhinoviruses is unclear, Secondary bacterial infection may occur.

B8.1 Acute sinusitis

Clinical features – facial pain, nasal discharge, localized tenderness over affected sinus
Causative organisms – common bacteria include *H. influenzae*, *S. pneumoniae*, β-haemolytic group A streptococci (*S. pyogenes*). Anaerobes may also be involved
Management – definitive diagnosis is by aspiration of pus from the affected sinus, but this is not usually performed. Amoxycillin is first-line therapy
Complications – chronic sinusitis. Rarely may lead to osteomyelitis or cerebral abscess (see Case 3), especially if frontal sinuses involved

- Exacerbations of asthma and chronic bronchitis. Recent studies suggest that the common cold viruses are responsible for a large majority of wheezy attacks in children. The pathogenetic mechanisms underlying this association are the subject of research.
- Lower respiratory tract infection, such as bronchiolitis or pneumonia, but this is rare.

Q What is croup, and who suffers from it?

A Croup is more properly known as acute laryngotracheobronchitis, and is therefore an URTI. It usually occurs in children aged 6 months to 3 years.

Q What are the clinical features of croup?

A Clinical presentation is with coryzal symptoms for 1–2 days, followed by the development of an inspiratory stridor (owing to the passage of air through an inflamed and partially obstructed larynx), and a 'croupy' or 'barking' cough which is worse at night. There is little constitutional disturbance, with only a mild pyrexia. On examination supraclavicular and sternal recession may be evident, as well as use of the accessory muscles of respiration.

Q What are the causes of croup?

A Several viruses can cause croup, of which the parainfluenza viruses are the commonest. Rhinoviruses, RSV, influenza and measles viruses may also give rise to this syndrome.

Q How is a child with croup managed?

A Hospital admission may be necessary, depending on the degree of stridor. Important differential diagnoses of stridor to consider are acute epiglottitis and inhalation of a foreign body. The child should be kept as settled as possible. Antibiotics, steroids, humidified air and routine oxygen are of no benefit. In severe cases, where exhaustion is imminent, intubation may be necessary. With expert care the overwhelming majority of cases of croup make an uneventful recovery.

Summary: URTI
Presentation
Variable, depending on age and anatomical site involved
Aetiology
Viral: rhino-, corona-, parainfluenza-, influenza, entero-, adeno- and respiratory syncytial viruses
Diagnosis
Clinical
Management
No specific antiviral therapy
Prognosis
Excellent

CASE 9
Peter, a 19-year-old student with a sore throat

Peter, a 19-year-old student, gives a 4-day history of a sore throat, difficulty in swallowing and general malaise. His past medical history is unremarkable and he is not taking any form of medication. On examination he has a temperature of 38.6°C. His pharynx is obviously inflamed and there is a whitish membrane over his tonsils (Figure 9.1). He has marked cervical adenopathy.

Q What is the differential diagnosis?

A This is a young man with severe pharyngitis. A number of acute infections can present in this way:

- Viruses: Epstein–Barr virus (EBV); cytomegalovirus; adenoviruses, enteroviruses
- Bacteria: Groups A, C and G streptococci; *Corynebacterium diphtheriae* (see Box 9.1); mycoplasma; chlamydia.

On closer examination it can be seen that Peter's conjunctivae have a tinge of yellow, and in addition to the cervical adenopathy, the axillary nodes and a spleen tip are palpable, but no liver.

Q How do these new findings influence the clinical diagnosis?

A Evidence of systemic disease with generalized lymphadenopathy

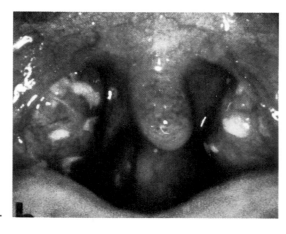

Fig. 9.1 Peter's pharynx.

has now been elicited. These clinical findings are best described as a 'glandular fever' or 'infectious mononucleosis' (IM) syndrome. Infection with EB virus, cytomegalovirus (CMV) and toxoplasma would now come top of the list, but malignancy of the reticuloendothelial system (lymphoma, leukaemia) should also be borne in mind. Acute infection with human immunodeficiency virus (HIV) may also present with an IM-like illness – the so-called sero-converting illness (see Case 30).

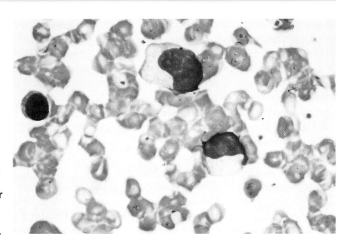

Fig. 9.2 Two atypical mononuclear cells (and one normal lymphocyte).

Direct questioning of Peter reveals no risk factors for HIV infection.

Q What investigations should be carried out?

A A full blood count, including differential and film, liver function tests, and blood for a 'Monospot' or Paul Bunnell test and viral serology will help to distinguish between the common causes of glandular fever listed above. A throat swab for bacterial culture is also indicated.

The next day the following results are received:
Hb 12.6 g/dl
WCC   **Lymphocytes 53%**
14.3×10⁹/l   **Monocytes 6%**
           Large unclassified
           cells (LUC) 11%
Plts 400×10⁹/l
Film shows atypical mononuclear cells (see Figure 9.2)
ALT 86 U/l (normal range 5–50)
Bilirubin 41 mmol/l (3–17)
Alk Phos 43 U/l (40–120)

Q How should these findings be interpreted?

A The blood count and film, showing a lymphocytosis with the presence of atypical mononuclear cells, confirm the clinical diagnosis of infectious mononucleosis. The liver function tests indicate hepatic involvement.

B9.1 Other causes of a severe sore throat

Diphtheria

- Severe sore throat with a 'false membrane' caused by *Corynebacterium diphtheriae*
- Exotoxin responsible for complications, which include polyneuritis, myocarditis/heart block, pneumonia, otitis media
- Laboratory diagnosis requires specialist media, e.g. tellurite, and confirmation of toxin production
- Toxoid part of 3-in-1 vaccine (DPT)

Streptococcal sore throat

- Lancefield Group A the commonest cause of bacterial pharyngitis. Group C + G less common and less severe
- Exudates often seen on the tonsils. Marked fever and cervical lymphadenopathy not unusual
- Penicillin is the treatment of choice but should be continued for 10–14 days to prevent relapse or complications (see Case 36)

Q What are the atypical mononuclear cells?

A Activated T lymphocytes. These occur in small numbers in many acute viral infections. However, if they constitute more than 10% of the total WCC, EBV infection (see Box 9.2) is the most likely cause.

Further results from Peter are:
Monospot – negative
Throat swab – commensals only

B9.2 Features of Epstein–Barr virus

Classification

A herpesvirus – human herpesvirus 4

Sites of infection

- Oropharyngeal epithelial cells, resulting in release of infectious virus in saliva
- Circulating B lymphocytes – the site of EBV latency. Note: infection of B cells *in vitro* results in polyclonal B-cell activation, i.e. antibody production, and transformation, i.e. immortalization of cells into a lymphoblastoid cell line

Transmission

Via saliva – 'kissing disease!'

Outcome of infection

- Asymptomatic seroconversion – the usual outcome in the first few years of life
- Acute infectious mononucleosis – a disease of teenagers and young adults
- Chronic infectious mononucleosis – a controversial diagnosis. Prolonged time to recovery may be part of the natural history of acute EBV infection

Q What is the basis of the Monospot test?

A The Monospot and Paul Bunnell (PB) tests detect the presence of heterophile antibodies (antibodies that react with antigens other than the specific inducing antigen) expressed on foreign red blood cells. EBV infection often results in the transient production of such antibodies, presumably as a result of EBV-induced polyclonal B-cell activation. Therefore the presence of these antibodies, as detected by either of the above tests, is highly suggestive of recent EBV infection. The PB test is slightly more sophisticated as it involves an absorption step to distinguish heterophile antibodies which react with different species of red blood cells.

Q Does a negative Monospot result exclude a diagnosis of acute EBV infection?

A No: 10% of individuals infected with EBV fail to produce heterophile antibodies, and are therefore Monospot and PB negative. Note that cytomegalovirus (CMV), toxoplasma and HIV-induced acute IM are all heterophile antibody negative, and therefore Monospot and PB negative.

Q What further tests should be ordered to confirm Peter's diagnosis?

A A diagnosis of EBV infection can be made by demonstrating the presence of EBV-specific IgM antibodies in an acute serum sample. A rise in antibody titre to CMV or toxoplasma in paired serum samples, or the presence of specific IgM against either organism, would confirm infection with those agents.

The EBV IgM result is positive. Peter was suffering from EBV-induced infectious mononucleosis.

Q What are the complications of acute EBV infection?

A Complications of acute infectious mononucleosis include:

- hepatitis: 5–10% of patients are jaundiced
- splenomegaly: splenic rupture may cause death

- central nervous system manifestations; e.g. encephalitis, meningoencephalitis, Guillain–Barré syndrome, cranial nerve palsies
- airway obstruction due to exudative pharyngotonsillitis: may also be fatal.

Hepatitis and CNS involvement can occur in the absence of other features of acute IM, especially in older patients, leading to diagnostic difficulties.

Four months later Peter returns complaining that he still feels lethargic and unable to resume many of his normal daily activities. He is worried that he may be suffering from some underlying disease, and also that his academic performance is declining. On examination, all the abnormal physical signs present during the acute illness have resolved. Investigations conducted in the previous month showed that his white cell count had returned to normal, and the atypical cells had disappeared.

Q What should be done next?

A Acute infectious mononucleosis is not a trivial illness. Many patients describe taking months or even a year or two before they feel fully fit again. Peter should be reassured that his prolonged lethargy does not indicate some dreadful disease process, but is relatively common. It should also be made clear to him that he will eventually recover. A report should be sent to his university tutor indicating the diagnosis, as his illness should be taken into account in relation to his poor academic performance.

Q What other diseases are associated with Epstein–Barr virus infection?

A EBV infection appears to be important in the development of a number of malignant diseases:

- lymphomas in the immunosuppressed, i.e. transplant recipients,

AIDS patients. Initially polyclonal B-cell proliferations that develop into monoclonal lymphomas. Pathogenesis related to loss of potent T-cell control of EBV-driven B-cell proliferation.

- Burkitt's lymphoma – discussed below.
- nasopharyngeal carcinoma – discussed below.
- Hodgkin's disease – the possible role of EBV in the generation of this disease is the subject of much current research.
- X-linked lymphoproliferative syndrome (XLP), formerly known as Duncan's syndrome. Rare. Inherited defective immunity to EBV in males results in uncontrolled lymphoproliferation following acute infection, with a high mortality.

Q What is the evidence linking EBV infection to the development of Burkitt's lymphoma and nasopharyngeal carcinoma (NPC)?

A

- The tumour cells – B cells in Burkitt's lymphoma and epithelial cells in NPC – contain multiple copies of the EBV genome (EBV was first isolated from a Burkitt's lymphoma biopsy).
- Sera from patients with these tumours contain very high titres of antibodies to EBV, often directed against unusual viral antigens.
- Antibody titres parallel clinical events, i.e. chemotherapy-induced remission is associated with a drop in antibody titres, whereas recurrence of the tumours may be heralded by a rise in titre.
- As a result, EBV serology can be used to screen patients for the presence of Burkitt's lymphoma and NPC, and to monitor response to therapy.
- EBV is tumorigenic in animal models (inducing lymphoma formation in tamarin monkeys), and can immortalize B cells *in vitro*.

However, EBV cannot be the only factor resulting in these malignancies, as 90% of the world's population are infected with EBV and yet these tumours are very geographically restricted in their distribution. Other cofactors must act together with EBV infection in the pathogenesis of such tumours. One such cofactor in the development of Burkitt's lymphoma is the presence of hyperendemic malaria. Possible cofactors for NPC have not yet been identified.

Q What other virus infections are associated with the development of malignant disease?

A

- Hepatitis B virus and hepatocellular carcinoma (see Case 22)
- Hepatitis C virus and hepatocellular carcinoma (see Case 22)
- HTLV-1 and adult T-cell leukaemia/lymphoma (see Case 61)
- Human papilloma viruses, particularly types 16 and 18, and carcinoma of the uterine cervix (see Case 32).

Summary: Infectious mononucleosis
Presentation
Fever, pharyngitis, lymphadenopathy
Causative agents
EB virus, CMV, HIV, toxoplasmosis, Group A streptococcus
Diagnosis
Full blood count and film; Monospot/Paul Bunnell tests; serology; culture of throat swab
Complications
Hepatitis, splenomegaly, neuropathy, respiratory obstruction
Management
Symptomatic; steroids if respiratory obstruction

A 1-year-old dehydrated female infant, Catriona, is brought to the Accident and Emergency department in respiratory distress. Her father reported that following a period of increased nasal discharge and a slight pyrexia, which lasted for 3 days, she began breathing fast and developed a paroxysmal cough.

Q What other information should be elicited from the parents?

A Apart from assessing whether other siblings were affected the significant question here concerns the vaccination status of the patient. In particular has the child been vaccinated against whooping cough?

Catriona is admitted to hospital and nursed in a side room. Vital signs are closely monitored and parenteral hydration is commenced. Over the next 2–3 days she becomes less distressed and the coughing resolves. It is subsequently learned that Catriona has not been vaccinated against whooping cough because her parents were concerned about reported side-effects.

Q What are the clinical features of whooping cough?

A Not all children with whooping cough have the 'whoop', the classic feature of this condition. The condition may present with severe cough, tachypnoea and cyanosis, but in many instances the presentation may not be dissimilar to other respiratory infections.

Q What is the mechanism by which the 'whoop' is produced?

A The 'whoop' is caused by a series of expiratory bursts followed by an inspiratory gasp. The whooping or spasmodic stage is preceded by the catarrhal stage, and is followed by a period of recovery when the paroxysms of coughing become less severe.

Q How may the diagnosis of whooping cough be confirmed?

A Whooping cough is a clinical syndrome most commonly caused by *Bordetella pertussis*, which can be cultured during the early stages of the illness, but the condition may also be caused by:

- *B. parapertussis*
- viruses
    respiratory syncytial
    parainfluenza
    adenovirus
- *Mycoplasma pneumoniae*.

Isolation of *Bordetella* is best from a pernasal swab (see Box 10.1 and Figure 10.1).

Q What is the antibiotic of choice to treat *Bordetella* infections?

A It is not clear whether antimicrobial treatment alters the natural history of infection, but ery-

B10.1 Laboratory diagnosis of *Bordetella pertussis* and *B. parapertussis*
Specimen
Pernasal preferred to nasal swab, sputum or nasopharyngeal swab. Cough plates may also be used but are less convenient
Media
Selective media such as Bordet and Gengou or charcoal–cephalexin. Specimen should be transported to the laboratory rapidly or transport medium used
Identification
Plates incubated for up to 5 days. Suspect colonies (mercury-like on charcoal, haemolytic on Bordet and Gengou) are tested for agglutination with polyvalent serum for confirmation

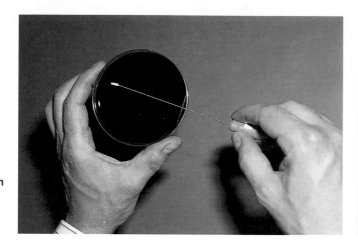

Fig. 10.1 Innoculation of pernasal swab onto charcoal blood agar.

B10.2 Pertussis vaccine

- Suspension of killed bacterial cells which includes three agglutinins adsorbed on to an adjuvant (aluminium hydroxide)
- Administered by deep intramuscular injection with diphtheria and tetanus in three doses, e.g. at 2, 3 and 4 months (booster 4–5 years later)
- Adverse reactions include swelling and redness at injection site, screaming and crying attacks and encephalopathy/convulsions leading to brain damage (1 in 310 000)

---

thromycin is usually prescribed in the hope of reducing infectivity. This may be important where there are non-vaccinated siblings. There is little place, if any, for treatment with immunoglobulin.

Q What are the complications of whooping cough?

A Complications are most likely in children less than 1 year, and these include:

- apnoea leading to convulsions and possibly brain damage
- pneumonia, lobar collapse and pneumothorax
- subconjunctival haemorrhage and epistaxis (due to convulsive coughing)
- hernias and rectal prolapse (due to convulsive coughing).

Q What are the contraindications to pertussis vaccination?

A The current vaccine (composed of a suspension of killed organisms) is 90% effective. Reasons for not vaccinating include:

- concurrent fever or acute illness (postpone vaccination)
- history of previous adverse local (severe) or general reaction.

A personal or family history of allergy (e.g. to aspirin or penicillin) is not a contraindication, nor are stable neurological conditions such as cerebral palsy or previous febrile convulsions.

Q What are the side-effects of the vaccine?

A These include local swelling at the site of injection and crying. The most controversial and serious, however, have been neurological, including encephalopathy and prolonged convulsions, resulting in severe brain damage and even death. In a number of cases it has not been possible to link the vaccine directly with the complications, and it is generally agreed that the risk of serious neurological complications arising from pertussis is greater than that from the vaccine. It is very likely that in the next few years a new generation of more purified components of *Bordetella pertussis* or acellular vaccines will become available to replace the whole-cell vaccine currently in use. These are much less likely to result in neurological complications.

Summary: Whooping cough
Presentation
Paroxysmal cough, respiratory distress
Diagnosis
Clinical features, pernasal swab for isolation of *Bordetella*
Management
Vaccination (prevention), rehydration, ventilation occasionally, erythromycin

CASE 11
Mrs Smith, 32 years old, with a cough and generalized muscle aches and pains

Mrs Smith, a 32-year-old woman, complains of a febrile illness that began abruptly 3 days ago, on Christmas day, with a marked fever, headache and shivering. Since then she has developed a non-productive cough, muscle aches all over her body, especially in the legs, and her eyes have become watery and painful to move. She is a non-smoker, previously fit and well, and on no regular medication. On examination she is febrile (38.2°C) and has difficulty in breathing through her nose, but there are no other abnormal physical signs.

Q What is the diagnosis?

A These are the classic symptoms and signs of influenza. Clinically, the terms 'flu' and 'flu-like illness' should refer to more than just a simple common cold (runny nose, headache, irritating cough), i.e. there should be evidence of systemic upset, with fever, myalgia and severe malaise. However, this terminology is often misused by the general public, who may regard any upper respiratory tract symptoms as evidence that they are suffering from 'flu'. Infection with influenza viruses A or B is the commonest cause of this clinical syndrome, other causes include RSV (particularly in the elderly), adenovirus, *Mycoplasma pneumoniae* and *Chlamydia* species (see Case 13).

Q What would the management of Mrs Smith consist of?

A Management is symptomatic only, e.g. paracetamol (not aspirin, because of the risk of Reye's syndrome particularly in young children), codeine linctus and bed rest. The infection usually resolves within 7 days, but patients may complain of feeling listless for some time afterwards.

Two days later Mrs Smith still has a fever (38.5°C) and is feeling worse. Her cough is more pronounced, although not very productive, and she complains of chest tightness and breathlessness on the slightest exertion. There are no signs of consolidation in the chest, but widespread rhonchi and crepitations are heard on auscultation.

Q What complication of influenza virus infection could this indicate?

A Pneumonia. This is the commonest life-threatening complication of influenza virus infection.

Q What aetiological types of pneumonia may follow influenza virus infection?

A Primary viral or secondary bacterial pneumonia (see Box 11.1).

Mrs Smith is admitted to hospital for further investigation and management.

Q What microbiological investigations should be performed?

A Confirmation of the influenza virus infection should be sought by sending an NPA or throat swab in viral transport medium for viral culture, and an acute serum sample for subsequent antibody assays. A sputum sample, for both bacterial and viral culture, is also mandatory. Blood cultures should also be taken to diagnose bacteraemic pneumonia.

In extreme cases, in patients failing to respond to therapy where no diagnosis has been reached, and where atypical pneumonia is a possibility (see Case 13), bronchoalveolar lavage fluid should be sent for study.

Q What tests would the virology laboratory perform on a nasopharyngeal aspirate, sputum or lavage fluid?

A In addition to inoculating appropriate tissue cultures for virus isolation, a rapid diagnosis can be attempted by immunofluorescent staining of cells obtained from the clinical material with monoclonal antibodies against, e.g. influenza A virus, influenza B virus, RSV, parainfluenza viruses, adenoviruses and chlamydia. The technique of immunofluorescence is explained in Case 15.

Mrs Smith's chest X-ray shows diffuse shadowing in both lung fields. Blood gases demonstrate hypoxia ($Pa o_2$ = 9.2 kPa) and a full blood count shows a normal white cell count and differential. The sputum was positive for the presence of influenza A virus by immunofluorescence. The next morning, bacterial culture of the sputum reveals commensals only.

B11.1 Pneumonia following influenza infection

Primary viral pneumonia

- Causative agent influenza virus
- Can occur in previously fit and healthy persons
- Follows on from acute infection
- Alveolar space becomes filled with fibrinous material
- Mononuclear cell infiltrate into alveolar walls

Secondary bacterial pneumonia

- Causative agents *Streptococcus pneumoniae*, *Haemophilus influenzae*, *Staphylococcus aureus*, for example
- More common than viral pneumonia, especially in the elderly
- Many patients have underlying disease, e.g. chronic bronchitis
- May follow a period of initial improvement of acute disease
- Alveolar space filled with polymorphonuclear cell infiltrate

---

Q What is your diagnosis?

A The clinical picture here is very suggestive of primary viral pneumonia, as evidenced by illness in a previously fit non-smoker; failure to mount a neutrophil response; virus but no bacterial pathogens in a sputum sample.

Q What antiviral agents are available for the treatment of influenza virus infection?

A Amantadine (and its derivative, rimantadine):

- interferes with uncoating of virus within infected cells; active only against influenza A virus, but has side-effects such as insomnia, confusion and restlessness, and is therefore poorly tolerated, especially by the elderly.

Ribavirin:
- interferes with processing of viral mRNA; active against both influenza A and B viruses and RSV, but must be administered by continuous inhalation for optimal effect.

Mrs Smith is treated with amantadine and cefuroxime (to cover undiagnosed bacterial pneumonia, including *Staph. aureus*), and observed carefully. Her chest gradually improves and she is well enough to be discharged 14 days after admission. No bacterial pathogen was ever isolated from her chest or blood cultures.

Q What is the pathogenesis of influenza virus infection?

A Influenza virus infects the epithelial cells lining the respiratory tract. All such cells, whether in the upper or the lower respiratory tract, are susceptible. Primary viral pneumonia arises from direct spread of virus to the lower respiratory tract.

Infected cells become rounded and swollen, and ciliation, an important defence mechanism to prevent the passage of particulate matter (including bacteria) into the lower respiratory tract, is lost. This can be seen in Figure 11.1.

The systemic symptoms of influenza are most likely due to virus-induced release of cytokines such as α-interferon. Viraemia is very difficult to demonstrate, even at the acute stage of the illness.

Q What other complications may arise from influenza virus infection?

A In the respiratory tract tracheobronchitis, bronchiolitis and pneumonia (primary or secondary) are the most common. Myocarditis may arise, a serious complication especially in individuals with pre-existing cardiac disease.

Neurological complications are postinfectious encephalitis (see Case 37 for a definition of this term), Guillain–Barré syndrome and Reye's syndrome (precipitated by aspirin ingestion).

Q How are influenza viruses classified?

A A schematic diagram of an influenza virus is shown in Figure 11.2. Influenza viruses are classified into types A, B or C (not a serious human pathogen) on the basis of the nature of the *internal* viral proteins. Influenza A viruses are further subdivided into subtypes on the basis of the nature of the two surface glycoproteins, i.e. the haemagglutinin (H) and neuraminidase (N). Influenza viruses are widespread throughout nature, and thus far nine distinct H and 13 N molecules have been identified in influenza A viruses. It is customary, therefore, when referring to an influenza A virus, to indicate which particular H and N molecules it possesses, e.g. influenza A H1N1.

Q What is understood by the terms 'pandemic' and 'interpandemic epidemic' influenza?

A The epidemiology of influenza is most unusual (see Figure 11.3). Epidemics occur every winter in temperate climates, to a greater or lesser extent. However, every 20 years or so a massive epidemic sweeps the globe, with hugely increased numbers of infected individuals and associated mortality rates. These occurrences are referred to as pandemics, and the smaller peaks of infection and morbidity occurring in between the pandemics are known as interpandemic epidemics.

Q What are the mechanisms underlying the emergence of influenza epidemics and pandemics?

A Antigenic *drift* (see Box 11.2) is responsible for the generation of new epidemic strains each winter, whereas antigenic *shift* (see Box 11.3) gives rise to the pandemic strains every 20 years or so. These terms refer to changes that take place in the surface glycoproteins

A

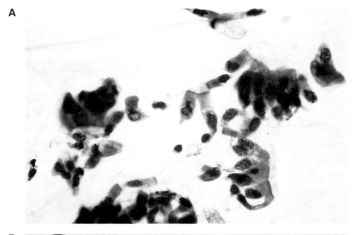

B

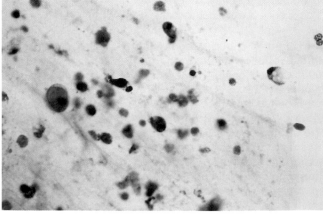

Fig. 11.1 Sputum epithelial cells from (A) normal and (B) influenza infected individuals. In the latter the cells are rounded and dying. The ciliated brush border is lost.

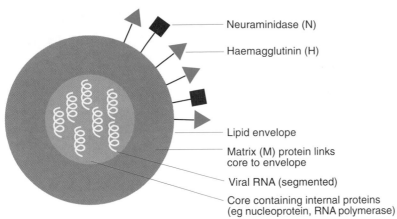

Neuraminidase (N)

Haemagglutinin (H)

Lipid envelope

Matrix (M) protein links
core to envelope

Viral RNA (segmented)

Core containing internal proteins
(eg nucleoprotein, RNA polymerase)

Fig. 11.2 Schematic diagram of influenza virus.

(i.e. the H and N proteins of
influenza viruses.

Since the last pandemic in 1976,
three human influenza viruses have
co-circulated each winter – influenza A viruses H1N1 and H3N2,
and influenza B. In any one season
one of these three viruses tends to
dominate, but the dominant virus
may change from season to season.

Q Is influenza virus infection
preventable?

A Yes, by means of inactivated
vaccines. Vaccines must contain
each of the three viruses that co-
circulate. Current vaccines are about
70% effective in protecting against
infection.

Q For how long are the vaccines
effective?

A One winter only, as the circulating viruses exhibit antigenic
drift from year to year. Thus, the
constituent vaccine viruses need to
be altered accordingly, and patients
need a dose of vaccine each
autumn. The WHO monitors the
antigenicity of circulating influenza
viruses, and recommendations are
made each year as to what would
be the most appropriate strains to
include in the vaccine.

Q Who should be vaccinated
against influenza?

A The current policy is to protect
those patients groups who are at
increased risk of serious complications of infection. Immunization is
strongly recommended for adults
and children with the following:

- chronic respiratory disease, including asthma

- chronic heart disease
- chronic renal failure
- diabetes mellitus and other endocrine disorders
- immunosuppression due to
  disease or treatment.

Immunization is also recommended
for residents of old people's homes

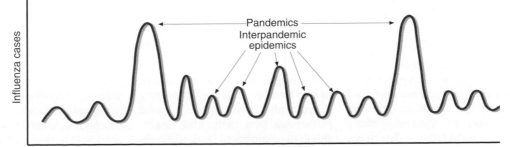

**Fig. 11.3
Epidemiology
of influenza.**

Influenza cases

Pandemics
Interpandemic
epidemics

Years

CASE 11

or other institutions, where rapid spread is likely to follow introduction of infection.

Q Is there any alternative to vaccination, e.g. in those allergic to eggs (a contraindication to vaccination)?

A Yes. Amantadine given as prophylaxis has been shown to be effective in preventing influenza infection, but is poorly tolerated by many patients. It is useful in an outbreak setting, where there may not be sufficient time to allow the vaccine to work.

Summary: Influenza
Presentation
Coryza, cough, headache, fever, generalized myalgia
Diagnosis
Clinical; serology; viral culture of NPA, throat swab
Complications
Pneumonia (primary viral or secondary bacterial); myocarditis; postinfectious encephalitis
Management
Symptomatic; amantadine; antibiotics if pneumonia
Prevention
Vaccination of high-risk groups

CASE 12
Sarah, a 55-year-old woman with rigors, cough and chest pain

Sarah, a 55-year-old pyrexial woman, is referred to the Accident and Emergency department with a 24-hour history of cough, left-sided chest pain and rigors. She has a cough productive of sputum most mornings, but this has become increasingly purulent. Until a myocardial infarction 2 years previously she smoked 40 cigarettes a day.

Q What physical findings might be elicited on respiratory examination?

A Physical signs of consolidation, i.e. dullness on percussion, an area of bronchial breathing with or without absent breath sounds, would suggest lobar pneumonia whereas reduced breath sounds accompanied by crepitations would be more characteristic of bronchopneumonia. These findings may also be relevant when considering likely aetiology.

On examination Sarah has a fever of 40°C, a tachycardia of 130/min and is tachypnoeic, but her blood pressure is normal. Auscultation of the respiratory system indicates probable consolidation.

Q What is the clinical diagnosis and how may this be confirmed?

A A high fever, chest pain, productive cough and the above findings on physical examination are very suggestive of pneumonia requiring admission to hospital for investigation and management. Chest X-ray, white cell count, sputum for microscopy and culture, blood cultures and arterial blood gases will help in assessing the likely aetiology and the severity of the illness.

The peripheral white cell count is elevated, at 22 000 × 10⁹/l (90% polymorph neutrophils) and numerous pus cells and Gram-positive diplococci are seen in the Gram stain of the sputum.

CASE 12

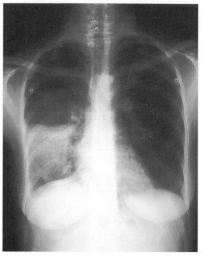

A

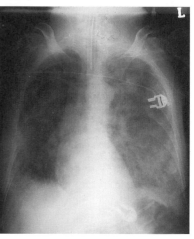

B

Fig. 12.1 Chest X-rays of (A) lobar and (B) bilateral bronchopneumonia.

Chest X-ray confirms right lobar pneumonia (Figure 12.1A).

Q What does the Gram stain tell us?

A The presence of pus cells in the absence of epithelial cells confirms that this is most likely a specimen obtained from the lower respiratory tract, and therefore culture is unlikely to reflect merely upper respiratory flora. It is not possible to distinguish definitely the different types of inflammatory cell (i.e. polymorphs, lymphocytes, monocytes) seen with a Gram stain, but in this instance these are likely to be poly-

B12.1 *Streptococcus pneumoniae*
Microbiology
Gram-positive coccus that may be in pairs or short chains α-haemolytic colonies on blood agar identified by sensitivity to optochin Virulence determinants include a capsule and pneumolysin
Diseases
Systemic 　pneumonia (also abscess and 　　empyema) 　bacteraemia (see Case 44) 　meningitis (see Case 1) 　arthritis (see Case 51), peritonitis 　　(primary) etc. *Localized* 　otitis media (see Case 7) 　sinusitis/mastoiditis 　bronchitis (see Case 14) 　conjunctivitis

morphs. The organisms seen are likely to be *Streptococcus pneumoniae* (pneumococcus, see Box 12.1). The isolation of α-haemolytic streptococci (see Case 36) with typical colonial features sensitive to optochin will confirm this. If culture is negative, owing, for example, to the patient having recently been given antibiotics, antigen detection techniques such as counterimmuno-electrophoresis (CIE) may confirm the diagnosis.

Q What other investigations may be helpful?

A Many patients with pneumococcal pneumonia are bacteraemic and therefore blood cultures are important, especially where sputum is not available, e.g. in the elderly patient. The presence of bacteraemia also heralds a poorer prognosis. Respiratory specimens obtained at bronchoscopy are also useful if there is no sputum, if the diagnosis is uncertain or if an atypical pathogen (see Case 13) is suspected. Finally, paired sera (10–14 days apart) and pleural fluid for culture may also be helpful and indicated in certain circumstances.

Q What are the most common causes of pneumonia?

A *S. pneumoniae* is by far the commonest cause of community-acquired pneumonia, followed by *Mycoplasma pneumoniae*, but the aetiology of hospital-acquired infection is different, with *S. pneumoniae* encountered much less frequently (see Table 12.1).

Q Why is the aetiology of hospital-acquired pneumonia so different?

A Gram-negative bacilli and *Staphylococcus aureus* predominate in hospital because of increased colonization of the upper airways following hospital admission, antibiotics and invasive procedures. Polymicrobial infection may follow aspiration and, in severely immuno-suppressed patients, viral (cytomegalovirus), fungal (*Aspergillus*) and protozoan (*Pneumocystis carinii*) causes must be considered.

Q What is the treatment of choice for pneumococcal disease?

A Benzylpenicillin (minimum inhibitory concentration to *S. pneumoniae* is 0.03 mg/l) is the treatment of choice unless the patient has a definite history of penicillin allergy or the isolate is resistant (common in certain parts of the world, such as South Africa and Spain). Where the aetiology is unclear, ampicillin, co-amoxyclav or a parenteral cephalosporin such as cefotaxime is preferred to cover *H. influenzae*, even though these antibiotics are less active against the pneumococcus.

Sarah is started on intravenous benzylpenicillin, but 12 hours later she is transferred to the ITU for ventilation because of persistent hypoxia. *S. pneumoniae* is isolated from two sets of blood cultures taken on admission as well as from sputum. Three days later she still requires ventilation and her antibiotic has been changed to cefotaxime, to cover against an ITU-acquired pneumonia. The white cell count is now over 35 000 × 10⁹/l and the chest X-ray shows deterioration, with increasing consolidation and a pleural effusion. Repeat respiratory specimens taken during bronchoscopy and blood cultures are sterile. On day 5 Sarah has a cardiac arrest and dies.

Q What factors are associated with an unfavourable prognosis?

A A high mortality from pneumococcal pneumonia is associated with:

- bacteraemia (20% vs. 5% in non-bacteraemic patients)
- accompanying extrapulmonary focus
- certain capsular types (typing of isolates not routine)
- underlying disease such as splenic dysfunction, cirrhosis.

Q How may pneumococcal disease be prevented?

A A polyvalent vaccine derived from 23 capsular types is available and has an efficacy of 60–70%,

Table 12.1 Aetiology of community- and hospital-acquired pneumonia	
Community-acquired	**Hospital-acquired**
S. pneumoniae *Mycoplasma pneumoniae* (young adults) *Haemophilus influenzae* *Moraxella catarrhalis* Influenza virus *Legionella* spp.	Enterobacteriaceae, e.g. *E. coli*, *Klebsiella* spp. *Pseudomonas aeruginosa* (ITU) *Staphylococcus aureus* Anaerobes, e.g. *Bacteroides fragilis* (aspiration) Fungi, e.g. *Candida*, *Aspergillus*

especially in non-immunosuppressed adults. A single dose is administered intramuscularly or subcutaneously. Indications for vaccination are:

- splenic dysfunction such as sickle cell disease; before elective or following emergency splenectomy
- chronic heart, lung, liver or renal disease
- diabetes mellitus
- immunosuppressed patients, including those with HIV infection.

Summary: Pneumococcal pneumonia
Presentation
Lobar (more characteristic) or bronchopneumonia with high fever, purulent sputum, chest pain, rigors and signs of consolidation
Diagnosis
Physical findings on examination, chest X-ray, sputum or bronchoscopy specimens for microscopy and culture and blood cultures
Management
Prevention by vaccination for at-risk groups; benzylpenicillin is the antibiotic of choice

CASE 13
Dermot, a 57-year-old smoker with increasing dyspnoea and confusion

Dermot, a 57-year-old man, is admitted to hospital because of increasing dyspnoea and confusion. Five days previously he developed a non-productive cough which has become worse, and he has become more housebound because of breathlessness. He smokes 20–30 cigarettes a day despite having had a myocardial infarction 3 years previously. His only medication is a thiazide diuretic for mild hypertension. On examination he is a little drowsy and disorientated in time. He has a respiratory rate of 22/min, a heart rate of 95/min and his temperature is 37.5°C. Scattered crepitations, more marked on the left, are heard on auscultation. Neurological examination is grossly normal.

Q What relevant initial investigations should be carried out?

A The previous medical history and presenting symptoms suggest a possible cardiac cause, and consequently an electrocardiogram (ECG) and chest X-ray should be carried out immediately. Blood gases will indicate whether he is hypoxic and/or hypercapnic, and in a distressed patient with pyrexia, sputum and blood should be taken for culture.

The ECG shows evidence of a previous posterior infarct and the arterial oxygen pressure is low at 8 kPa (11–13). **Chest X-ray reveals a normal heart size but patchy consolidation in the left-mid and upper zones. Full blood count, urea and electrolytes, serum glucose and calcium are normal. Despite nasal oxygen, he remains hypoxic and within 18 hours of admission requires ventilation in the intensive therapy unit. His wife, Maura, is interviewed and she remarks that he has become more disorientated and confused in recent days, but that he had been well throughout their holiday in Spain, from which they returned** a week ago. She also remarks that the illness started with a viral-type respiratory illness, i.e. generalized lethargy, nasal discharge and a mild cough.

Q What diagnosis comes to mind following the collateral history from his wife?

A The clinical and radiological features of this case strongly suggest pneumonia, but the absence of a high fever, a productive cough and marked physical findings on examination of the chest point to a diagnosis of 'atypical pneumonia'.

Q What is 'atypical' compared with 'typical' pneumonia?

A The term 'atypical' is usually meant to refer to the less common aetiological agents which do not present with classical pneumonia. It is best, however, to consider this clinical syndrome and how the term 'atypical' originates under a number of headings:

- *Presentation*: flu-like illness, sometimes with few if any respiratory symptoms. Productive cough and a high fever, which are characteristic of pneumonia, are often absent.
- *Diagnosis*: the organisms responsible are largely non-bacterial and therefore culture of sputum and blood will only serve to exclude more conventional causes of pneumonia, such as *Streptococcus pneumoniae* (see Case 12). Respiratory specimens obtained during bronchoscopy, specialized culture techniques, antigen detection and serology are part of the work-up of such a patient.
- *Aetiology*: bacterial, viral, chlamydial and rickettsial causes have all been implicated, and many of these are associated with specific clinical and/or epidemiological features (Table 13.1).
- *Treatment*: failure to respond to β-lactam antibiotics.

Table 13.1 Aetiology and features of atypical pneumonia

Class of microbe	Organism	Features of infection
Bacteria	*Legionella pneumophila*	Ubiquitous in aquatic environment Associated with travel abroad, air-conditioning system (e.g. in hotels)
	Mycoplasma pneumoniae	Cell wall-deficient bacteria Commonest cause of pneumonia in young adults
Chlamydia	*Chlamydia psittaci*	May be associated with psittacine birds. Causes a severe pneumonia
	Chlamydia pneumoniae	Occurs in children or young adults May recur
Rickettsiae	*Coxiella burnetti*	May be occupation related, e.g. farmers. Also causes endocarditis (see Case 46). Also known as Q fever
Viruses	Influenza A, B, C	Occur during epidemics, especially A
	Adenovirus	Important cause in the young, especially in institutions such as military barracks

On admission to the ITU a bronchoscopy is carried out and the bronchi are noted to be inflamed, with increased secretions, especially on the left side. Following instillation of normal saline, lavage fluid is obtained and sent to the laboratory for culture, *Legionella* isolation and direct antigen detection by immunofluorescence. Immunofluorescence is negative for *Legionella*, *Mycoplasma pneumoniae*, *Chlamydia* spp., adenoviruses and influenza viruses.

Q Does a negative immunofluorescence result rule out infection with *Legionella*?

A Immunofluorescence is a highly specific test in the diagnosis of *Legionella* infection, but it is less sensitive than culture because only a smaller volume of specimen can be examined. Patients who have recently been treated with antimicrobial agents active against *Legionella* may be negative on culture but positive for immunofluorescence, since the latter is not dependent on viable organisms. Recent evidence suggests that antigen detection in the urine may be useful in making a diagnosis early in the course of the illness. It is possible that DNA probes which detect gene-specific ribosomal RNA will increasingly be used in diagnosis. Culture has the added advantage

that it will not only isolate *L. pneumophila* serogroup 1, but also other serogroups or species.

***L. pneumophila* serogroup 1, however, is isolated and although antibodies to Legionella are 1/16 on admission these rise to 1/128 10 days later when repeated. It is therefore concluded that Dermot has acquired Legionnaires' disease.**

Q How useful is serology in making a diagnosis?

A Serology is negative – i.e. there is a failure to demonstrate a four fold rise in titres – in up to 25% of cases, and therefore a range of diagnostic approaches must be considered when investigating cases of legionella pneumonia or other causes of atypical pneumonia.

Q What other clinical features may be seen with Legionnaires' disease?

A Diarrhoea is present in about a quarter of cases. Changes in mental status, including encephalopathy, and peripheral neuropathy, may also be seen. A number of laboratory parameters are often abnormal, including liver function tests and, in particular, serum sodium.

Q What is the antibiotic of choice for treatment?

A Legionellae, like chlamydia and rickettsiae, are resistant to the β-lactam antibiotics (penicillins and cephalosporins). Erythromycin is the agent of choice, with rifampicin added for severe cases requiring ventilation or organ support. Other macrolides such as clarithromycin and azithromycin have been advocated for treatment, as have been the quinolones, e.g. ciprofloxacin, but studies demonstrating a better outcome have not been carried out. Erythromycin is also the drug of choice for *Mycoplasma pneumoniae* infections, but a tetracycline is preferred for the treatment of chlamydial and rickettsial infections. Because of the relative infrequency of many of these causes of pneumonia, large-scale comparative antibiotic trials have not been conducted and recommendations on treatment have arisen from individual and collective experience, *in-vitro* studies on antimicrobial activity and by general consensus.

Dermot is started on intravenous erythromycin and improves after 48–72 hours. Two days later he is transferred back to a general medical ward, and later the erythromycin is changed to oral administration for the second week of his 2-week course. Dermot is subsequently discharged from hospital having made a full recovery. Maura, his wife, continues to remain asymptomatic.

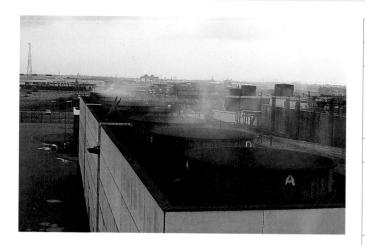

Fig. 13.1 Cooling towers – a possible source of *Legionella* infection.

Summary: Legionnaires' disease
Presentation
Fever, dry cough, dyspnoea, but without rigors or purulent sputum. Respiratory failure may be a feature in patients with underlying lung disease
Diagnosis
Clinical suspicion in a patient with 'atypical' features, bronchoscopy specimens for culture and antigen detection and paired sera for antibody production
Management
High-dose erythromycin with or without rifampicin in severe cases. Patients may require ventilation in an intensive therapy unit.

Q How may infection with *Legionella* be acquired?

A Legionellae are Gram-negative rods which are widely distributed in nature (see Box 13.1), especially in aquatic environments. They flourish in the water systems of buildings, such as potable water and water systems (see Figure 13.1). It is possible that Dermot acquired the infection while on holiday in Spain, especially if the hotel in which the couple were staying had air conditioning. Most community-acquired cases of *Legionella* infection are sporadic and no definite source is ever identified. Nosocomial infection is well described, is most likely to occur during the summer months, and is associated with widespread and heavy contamination of water sources, conducting systems such as piping, or inadequately heated hot water. The facility of *Legionella* to survive inside protozoa which may be found in many water supplies partly explains their ability to persist in domestic and other water supplies.

Q What precautions should nursing and medical staff take while caring for this patient?

A Person-to-person spread of *Legionella* is not known to occur and therefore special precautions are not required to prevent transmission to other patients or staff.

There is a possibility that the patient's wife may have contracted *Legionella*, as she is likely to have been exposed to the same sources as her husband. She may not, however, develop symptoms because of having been exposed to a smaller inoculum, previous exposure to *Legionella* and some degree of immunity, or the absence of underlying disease such as emphysema due to smoking.

B13.1 Legionella
• Gram-negative rods poorly visualized on routine microscopy. Natural habitat is water, such as hot water systems, nebulizers, showers and air conditioning systems; 36 species, the most important being *L. pneumophila*
• Cause Pontiac fever (a mild flu-like illness) and pneumonia, which is more severe in patients with pre-existing lung disease
• Will not grow on routine laboratory media. Bronchoscopic specimens or tissue superior to sputum for culture and antigen detection. Serology important in the absence of respiratory specimens

CASE 14
Dyspnoea, wheeze and a productive cough in Tony, a 55-year-old smoker

Tony is a 55-year-old man who complains of increasing breathlessness, wheeze and a productive purulent cough for the last 3 days. He smokes 20 cigarettes a day, down from 30–40 a day since a previous admission to hospital 2 years ago for pneumonia, expectorates clear sputum most mornings, and is on no medication apart from a salbutamol inhaler, which he uses occasionally. He is examined by his GP, who notes that he has a pyrexia of 38°C and that he has scattered rhonchi throughout both lung fields.

Q Has Tony got chronic bronchitis?

A Most probably. A diagnosis of chronic bronchitis is a clinical one and is made on a history of sputum produced on most days for at least 3 consecutive months for more than 2 consecutive years. Chronic bronchitis is usually characterized by bronchial oedema, epithelial hyperplasia, increased mucus-secreting cells and bronchospasm. It is closely associated with cigarette smoking; in some patients emphysema is predominant, in others an asthmatic component, as described here, largely explains the symptomatology. This patient most likely has an acute exacerbation of chronic bronchitis superimposed upon chronic obstructive lung disease.

Q What clinical features would suggest an infective component?

A Acute bronchitis of infective aetiology is usually characterized by fever and a cough, with or without productive sputum, but acute exacerbations of chronic obstructive airways disease are not always necessarily due to infection. Increased sputum, accompanied by a change in colour from clear or mucoid to purulent (see Figure 14.1), indicates a probable infective component. A complaint of fatigue or other systemic symptoms also points towards infection. Non-infective causes include increased cigarette smoking and environmental factors such as smog.

Tony's GP advises him to reduce the number of cigarettes smoked, or preferably stop altogether, and prescribes inhaled salbutamol four times daily to reduce wheezing, and inhaled atropine to improve bronchospasm and inhibit the formation of mucus. She also prescribes a 5-day course of oral amoxycillin, but 1 week later the patient's cough is no better, despite his now smoking only 10 cigarettes a day. The sputum has also become more purulent.

Q What investigations, if any, are now required?

A A chest X-ray will help exclude other pathology in a smoker, including a lung neoplasm, pneumothorax, consolidation or possible tuberculosis. If none of these is present the X-ray may reveal signs

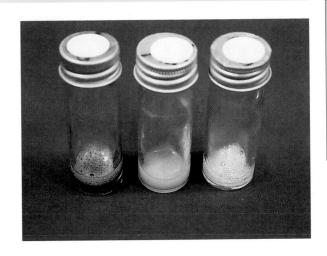

Fig. 14.1 Examples of blood-stained, purulent and mucoid sputa.

of chronic chest disease, such as emphysema and increased bronchiolar markings, but there are no characteristic radiological features of acute exacerbations of chronic obstructive airways disease.

Microscopy and culture of sputum is probably indicated because the sputum has become more purulent despite antibiotic treatment. A good-quality sputum should reveal numerous pus cells, few if any epithelial cells (usually from the buccal mucosa), and bacteria, some of which may be responsible for Tony's symptoms.

Q What microbes are responsible for acute exacerbations of emphysema and chronic bronchitis?

A Potential respiratory pathogens can be cultured from the sputum of most of these patients, unlike non-bronchitic patients. It may, however, be difficult to distinguish microbes representing colonization secondary to respiratory epithelial damage from those responsible for symptoms. *Streptococcus pneumoniae* and *Haemophilus influenzae* are the two most frequently implicated bacteria (see Table 14.1).

Table 14.1 Microbial pathogens responsible for acute exacerbations of chronic bronchitis and emphysema

Organism	Comment
Streptococcus pneumoniae	
Haemophilus influenzae	Non-encapsulated
Moraxella catarrhalis	Previously known as *Branhamella catarrhalis*
Staphylococcus aureus	Less common
Enterobacteria, e.g. *Escherichia coli*, *Klebsiella*	Less common, may represent colonization following antibiotics
Mycoplasma pneumoniae	Occasional cause. Diagnosis by serology
Viruses, e.g. influenza, coronavirus, parainfluenza, rhinovirus, respiratory syncytial virus	More common than appreciated and often precede bacteria

A chest X-ray is unremarkable, but *Moraxella catarrhalis* is isolated in heavy growth from sputum. The isolate is reported as resistant to ampicillin/amoxicillin and trimethoprim but sensitive to co-amoxyclav, cefaclor, cefuroxime and ciprofloxacin. Following a 5-day course of co-amoxyclav (see Case 7) Tony's cough improves and the sputum becomes much less purulent. Subsequently, however, Tony returns to smoking over 20 cigarettes a day!

Q What is *M. catarrhalis*?

A This bacterium is a Gram-negative coccus, previously known as *Neisseria* and subsequently as *Branhamella catarrhalis*. It may be distinguished from *Neisseria* in the laboratory by a number of bio-chemical reactions and the pro-duction of DNA-ase. It may be part of the normal upper respiratory tract flora but in recent years it has been increasingly recognized as a cause of upper (e.g. otitis media) and lower (e.g. pneumonia, bronchitis) respiratory tract infection, especially in patients with pre-existing chest disease. When playing a significant role as a pathogen it is usually isolated in heavy pure growth from purulent sputum, and characteristic Gram-negative cocci are seen in the Gram film. Scanty growth or iso-lation from mucoid or non-purulent sputum should not be considered clinically significant. 50% or more of isolates are β-lactamase producers and consequently will be resistant to penicillin or ampicillin.

Q What is the antimicrobial agent of choice for the initial treatment of exacerbations of chronic chest disease such as this?

A There are a number of options available, but most would consider a penicillin such as amoxycillin initially (better absorption than ampicillin following oral adminis-tration). Factors influencing the choice of one agent over another are a history of recent antibiotic use, treatment failure, side-effects and the results of antibiotic sus-ceptibility tests. Where β-lactamase production among *H. influenzae* isolates is common (>20%) amoxycillin may not be appropriate. Options for antimicrobial therapy are outlined in Box 14.1.

Q What other measures should be considered to reduce infective exacerbations of chronic bronchitis?

A Apart from reducing smoking, losing weight and regular exercise

to improve general health and pul-monary function, vaccination against pneumococcal disease (see Case 12) and influenza (see Case 11) should be considered, especially if the patient is over 65. Prophylactic antibiotics have no role to play in minimizing either the frequency or the severity of exacerbations, and indeed may result in the emergence of resistance. It may be appropriate for some patients, however, to have a course of antibiotics at home to take early during an exacerbation when the sputum changes colour, especially if there is likely to be a delay in seeing the GP.

B14.1 Oral antibiotics used to treat exacerbations of chronic bronchitis	
Ampicillin/amoxycillin	Active against *S. pneumoniae* and most isolates of *H. influenzae*. 50% *M. catarrhalis* resistant
Co-amoxyclav	Also active against β-lactamase-producing *H. influenzae* and *M. catarrhalis*
Erythromycin	Poor activity against *H. influenzae* but the agent of choice for *M. pneumoniae* and *Legionella*
Trimethoprim	Less commonly used now. Fewer side-effects than co-trimoxazole but inactive against *M. catarrhalis*
Cefaclor/cefadroxil/cefixime	Broad-spectrum cephalosporins with enhanced activity against *Haemophilus*. Expensive
Ciprofloxacin/ofloxacin	Second-line agents. Ciprofloxacin has poor activity against *S. pneumoniae*
Tetracycline	Rarely used now. Indicated if penicillin allergy or mycoplasma/chlamydia infections likely
Clarithromycin/azithromycin	New macrolides as alternatives to erythromycin. Better activity against *Haemophilus* but expensive

Summary: Infective exacerbations of chronic bronchitis
Presentation
Increased sputum production with change in colour, wheeze and breathlessness
Diagnosis
Essentially clinical. Chest X-ray to exclude other pathology and sputum microbiology to guide choice of antibiotic
Management
Cessation of smoking, bronchodilators, antibiotics (e.g. amoxycillin, co-amoxyclav or cefadroxil) and vaccination against pneumococcus and influenza

CASE 15
Shula, 5 months old, off colour and feeding poorly

Shula, 5 months old, is brought to Paediatric Casualty during the week before Christmas. Her parents have noticed that she has been off colour for the past 72 hours, with a runny nose, not eating well, and waking during the night with a non-productive cough. Her cough has become more pronounced in the past 24 hours. Her temperature last night was 38.5°C, so her parents gave her paracetamol syrup. This morning they have noticed that her breathing is very rapid.

Shula was born by normal vaginal delivery, weighed 7lb, and has subsequently hovered around the 30th centile for weight. She has received three doses of DPT, polio and Hib vaccines, the last set being

given 3 weeks previously. She has two older siblings, aged 3 and 5 years, both of whom are well.

On examination Shula is restless and distressed. She is febrile (38.4°C), has a pulse of 160 and a respiratory rate of 70. There is visible indrawing of the chest wall during inspiration. Diffuse wheezes and crackles are heard throughout both lung fields. Apart from the tachycardia there are no other abnormal signs in the cardiovascular system. The rest of the physical examination is also normal.

Q What is the likely diagnosis?

A The acute onset, the presence of fever and the abnormal respiratory signs all suggest an acute respiratory tract infection. The grossly elevated respiratory rate and the use of accessory muscles of respiration suggest lower respiratory tract involvement (i.e. bronchiolitis or pneumonia).

Q What investigations should be undertaken?

A A chest X-ray and pulse oximetry are useful in assessing the severity of infection. A nasopharyngeal aspirate (NPA), taken by passing a fine tube into the nasopharynx and applying suction (Figure 15.1), should be sent for identification of the causative pathogen.

Shula's chest X-ray shows evidence of hyperinflation and increased peribronchial markings. Her oxygen saturation is 82% (normal >95%). Shula is admitted to hospital where she can be nursed in a head-box with 30%

oxygen, and adequate hydration achieved via a nasogastric tube.

Q What is the most likely causative pathogen?

A There are two clues here – the age of the patient and the time of year. Respiratory syncytial virus (RSV) infection accounts for up to 90% of cases of bronchiolitis in infancy. RSV epidemics occur annually in temperate climates, and show sharp peaks of about 3 months duration, beginning in November/December. Lower respiratory tract infection in small children may also be due to parainfluenza viruses (occur throughout the year), adenoviruses (see Case 39), influenza viruses (seasonal, see Case 11) and *Mycoplasma pneumoniae* (epidemics occur every 5 years or so, see Case 13).

Q How will the laboratory identify the causative agent?

A The most commonly used rapid diagnostic technique is that of immunofluorescence. The principle underlying this is that cells (present in the NPA) infected with a virus will express virus-derived antigens on their surface. The presence of these antigens can be demonstrated by staining the cells with monoclonal antibodies to a variety of possible pathogens (e.g. against influenza A and B viruses, RSV, parainfluenza viruses or adenoviruses) to which a fluorescein dye has been chemically linked. Cells infected with a given organism will fluoresce under ultraviolet light if they are stained with the monoclonal antibody directed against that particular organism (Figure 15.2) Appropriate tissue cultures will also be inoculated for virus isolation, although these may take up to 2 weeks to become positive. RSV produces a characteristic cytopathic effect in cell culture, causing the formation of giant syncytial cells (this is how the virus acquired its name).

Q What are the possible clinical consequences of RSV infection?

A

- Most infections are asymptomatic, or result in only mild disease (75–100% of all infants are antibody positive by the age of 2 years).
- Lower respiratory tract disease (bronchiolitis and pneumonia), peak incidence in the first 6 months of life, resulting in hospitalization of around 1 in every 100 infants. Mortality is less than 1%.
- Infection in infants less than 1 month old may be atypical, dominated by non-specific signs such as poor feeding and lethargy. Apnoeic attacks may be the first indication of respiratory infection. RSV infection is detected in a proportion of victims of the sudden infant death syndrome.

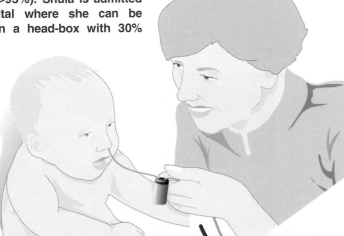

Fig. 15.1 Taking an NPA.

To suction

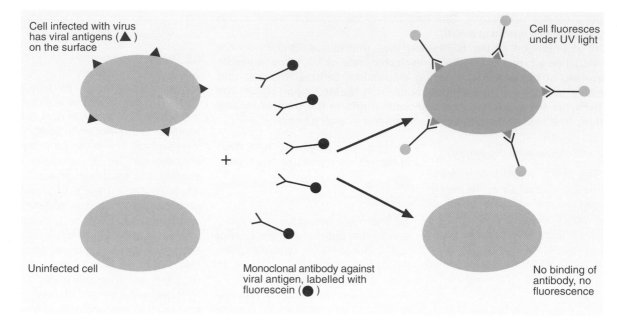

Cell infected with virus has viral antigens (▲) on the surface

Cell fluoresces under UV light

+

Uninfected cell

Monoclonal antibody against viral antigen, labelled with fluorescein (●)

No binding of antibody, no fluorescence

Fig. 15.2 Principle of immunofluorescent antigen detection.

- Repeat infections occur throughout life. These present as upper respiratory tract infections in older children and adults, with cough a marked symptom. Outbreaks of flu-like illness (see Case 11 for a definition of this) due to RSV infection may occur in the elderly, e.g. in nursing homes.

Q What are the complications of RSV infection?

A

- Otitis media. RSV can be recovered from middle-ear aspirates, either alone or together with bacterial agents.
- Severe RSV infection in infancy is associated with prolonged alterations in pulmonary function, and with further bouts of wheezing during childhood, which may be difficult to distinguish from asthma.

Q Which groups of children are at particular risk of severe disease or death from RSV infection?

A The mortality of RSV infection in infants with congenital heart disease, with underlying lung disease, and those who are immunosuppressed, is over 25%.

The virology laboratory rings later the same day, with a positive RSV immunofluorescence result from the NPA. Shula is being nursed on the paediatric oncology ward.

Q Is this the most appropriate ward for Shula to be nursed in?

A No. Nosocomial RSV infections are unfortunately all too common. The risk of acquiring RSV infection in this way is directly correlated with the length of hospitalization. Given the devastating consequences of RSV infection in immunosuppressed hosts, great care should be taken to avoid admitting RSV-infected infants on to wards where such children may be found. The same applies to wards where infants with congenital heart defects may be present.

Q What precautions should be taken to prevent the nosocomial spread of RSV?

A Spread of RSV is by inhalation of droplets, but also by direct inoculation into the pharynx of virus picked up from inanimate surfaces, e.g. via nurses' hands. All known

Fig. 15.3 Baby in head-box receiving Ribavirin.

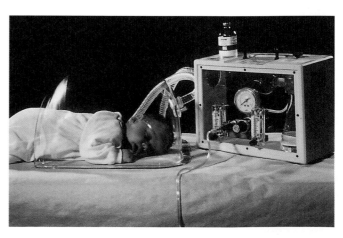

infected patients should be grouped on the same ward, or the same part of a ward; if possible, nurses should be assigned to look after either the RSV patients or the remaining patients, but not both (i.e. cohort nursing); the importance of strict handwashing after handling patients cannot be overemphasized.

Shula is immediately transferred to the general paediatric ward. Her oxygenation improves to normal over the following 48 hours, and she is discharged home on the fourth hospital day.

Q What antiviral agent might have been used to treat Shula?

A Tribavirin (also known as ribavirin) is a broad-spectrum antiviral agent which interferes with the processing of viral messenger RNA. Tribavirin therapy of infants hospitalized with RSV infection results in enhanced elimination of virus excretion, symptomatic improvement and a shorter duration of hospitalization. However, the drug has to be administered by inhalation of fine particles for at least 18 hours a day. A small-particle aerosol generator is thus needed and the infant must be nursed in a head-box (see Figure 15.3). For an otherwise uncomplicated case the disadvantages (cost and inconvenience) of therapy outweigh the benefits. Tribavirin does, however, reduce the mortality of RSV infection in high-risk patients (see above), and should be used in their management.

Summary: RSV bronchiolitis
Clinical features
1–6-month-old child with fever, cough and increased respiratory rate in winter months
Diagnosis
Clinical; antigen detection in NPA
Management
Adequate hydration and oxygenation; tribavirin if severe disease
Prognosis
Full recovery usual; high mortality if underlying lung or cardiac disease, or immunodeficiency

The resulting abnormalities in mucus and other secretions of the exocrine glands result in most of the clinical complications.

Q What are the complications of cystic fibrosis?

A Cystic fibrosis is a multisystem disorder and complications include:

- Respiratory:
  recurrent infections
  nasal polyps
  haemoptysis
  pneumothorax
- Gastrointestinal:
  meconium ileus at birth
  pancreatic insufficiency
  cirrhosis
  diabetes mellitus
- Genitourinary:
  male infertility
  amenorrhoea.

At the clinic Benjamin is apyrexial but has widespread rhonchi and crepitations throughout both lung fields. His pulmonary function tests are as follows: forced vital capacity (FVC) 45%, forced expiratory volume in one second (FEV$_1$) 50%. A chest X-ray reveals diffuse shadowing with bronchiectatic changes throughout both lung fields (Fig 16.1). A sample of sputum is obtained for culture and he is admitted to the cystic fibrosis unit for further management.

Q What is bronchiectasis?

A This is chronic dilatation of the bronchi which results in collections of bronchial secretions. Repeated bacterial infections follow and, occasionally, haemoptysis. The below-normal pulmonary function tests are characteristic of generalized bronchiectasis, especially during acute infections.

Q What pathogens are likely to be grown from the sputum?

A A number of respiratory pathogens may be isolated from the sputum of cystic fibrosis patients

CASE 16
Productive cough in Benjamin, a 14-year-old with cystic fibrosis

Benjamin, a 14-year-old youth, returns to the adult cystic fibrosis clinic after a 2-year absence complaining of increased cough productive of thick green sputum, breathlessness, generalized lethargy and weight loss. Cystic fibrosis was diagnosed at 2 years of age and, apart from occasional respiratory infections, he has remained well in the intervening period. He is one of a family of four children and his 16-year-old brother also has cystic fibrosis.

Q What is the underlying defect in cystic fibrosis?

A Cystic fibrosis is the commonest genetic disease among Caucasians. It is an autosomal recessive disorder and the carriage rate is approximately 1 in 20. The genetic abnormality is on the long arm of chromosome 7 in a gene coding for a chloride channel protein (cystic fibrosis transmembrane conductance regulator). This leads to altered secretions (sweat, mucus), which in turn leads to blocked ducts and retained mucosal secretions.

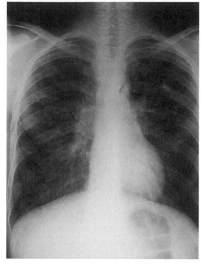

Fig. 16.1 Chest X-ray with bronchiectatic changes.

Table 16.1 The major respiratory pathogens in cystic fibrosis

Respiratory pathogen	Comments
Staphylococcus aureus	Colonizes and infects before the age of 2. Often fatal before effective antibiotics became available
Haemophilus influenzae	Non-capsulated types and hence not protected by Hib vaccine (see Case 7). Rarely fatal
Pseudomonas aeruginosa	Colonizes in late childhood or early adulthood. Mucoid strains (due to production of extracellular polysaccharide) difficult to eradicate (see also Box 16.1)
Burkholderia cepacia	Recognized recently but clinical significance often unclear. Usually multiply antibiotic resistant
Others	Include *S. pneumoniae, M. catarrhalis, Stenotrophomonas maltophilia, Mycoplasma pneumoniae, Aspergillus fumigatus*, but pathogenic role not certain

(see Table 16.1). It is not unusual to recover more than one pathogen. Previous admissions to hospital for treatment of acute respiratory infections, recent antibiotics, contact with other cystic fibrosis patients or siblings, may all influence which pathogens are recovered and their antimicrobial susceptibility. Sputum culture will assist in choosing the most appropriate antibiotics, but clinical improvement despite the persistence of pathogens, especially *Pseudomonas*, following a course of antibiotics is not unusual.

Q Which antibiotic or antibiotics should be started while the results of culture are awaited?

A Most episodes of respiratory infection are bacterial in aetiology, either as a primary or a secondary (i.e. following an initial viral infection) event. Often the patient is afebrile but nonetheless appropriate, and usually intravenous, antibiotics should be started promptly. The choice will be governed by the presence of the pathogens listed above and their antimicrobial susceptibility. Antibiotic cover against *P. aeruginosa* and *H. influenzae* should be instituted and an aminoglycoside (e.g. gentamicin, tobramycin, netilmicin) combined with an anti-pseudomonal penicillin (e.g. piperacillin, azlocillin) or a cephalosporin active against *Pseudomonas* (e.g. ceftazidime) is indicated. It is preferable to use combination antimicrobial chemotherapy when treating *Pseudomonas* infections because of possible antibiotic synergy (enhanced activity). This is especially important if the patient has received repeated courses of antibiotics in the recent past, as isolates may be resistant to one or more agents. This combination will also be active against *Haemophilus*.

B16.1 *Pseudomonas aeruginosa*

- Motile oxidase-positive Gram-negative bacillus capable of producing pigments, e.g. pyocyanin
- Isolated from moist environments such as sinks, disinfectants. Part of the normal gastrointestinal flora
- Causes hospital-acquired infections, e.g. urinary tract infection, bacteraemia, pneumonia, eye and skin infections.
- Is resistant to many commonly used antibiotics. Active agents include the aminoglycosides, piperacillin/azlocillin, ciprofloxacin, ceftazidime and imipenem
- Hospital-acquired infection may be prevented by reversing the underlying condition, e.g. neutropenia, hand-washing (prevents cross-infection) and the correct use of disinfectants

Benjamin was started on i.v. gentamicin and ceftazidime, nebulized salbutamol and twice-daily physiotherapy. A mucoid *P. aeruginosa* (see Figure 16.2), sensitive to gentamicin, azlocillin, ceftazidime and ciprofloxacin and *H. influenzae* sensitive to ampicillin, azlocillin and ceftazidime, were recovered from his sputum. Following a 14-day course of i.v. antibiotics he was considerably less breathless, his pulmonary function tests had significantly improved, he was feeling much better and his cough was less purulent. A repeat sputum was clear of *Haemophilus* but the *Pseudomonas* persisted.

Benjamin was discharged on no antibiotics as he was clinically much better, was advised about exercise and instructed on how to perform daily postural drainage to reduce the incidence of further exacerbations and help improve lung function. His pancreatic supplement, creon, was increased, levels of vitamins A and E were measured and, because of weight loss, diabetes mellitus was excluded. Finally, he

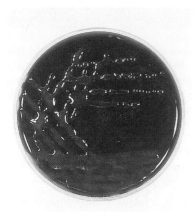

**Fig. 16.2 Mucoid isolate of
P. aeruginosa on blood agar.**

was asked to attend the cystic
fibrosis clinic monthly for further
follow-up.

Q Could ciprofloxacin have been
used to treat the chest infection?

A Preferably not. Ciprofloxacin, a
fluoroquinolone, has an important role
in the management of *Pseudomonas*
infections (see Box 16.1). A major
advantage is that it can be administered both orally and intravenously.
In cystic fibrosis it is often reserved
for outpatients but is relatively contraindicated in children because of
possible damage to growing cartilage
and bone. This has to be weighed
against the valuable contribution it
can make in management, and in
practice it is prescribed not infrequently in this setting. When used
alone, however, resistance may
emerge, especially following prolonged or repeat courses.

Q What role does nebulized colistin
have in management?

A Colistin (polymyxin E) is an antibiotic active against most Gram-
negative bacilli but because of its
toxicity it is confined to topical or
local use. In some centres nebulized
colistin is used in chronic *Pseudomonas* carriers to reduce exacerbations, but not as part of the acute
management in hospital.

Q How may the incidence and
severity of chest infections in cystic
fibrosis patients be reduced?

A This may be achieved by
attention to nutrition, instruction on
postural drainage, early and
aggressive treatment of infections
and vaccination against the usual
childhood illnesses, such as
diphtheria, *H. influenzae* type B etc.
By reducing the incidence of these
infections vaccination will also
prevent their complications, e.g.
pneumonia following whooping
cough.

Q Should patients with cystic fibrosis
be offered pneumococcal vaccine?

A The use of pneumococcal vaccine in cystic fibrosis is controversial
because the pneumococcus is
encountered relatively infrequently,
and consequently vaccination policies
vary from unit to unit.

Q Which other conditions predispose to the development of
bronchiectasis?

A The causes of bronchiectasis
may be summarized as:

- Congenital:
    cystic fibrosis (approximately
    50% of all cases)
    immotile ciliary syndrome
    complement deficiencies
- Previous lung infections:
    adenovirus pneumonia
    whooping cough
    measles
    tuberculosis (upper lobe)
    lung abscess (upper lobe)
- Aspiration/foreign body
- Tumour.

In many of these conditions the
bronchiectasis may be localized
and the symptoms less severe than
in cystic fibrosis. The microbiology
of acute infective exacerbations is
similar to that of cystic fibrosis.
Occasionally, a lung abscess or
empyema of polymicrobial aetiology
may develop which requires aspiration or drainage.

Q What factors predispose to the
development of lung abscess?

A Lung abscess (that is, a collection of pus within the lung
parenchyma which may be polymicrobial in aetiology) is less common than previously because of
more effective treatment for pneumonia and other suppurative lung
conditions. Many abscesses are
idiopathic but the remainder may
arise because of:

- Necrotizing lung infection:
    pneumonia (*S. aureus*)
    tuberculosis
- Aspiration:
    dysphagia
    alcohol
    general anaesthetic
    cerebrovascular accident
- Dental disease/gingivitis
- Lung tumours
    lymphoma
    carcinoma
- Lung infarction following embolus
- Bacteraemia:
    septic emboli settle in lungs, e.g.
    following infective endocarditis

Summary: Infective bronchiectasis
Presentation
Productive cough with purulent, often foul-smelling, sputum, dyspnoea and wheeze against a background of cystic fibrosis or other condition
Microbiology
Haemophilus, *S. aureus* and *P. aeruginosa* are the most common pathogens but viruses and other common (*S. pneumoniae*) and less common bacteria (*B. cepacia*) must be considered
Management
Aggressive i.v. antimicrobial therapy to cover *Pseudomonas*, especially during acute exacerbations, postural drainage, adequate nutrition and vaccination against common respiratory pathogens (tuberculosis, diphtheria etc.)

CASE 17
Bertrand, a 35-year-old Frenchman with nausea, abdominal pain and diarrhoea

Bertrand, a 35-year-old French computer programmer, is seen in the Accident and Emergency Department at 11 a.m. on a Saturday complaining of nausea, diarrhoea and abdominal pain. The diarrhoea woke him earlier that morning and appears to be getting worse. The abdominal pain is central in location and 'crampy' in character. He is on no medications, has never been seriously ill or previously required admission to hospital.

Q What further information might help in identifying the cause of his symptoms?

A Once medications have been excluded as a cause of gastrointestinal upset, the patient should be asked whether he has been abroad recently, whether other members of his household have also been unwell, and whether he can identify anything he has eaten in the last few days that might account for his illness.

Bertrand has been living in England for the past 5 years, and apart from a return trip to visit his elderly parents in Bordeaux a month ago has not been abroad recently. His girlfriend, Michelle, with whom he shares a flat, does not have any gastrointestinal symptoms. He is uncertain about any details of what he has eaten in the last 3 days, but remarks that he attended a retirement party for a colleague at Friday lunchtime at a local hotel. On examination he is apyrexial and his pulse and blood pressure are normal. There is no abdominal tenderness or masses.

Q What is the most likely diagnosis here?

A The patient has 'gastroenteritis', probably due to food poisoning. The absence of previous gastrointestinal disease, the recent onset of symptoms and a normal physical examination also point to this. The terms 'gastroenteritis' and 'food poisoning' are often used rather loosely, but the latter term is perhaps more likely to suggest an infective aetiology.

Q How relevant might the retirement party be?

A The provision of food for parties, receptions, weddings etc. is often associated with problems of preparation and storage, as food is being provided for larger numbers of people than is the case domestically. Details on what foods were eaten, what quantities of individual dishes were consumed, and whether any colleagues from work have been similarly affected will help in identifying the cause.

Q What are the mechanisms by which organisms cause food poisoning?

A These may be either by toxins, preformed and present in the food or produced with multiplication, or by tissue invasion (see Table 17.1). For example *Bacillus cereus* may cause two clinical forms of food poisoning: that characterized by vomiting (preformed toxin in the food) and that where diarrhoea is more prominent (toxin production *in vivo*). The different mechanisms may be reflected in the incubation period, with food poisoning mediated by toxin production having a short interval between ingestion and symptoms, as suggested in the case described here.

Q What else may cause food poisoning apart from bacteria?

A Viruses such as the Norwalk agent (a small round structured virus) may cause outbreaks characterized by explosive diarrhoea (see

Table 17.1 Aetiology and pathogenesis of bacterial food poisoning

Preformed toxin	Toxin production *in vivo*	Tissue invasion
Bacillus cereus *Staphylococcus aureus* *Clostridium botulinum* (See also Case 4)	*Clostridium perfringens* *Bacillus cereus* Enterotoxigenic *E. coli* *Vibrio* spp.	*Campylobacter jejuni* *Salmonella* spp. Invasive *E. coli*

Cases 18 and 65). Also, chemicals such as heavy metals, histamine and neurotoxins may be ingested with food (e.g. fish) and result in gastrointestinal and other symptoms.

Q Are particular foods associated with certain pathogens?

A A variety of different foods may cause food poisoning (see Figure 17.1).

- *Clostridium perfringens* often occurs in meat or gravy, especially when reheated, when suitable anaerobic conditions occur.
- Food with a high protein content, such as ham, poultry and egg salads, are often implicated in staphylococcal food poisoning, where the organism may have come from the nose or hand of a food handler after initial cooking or preparation.
- Cooked but inadequately stored rice may be responsible for *B. cereus*.
- *Salmonellae* are associated with poultry or raw or inadequately cooked eggs.
- *Campylobacter jejuni*, only recognized as a human intestinal

pathogen in the last 15 years, is associated with unpasteurized milk and poultry.
- The Norwalk virus causes food poisoning through contaminated shellfish or salads.

Q How might one confirm which pathogen is responsible?

A Microscopy and culture of vomitus is rarely helpful in identifying the aetiology of food poisoning. A stool for culture may grow *Salmonella*, *Shigella* or *Campylobacter* spp. Most microbiology laboratories do not report the isolation of *E. coli* from all stool samples as it is part of the normal flora, but in certain circumstances the presence of enterotoxigenic strains (see Case 19) which cause bloody diarrhoea with renal failure as part of the haemolytic–uraemic syndrome may be sought. These strains do not ferment sorbitol, a feature that can be easily recognized in the laboratory, and they also produce a heat-labile toxin. Isolation of the organism from food is preferred when diagnosing *S. aureus* or *C. perfringens* food poisoning, as these bacteria are

also part of the normal bowel flora. However, confirmation that an outbreak is due to *C. perfringens* is obtained if there is a heavy growth from the faeces of affected patients, if all the strains from the patients are the same type, and if isolates from food and stools are similar.

Q What other line of investigation might help in identifying the cause?

A In the absence of remaining food from the incriminated meal, it may be possible to make a presumptive diagnosis about the cause following epidemiological investigations. This involves following up those who attended the retirement party or wedding reception, with a questionnaire to investigate how many developed symptoms and what foods they ate. If symptoms are subsequently shown to be associated with eating, e.g. a mousse or mayonnaise, and a *Salmonella* is recovered from the stools of many of those affected (see Box 17.1), then further questioning may reveal that raw eggs were used during preparation. This type of investigation is usually coordinated by the local or public health authorities, and therefore it is essential that food poisoning is notified.

B17.1 Salmonella food poisoning

- Due to non-enteric *Salmonella* (not *S. typhi* or *S. paratyphi*, see Case 21), such as *S. enteriditis*, *S. typhimurium*, *S. dublin*, *S. agona* etc., most of which are from animal sources
- *S. enteritidis* phage-type 4 is responsible for much of the recent increase in salmonellosis due to contamination of egg contents
- Usually mild and self-limiting without systemic invasion, but can cause severe illness and even death in the very young (neonatal meningitis) and the very elderly (septicaemia)
- Prevention is by monitoring and sampling laying hens and eggs, slaughter of infected flocks and advice to the public about cooking eggs and poultry adequately

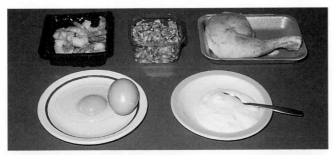

Fig. 17.1 Foods (shellfish, poultry, raw eggs, homemade mayonnaise) implicated in food poisoning.

Bertrand was discharged from the Accident and Emergency department and subsequently improved in the next 24 hours. He was able to return to work on the Monday. It transpired that a number of Bertrand's colleagues had similar symptoms over the weekend, and the public health authorities, together with the local Public Health Laboratory, undertook an investigation. There was some food remaining from the reception, and following anaerobic culture *C. perfringens* was recovered from roast beef, which had been eaten by 80% of those with symptoms.

Q What is the commonest recognized cause of food poisoning?

A *C. jejuni*, a spiral-shaped Gram-negative bacillus, is the commonest identified cause of food poisoning, which may be accompanied by severe abdominal pain that can be mistaken for an acute abdominal emergency requiring surgical investigation, and even bloody diarrhoea. *Salmonella* spp. are the next most important cause.

Q How is shigellosis spread and how do *Shigella* spp. cause diarrhoea?

A Most cases of shigella in the developed world arise from person-to-person spread and *Shigella sonnei* is the most common species isolated. In the less developed parts of the world, where classic dysentery (bloody diarrhoea) is more common, *S. dysenteriae* is relatively more common and both water and food are implicated in spread. These bacteria invade the intestinal mucosa, but most species are capable of producing an enterotoxin which is probably responsible for the watery diarrhoea seen early on in the illness.

Q What are the principles of the management of food poisoning?

A Most cases are self-limiting and therefore fluid replacement is the mainstay of treatment. This is especially important where there has been severe dehydration. In these circumstances intravenous fluids such as Hartmann's solution may be necessary. Antidiarrhoeal agents such as loperamide should be avoided if at all possible because they may affect the natural history of the disease by impairing the bowel's efforts to excrete the pathogen.

Q When, if ever, are antibiotics indicated?

A Antibiotic treatment of diarrhoea due to food poisoning or gastroenteritis is rarely indicated as there is little evidence that it will improve symptoms, and indeed it may prolong carriage or result in antibiotic-associated diarrhoea (see Box 17.2). Exceptions to this include:

- salmonella infection which has invaded the bloodstream, meninges, bone etc.
- salmonella in the elderly accompanied by severe gastrointestinal symptoms
- severe shigellosis

- campylobacter infection with colitis or bloody stools
- salmonella, shigella or campylobacter infection in an immunocompromised patient or a patient with relevant underlying disease, e.g. ulcerative colitis with moderate to severe symptoms.

A newer quinolone such as ciprofloxacin is probably the agent of choice for the above, except for campylobacter, where erythromycin is recommended.

Q Which organisms causing gastrointestinal symptoms are water borne, apart from *Shigella*?

A The distinction between food-borne and water-borne disease is not always clear, especially where food has been washed in contaminated water. Recognized water-borne organisms include:

- Bacteria: *Campylobacter* spp., salmonella causing enteric fever (*S. typhi, S. paratyphi*), *Vibrio cholerae, Vibrio* spp., *E. coli*
- Viruses: Hepatitis A, Norwalk-like viruses, rotavirus (see Case 18)
- Protozoa: *Giardia lamblia, Cryptosporidium, Entamoeba histolytica*.

B17.2 Antibiotic-associated diarrhoea

- Usually due to toxin-producing *Clostridium difficile* in a patient who has been on antibiotics in the recent past resulting in disruption to the normal gastrointestinal flora. Most, if not all, antibiotics have been implicated
- Varies from mild to severe life-threatening disease, such as pseudomembranous colitis, megacolon and bowel perforation
- Diagnosis is confirmed by detection of cytotoxin in faeces which is neutralized by *C. sordelli* antitoxin
- Management includes patient isolation/segregation, fluid replacement, discontinuation of antibiotics and, if symptoms still persist, oral metronidazole or vancomycin

---

Summary: Food poisoning

Presentation

Vomiting (especially *S. aureus, B. cereus*), abdominal pain and diarrhoea. Sporadic in the majority of cases, where no food is ever incriminated

Diagnosis

Clinical diagnosis having excluded other possibilities such as appendicitis. Stool for culture and other appropriate tests with epidemiological investigations if part of an outbreak

Management

Fluid replacement. Antibiotics rarely required

CASE 18
Damian, a 13-month-old baby with vomiting and diarrhoea

Damian, a 13-month-old baby, is brought in by his mother in the week before Christmas. For the past 2 days Damian has been vomiting, and this morning he has already soiled four nappies with profuse watery diarrhoea. He has not eaten anything unusual over the last 4 days. He attends a day-care nursery when his mother is working. He has reached all his developmental milestones at the appropriate ages, and has received full courses of DTP, polio and Hlb vaccines. On examination Damian is febrile (38.5°C), and assessment of skin turgor suggests that he is moderately dehydrated.

Q What is the diagnosis?

A Damian has acute gastroenteritis. The acute onset, the presence of fever and the lack of any relevant past medical history make infection the most likely cause. Viruses are more frequent than bacterial pathogens as causes of infantile gastroenteritis in temperate climates.

Q Name four groups of viruses that cause gastroenteritis.

A

- Rotaviruses – the commonest cause in young children
- Enteric adenoviruses (serotypes 40 and 41, see Case 39)
- Astroviruses, so called because of their starlike morphology. Astrovirus gastroenteritis is usually mild and rarely necessitates hospitalization
- Caliciviruses and the small round structured viruses (SRSVs, also known as Norwalk-like agents; see Box 18.1).

Coronaviruses, enteroviruses, and small round viruses (SRVs, also known as small featureless viruses) are also found in human stools, but their role as causative agents of diarrhoea is unproven.

Q How would this diagnosis in Damian be confirmed?

A A stool sample should be sent as soon as possible for electron microscopy (EM) (Fig. 18.1). None of the above-mentioned viruses will grow in the tissue culture cell lines maintained in a routine diagnostic laboratory, so virus culture is not possible. However, all are excreted in extremely large amounts in infected stools (>10^6 particles per ml) during the early phase of acute gastroenteritis, and therefore they can be visualized with an EM. Virus excretion does, however, fall off rapidly with time, hence the need for specimens to be taken as soon as possible. Each virus is recognized by its characteristic morphology (see Figure 18.2). A bacterial cause (e.g. *Salmonella*) of Damian's illness must also be excluded by appropriate culture of his stool.

Electron microscopy is a rapid diagnostic technique (a positive result can be available within 3 hours) and is also comprehensive, i.e. it will detect whatever virus is there, provided the virus is present in sufficient quantity. However, it is expensive and alternatives are being developed, including antigen detection by ELISA or latex particle agglutination. These are rapid and cheaper techniques, but will only detect specific viruses: a rotavirus ELISA will not pick up adenoviruses, for example.

Q What are the short-term complications of viral gastroenteritis?

A Excessive fluid loss may result in dehydration and electrolyte imbalance, most commonly a metabolic acidosis.

B18.1 Caliciviruses and SRSVs

Caliciviruses

- So called because of the cuplike hollows on their surface (Greek *calyx*)
- Cause winter vomiting and diarrhoea in children

Norwalk virus, Norwalk-like agents and SRSVs (see also Case 65)

- Named after identification in association with outbreak of gastroenteritis in Norwalk, Ohio, USA
- Genome analysis suggests that all these viruses are related to each other, and to the caliciviruses
- These agents are particularly associated with outbreaks of gastroenteritis, which affect people of all ages
- Spread by food (especially shellfish) and water
- Aerosols, generated by forceful vomiting, also important in transmission

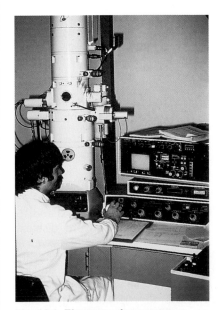

Fig. 18.1 Electron microscope.

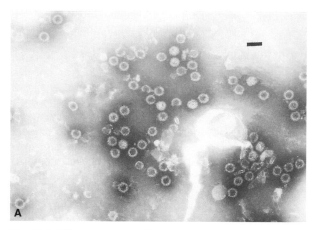
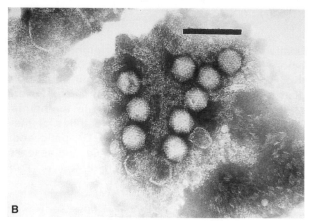

Fig. 18.2 (A) rotaviruses; (B) adenoviruses; (C) SRSV.

Damian is referred to the local hospital because of his profuse diarrhoea and signs of dehydration. A stool sample is sent to the laboratory, where rotaviruses are seen on EM. On the ward an initial attempt at oral rehydration is made, but this is abandoned after persistent vomiting and an intravenous drip is set up. After 48 hours of i.v. fluid replacement Damian's stool output declines, and over the next 48 hours oral feeding is gradually re-established.

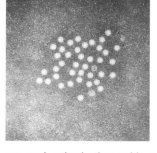

Q Should Damian be nursed on an open ward?

A There is a significant risk of nosocomial spread of rotavirus infection, and ward staff must be aware of this. Adherence to strict hand-washing protocols is the single most useful measure to reduce the risk of spread. Patients should ideally be nursed in single rooms, but this is not always practicable or possible.

Q Can this be described as a typical case of rotavirus gastroenteritis?

A Yes. The features of rotavirus infection in temperate climates are listed below:

- Commoner in autumn/winter
- Peak incidence between 3 and 15 months of age, severe disease unusual after the age of 3 years
- Transmission mainly by faecal–oral route
- Severity varies from a 24-hour illness to overwhelming gastro-enteritis, with occasional deaths

- Vomiting, a prominent feature, may precede diarrhoea by 48 hours
- Fever >38.5°C almost universal
- Watery diarrhoea persists for 5–7 days on average. Blood or pus in stools suggests concurrent bacterial infection.

Q Which patients are at risk of chronic rotavirus infection?

A Immunosuppressed children or adults may suffer from chronic diarrhoea (>3 months). Management is difficult, but there are reports of successful treatment with human immunoglobulin containing antibodies to rotavirus.

Q How does rotavirus infection differ outside the developed countries?

A Rotaviruses are the commonest single cause of diarrhoeal illness worldwide, with an estimated annual incidence of 125 million cases and 8–900 000 deaths, most of which occur in poorer countries. No specific antiviral agents are available, and management is dependent largely on oral rehydration with solutions containing glucose and electrolytes. Breastfeeding significantly reduces the chances of diarrhoeal illness, presumably via passive immunization. Much effort has been expended in the development of rotavirus vaccines, but these remain experimental at present.

Summary: Rotavirus gastroenteritis
Presentation
Vomiting and profuse watery diarrhoea, usually in a small child
Diagnosis
Examination of faecal sample by electron microscopy (will also allow diagnosis of other causes of gastroenteritis, e.g. adenoviruses (children), caliciviruses (cause outbreaks in adults), astroviruses
Management
Supportive, fluid replacement

CASE 19

Fraser, a 37-year-old business executive with abdominal pain, diarrhoea and flatulence

Fraser, a 37-year-old business executive, complains of central abdominal pain, moderate to severe diarrhoea and flatulence for 4 days. He has no relevant previous medical history, is on no medications and neither his wife nor his two children have any gastrointestinal symptoms. Physical examination is unremarkable. On further questioning it transpires that Fraser has spent a week in Central America, returning 2 days ago.

Q What else would it be useful to know about his recent trip abroad?

A It is certainly likely that his symptoms relate to his trip abroad, but details of where he was in Central America, whether his trip was confined to cities, what foods or liquids he consumed and whether he took any drugs, such as antibiotics, before, during or after returning home, are very relevant.

Fraser's trip was to Nicaragua and he spent most of the time in cities, but there were a few field trips. He avoided drinking anything except bottled liquids where at all possible, and most of the food he ate was freshly cooked. He did not take any medication before travelling, although he remarked that a number of his colleagues who had been on the trip with him had been on medication since returning.

Q What is the general term for this condition and how common is it?

A This man has probably acquired traveller's diarrhoea, the most common medical condition among people travelling to tropical or subtropical parts of the world. It occurs in about 20–50% of travellers.

Q What are the causes?

A About 70% of episodes are due to an infective agent of one kind or another (see Table 19.1). However, a proportion may be due to overindulgence in alcohol or food, and some cases may be accounted for by chemical poisoning, e.g. scombrotoxin. Bacterial pathogens account for about 70% of infective cases.

Q What initial investigations should be made?

A A sample of faeces should be sent for culture. In addition, microscopy for ova, trophozoites (in fresh liquid faeces) and parasite cysts should be requested, and full clinical details plus information on where the patient has been, and whether he has been on antibiotics, should be included on the request form, so that less common parasitic causes in particular will be considered.

Cysts of *Giardia lamblia* (see Box 19.1 and Figure 19.1) are seen under light microscopy in two consecutive stool samples. Culture for bacterial pathogens, including *Vibro* spp., is negative. Fraser is put on appropriate treatment and makes an uneventful recovery.

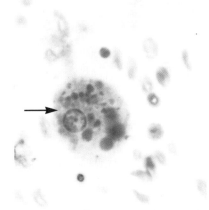

A

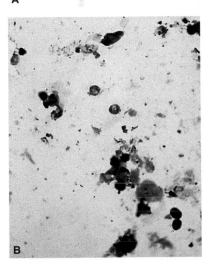

B

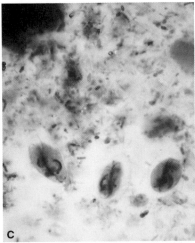

C

Fig. 19.1 Protozoan causes of traveller's diarrhoea. (A) *Entamoeba histolytica* (trophozoites); (B) Cryptosporidia (cysts); (C) Giardia lamblia (cysts).

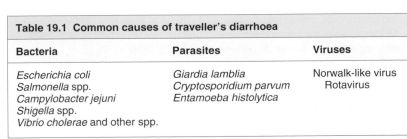

Table 19.1 Common causes of traveller's diarrhoea		
Bacteria	**Parasites**	**Viruses**
Escherichia coli *Salmonella* spp. *Campylobacter jejuni* *Shigella* spp. *Vibrio cholerae* and other spp.	*Giardia lamblia* *Cryptosporidium parvum* *Entamoeba histolytica*	Norwalk-like virus Rotavirus

B19.1 Important features of *Giardia lamblia*

Organism

Flagellated enteric protozoan
Trophozoite is free-living, encystation occurs in intestine

Transmission

Faecally contaminated water
Person-to-person spread, e.g. day-care nurseries
Sexual, i.e. homosexual

Pathogenesis

Disruption of brush border of the small intestine
Disaccharidase deficiencies

Clinical disease

Asymptomatic
Self-limiting diarrhoea (25–50%)
Chronic diarrhoea and malabsorption

Diagnosis

Faeces for trophozoites (early stages of disease) or cysts following ether concentration
Duodenal aspirate for microscopy

B19.2 *Entamoeba histolytica*

Clinical illness

Diarrhoea and abdominal pain, dysentery (bloody diarrhoea), toxic megacolon, extraintestinal spread (liver abscess, lung, brain)

Diagnosis

Stool for cysts (trophozoites seen in fresh specimens only), colonoscopy, serology and CT/MRI scans if invasive

B19.3 *Cryptosporidium parvum*

Clinical illness

Self-limiting diarrhoeal illness in immunocompetent host, severe watery diarrhoea in HIV patients with, occasionally, cholecystitis. No antimicrobial therapy effective

Diagnosis

Modified Ziehl–Neelsen stain on stool sample

Q What is the appropriate therapy for giardiasis?

A Rehydration and oral metronidazole for 10 days.

Q What should the patient be told before taking metronidazole?

A Metronidazole may cause a disulfiram-like reaction, with flushing and hypotension following alcohol ingestion, and therefore alcohol should be avoided during treatment. Prolonged use of metronidazole may result in peripheral neuropathy, and although it has been used frequently during pregnancy for the treatment of vaginal discharge it should be avoided if possible, especially during the first trimester. Metronidazole is also the treatment of choice for amoebiasis caused by *Entamoeba histolytica* (Box 19.2; see also Case 23) but is ineffective against cryptosporidiosis (see Box 19.3)

Q Is giardia the commonest cause of traveller's diarrhoea?

A No. Enterotoxigenic strains of *E. coli* are more common and account for approximately 50% of cases. Diarrhoea-producing *E. coli* may be subdivided into:

- *enteropathogenic* – strongly adherent to intestinal epithelial cells. Cause infantile gastroenteritis in the tropics and sometimes in hospitals
- *enterotoxigenic* – produce either a heat-labile or heat-stable toxin, together with adhesive factors. Major cause of traveller's diarrhoea
- *enteroinvasive* – cause an illness similar to shigella dysentery in patients of all ages
- *cytotoxin-producing* – *E. coli* 0157 is the commonest serotype and the toxin is closely related to the shiga toxin of *Shigella dysenteriae*.

Causes a variety of diarrhoeal diseases, including colitis and the haemolytic uraemic syndrome.

Q How may traveller's diarrhoea be avoided?

A Improved food hygiene practices in warmer climates may in time reduce the incidence, but in the meantime travellers should eat only freshly prepared foods that are served hot and fruit or vegetables that can be peeled. Salads in particular should be avoided. Hot tea or coffee, recently boiled drinks or bottled beverages are safe but tap water and ice cubes should be avoided. Travellers to a cholera-endemic area may receive whole-cell cholera vaccine (of questionable efficacy) before travelling (see Case 24). It is not clear what precise role prophylactic antibiotics (mainly to prevent infection caused by *E. coli*) have in preventing this condition, but if used they should be started on arrival and continued for 2–3 days after returning. Travellers for whom prophylaxis should be considered are:

- those with inflammatory bowel disease
- diabetics
- the elderly
- patients with AIDS
- those travelling to the tropics for a brief but very important visit.

The potential side-effects of the agents listed below, plus their loss as a therapeutic option due to resistance, are arguments against routine prophylaxis. The agents most commonly prescribed are:

- co-trimoxazole: resistance increasingly emerging
- doxycycline: less frequently used now. To be avoided in children or during pregnancy
- quinolones: e.g. norfloxacin, ciprofloxacin etc. if antibiotic resistance prevalent
- Bismuth compounds: used more frequently by travellers from North America.

Q What are the principles of management of traveller's diarrhoea?

A The key features are:

- fluid and electrolyte replacement
- antimotility drugs such as loperamide (used with caution)
- a short course of ciprofloxacin or co-trimoxazole (only if symptoms persist and giardiasis or amoebiasis excluded).

Summary: Traveller's diarrhoea
Presentation
Diarrhoea and abdominal pain shortly after arriving or returning from a visit to a tropical or subtropical area
Diagnosis
One or more stool samples, preferably fresh, for culture and microscopic examination for ova, cysts etc. Important to inform the laboratory of areas visited to ensure all potential pathogens are looked for
Management
Likelihood of contracting diarrhoea when travelling may be reduced by careful attention to foods consumed, and occasionally, prophylactic antibiotics. Treatment involves fluid replacement, loperamide and either ciprofloxacin or co-trimoxazole if bacterial

CASE 20
Bob, a 55-year-old retired coal miner with abdominal pain

Bob is a 55-year-old retired coal miner who is referred to the Accident and Emergency department by his family doctor with a 10-day history of increasing crampy abdominal pain, vomiting and constipation. The abdominal pain has become severe in the preceding 24 hours. On examination Bob has a temperature of 39.5°C and is clinically toxic. He is tender in the right lower quadrant with rebound tenderness, and has absent abdominal bowel sounds.

Q What is the diagnosis?

A The history and physical findings are suggestive of peritonitis, most likely due to a perforated viscus. Although peritonitis *per se* does not automatically mean infection, it is likely that spillage of bowel contents will result in infection. This might be caused by a perforated appendix (the patient is a little old for this), diverticulitis, large-bowel neoplasm, inflammatory bowel disease or a perforated peptic ulcer.

Q What microbes may be causing the peritonitis?

A This depends on the site of perforation. The number of commensal organisms increases as one descends through the gastrointestinal tract (see Table 20.1). Anaerobes such as *Clostridium*, *Fusobacterium* and *Bacteroides* spp. become the dominant bacterial flora in the large bowel. Potential pathogens such as *Escherichia coli*, *Proteus mirabilis* and *Pseudomonas aeruginosa* are less numerous, but become more so following instrumentation or broad-spectrum antibiotic therapy.

Shortly after admission Bob is taken to theatre for a laparotomy, which reveals a tumour and a perforated descending colon with a walled-off abscess and localized peritonitis. The tumour is resected but the procedure is technically difficult and there is spillage of pus into the peritoneum. An anterior resection with de-functioning colostomy is performed. A swab of the pus is obtained for culture and Bob, who is allergic to penicillin, is started on intravenous antibiotics

Q Was a swab the best specimen to send for culture?

A Unless there is insufficient material to collect or it is difficult to aspirate, actual pus or tissue is always preferable to a swab, especially when isolating anaerobes. In addition, a Gram stain of the pus may give an early idea of the likely pathogens. Pus may be collected and forwarded to the laboratory in a sterile container or a syringe sealed with a rubber plug.

Table 20.1 Normal flora of the gastrointestinal tract

Site	No. of organisms (cfu/g)	Common microbes	Comment
Stomach	$<10^3$	Lactobacilli, streptococci, yeasts	Numbers increase with age, achlorhydria
Small bowel	10^3–10^9	As above plus clostridia, enterobacteriaceae, enterococci	Increase distally Antibiotics affect relative numbers
Large bowel	10^8–10^{12}	As above plus protozoa (*Chilomastix*, *Trichomonas*), yeasts	Anaerobes outnumber facultative organisms by 1000– 10 000: 1

Q What antibiotic or antibiotics are indicated here, and ideally when should they be started?

A The details of this patient's condition suggested intra-abdominal sepsis and therefore antibiotics should have been administered before laparotomy. This will also ensure that the patient is protected when the first incision is made, or if pus or the contents of a viscus is spilled into the peritoneum, resulting in possible bacteraemia.

Metronidazole will cover anaerobes, including *Bacteroides fragilis*, which are often resistant to penicillin. If there is a history of penicillin allergy every effort should be made to confirm this, as otherwise the patient will be deprived of some of the best antibiotics available. A genuine history of allergy may be indicated by a history of a skin rash, anaphylaxis or angioneurotic oedema. Diarrhoea or a fainting attack following an intramuscular injection do not represent allergy. Gentamicin, or a cephalosporin such as cefuroxime or cefotaxime, should be given here as these will cover most coliforms. There is approximately a 10% chance of cross-allergy to cephalosporins, but this should be balanced against the severity of the patient's condition and the nature of the original allergic reaction. Erythromycin has poor activity against Gram-negative bacilli and results in thrombophlebitis when given intravenously.

Q How does the use of antibiotics as part of surgical chemoprophylaxis differ from that of treatment?

A Chemoprophylaxis implies the use of antibiotics to prevent infection arising from the surgical procedure, rather than to treat established infection. In particular, the timing of the first dose and duration are critical in chemoprophylaxis (see Box 20.1).

Bob is transferred to the intensive therapy unit (ITU) after

B20.1 Principles of surgical antimicrobial prophylaxis

Identify patients at risk, e.g. large-bowel resection, amputation of ischaemic limb, prosthetic joint implantation
Match antibiotics with pathogens, e.g. cefotaxime+metronidazole – abdominal surgery
co-amoxyclav – gynaecological surgery, flucloxacillin – joint implant
First dose before incision: at induction or with premedication but *not* days before surgery, during or after operation
Discontinue after surgery: NB: at most 2–3 doses or 24 hours in total. Continuation beyond this has no prophylactic benefit. Treatment as opposed to prophylaxis may require different antibiotics

---

surgery, for ventilation and monitoring. He develops the adult respiratory distress syndrome (ARDS), acute renal failure (serum creatine 250 μg/ml), and requires positive pressure ventilation to maintain satisfactory blood gases and inotropes, i.e. multiorgan failure. Blood cultures subsequently grow *E. coli*, resistant to cephradine and ampicillin but sensitive to gentamicin, cefuroxime and cefotaxime, and *B. fragilis*. The swab taken at laparotomy also grows the same two organisms plus enterococci.

Gentamicin is added to the metronidazole and cefotaxime (a third-generation cephalosporin) started postoperatively.

Q What is the significance of the enterococci isolated from the swab?

A Although enterococci are part of the normal bowel flora and frequently recovered from intra-abdominal and wound specimens, they are usually less pathogenic than anaerobes or coliforms such as *E. coli* unless they cause intravascular line infection or bacteraemia.

Q Was it wise to add gentamicin in light of the poor renal function?

A The aminoglycosides (gentamicin, tobramicin, netilmicin, amikacin etc.) are among the most active agents against Gram-negative bacteria. Their use is not contraindicated in deteriorating renal function or failure but the dose and dosage interval need to be modified and frequent, if not daily, serum assays carried out (see Box 20.2). A once, or at most twice, daily dose will probably be adequate here. Aminoglycosides are increasingly being administered in a single daily dose as this results in higher peak serum concentrations, is less expensive, saves time and may even reduce toxic side-effects. The

---

B20.2 Serum aminoglycoside assays

- Should be carried out in *all* patients who receive more than three doses. Toxic: therapeutic ratio is low and there is considerable variation in pharmacokinetics between patients
- Imperative in the elderly, neonates, patients with declining renal function or patients on other nephrotoxic agents
- First set of levels should be done around the third or fourth dose and include a pre-dose, i.e. just before a dose (trough) and post-dose level, i.e. 1 hour after an i.v. dose (peak). Blood samples should not be taken through the intravascular line in which the aminoglycoside is given
- Should be repeated every 48–72 hours at least, and more frequently if initial levels are toxic, if the patient is extremely ill or if renal function declines
- Acceptable levels for 8 or 12 hourly administration are:
  - Gentamicin Trough   <2 μg/ml
  -                Peak   5–10 μg/ml
  - Tobramycin as for gentamicin
  - Netilmicin Trough   <3 μg/ml
  -                Peak   5–10 μg/ml
  - Amikacin   Trough   <10 μg/ml
  -                Peak   20–40 μg/ml

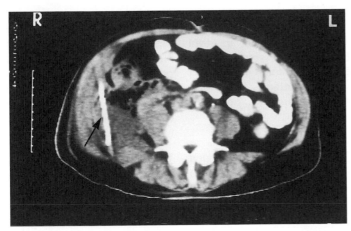

Fig. 20.1 CT scan demonstrating right-sided abdominal abscess with drain in situ (see arrow).

addition of gentamicin to cefotaxime (*E. coli* sensitive to both) is justified because of the uncontrolled Gram-negative sepsis with multiorgan damage.

Five days after admission to the ITU Bob remains pyrexial, has a white cell count of 24 000/×10⁹/l and requires inotropic support. CT reveals a residual paracolic abscess, which is drained using a percutaneous catheter under radiological control (see Figure 20.1) and a drain is left *in situ*. 20 ml of sterile pus is aspirated initially. Pus in decreasing amounts continues to drain for 4 days. Bob's pyrexia settles and his general condition improves over the next week. He remains on intravenous antibiotics for 14 days, but is eventually discharged from the unit despite developing a number of superinfections.

Q What is a superinfection?

A A 'superinfection' is a new infection that arises as a complication of antimicrobial therapy to treat an existing infection. Examples include:

- Oral thrush: Occurs in immunosuppressed patients or patients on corticosteroids who have recently been on broad-spectrum antibiotics such as ampicillin or cephalosporins.

- Antibiotic-associated diarrhoea: Most commonly due to enterotoxin produced by *Clostridium difficile* (see Case 17).
- Enterococcal UTI: *Enterococcus faecalis* and *E. faecium* are low-grade pathogens but symptomatic infection may occur in a catheterized patient (see Case 26) on antibiotics with little antienterococcal activity, used to treat another infection, e.g. ciprofloxacin, cephalosporins.

Summary: Peritonitis
Presentation
May be localized or generalized but usually presents with an 'acute abdomen'
Diagnosis
Usually clinical and confirmed at surgery. Ultrasound is helpful in localizing intra-abdominal abscesses and in removing pus. Blood cultures should also be taken as bacteraemia may occur
Management
Surgery is usually required to correct the underlying disease, e.g. removal of perforated tumour and for drainage. Broad-spectrum antibiotics (to cover Gram-negative bacilli and anaerobes) also indicated and admission to ITU if evidence of organ failure

CASE 21
Belinda, a 25-year-old non-Caucasian with malaise, myalgia and fever

Belinda, a 25-year-old non-Caucasian woman, is referred to the Accident and Emergency department of a local hospital by her GP. She has been unwell for a week and complains of malaise, headache, myalgia and some minor upper respiratory symptoms. Belinda is on no medications, has no relevant previous medical history, and her husband and two children are well. Apart from a temperature of 38°C, physical examination is unremarkable.

Q What aspects of Belinda's background require clarification?

A Some infections, e.g. tuberculosis are more common in certain ethnic groups or immigrants from the underdeveloped world, even when they have lived for some years in the developed world. Other infections e.g. malaria (see Case 47) and enteric fever, may be contracted during visits to see relatives. Consequently it is essential to ask about family history, whether there has been recent travel abroad (e.g. a history of recent travel to West Africa might suggest Lassa fever) and if so, what areas were visited and whether the patient was immunized before travel.

Further questioning reveals that Belinda was born in Bombay but she and her family moved to Britain when she was 5 years of age. Family history is unremarkable. She had visited her grandmother in India 2–3 weeks previously and had returned 6 days before presentation. Neither her husband nor her children had accompanied her. Apart from the routine vaccinations received as a child for tetanus, diphtheria etc., she had not been vaccinated before travel. Belinda did, however, take mefloquine prophylaxis for malaria.

Q What organ system apart from the respiratory tract should you ask about?

A It is possible that she has a minor viral-type illness contracted since her return but travel-associated illness must be excluded, in particular that affecting the gastrointestinal system. A history of diarrhoea, vomiting and abdominal pain may suggest traveller's diarrhoea (see Case 19). Notwithstanding the malaria prophylaxis (see Case 47) she could still have malaria, especially if prophylaxis was not started before travel and continued for 2 weeks following return.

On further questioning the respiratory symptoms are considered minor, but she admits to a short bout of nausea and diarrhoea shortly after arriving in India. This settled quickly and she is now if anything a little constipated.

Q What might the combination of pyrexia, evidence of a systemic illness (malaise, myalgia) and a history of recent gastrointestinal upset suggest?

A Enteric fever. Enteric or typhoid fever is an illness caused by infection with *Salmonella typhi* or *S. paratyphi* (paratyphoid fever) and may be contracted by people resident in temperate climates following travel abroad to tropical or subtropical areas. The clinical features are:

- pyrexial illness in a returned traveller
- malaise, headache, anorexia, myalgia, mild respiratory symptoms such as a cough
- diarrhoea or constipation, but *neither* may be present

- fever with relatively slow pulse
- rose spots – maculopapular lesions which blanch on pressure – are a late manifestation and are present in <20% of cases
- abdominal tenderness and hepatosplenomegaly may be present.

Q How may the diagnosis be confirmed and what should be included in the differential diagnosis?

A The diagnosis is made when there are clinical features such as those described above, together with isolation of the bacterium from appropriate sites such as blood, faeces etc. (see Figure 21.1). Laboratory abnormalities which may point towards enteric fever include leukopenia due to neutropenia, disseminated intravascular coagulation with low platelets, and elevated hepatic enzymes such as SGOT, (serum glutamic-oxaloacetic transaminase). The differential diagnosis includes malaria, intra-abdominal pathology such as appendicitis or a paracolic abscess, amoebic colitis, brucellosis, and even respiratory tract infection where respiratory symptoms are more prominent.

Q What other laboratory test is often requested when making a diagnosis of enteric fever?

A The Widal test determines the presence of antibodies to H (flagellar) and O (cell wall) salmonella antigens. The results, however, are not always easy to interpret and there may be some cross-reactions with non-enteric salmonellae. The Widal test is often not especially helpful in diagnosing infection caused by *S. paratyphi* because it is affected by vaccination against typhoid fever; there may also be false positive results in patients with connective tissue diseases.

Q What are the complications of enteric fever?

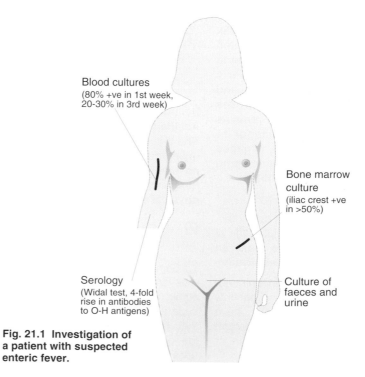

Blood cultures
(80% +ve in 1st week,
20-30% in 3rd week)

Bone marrow culture
(iliac crest +ve in >50%)

Serology
(Widal test, 4-fold rise in antibodies to O-H antigens)

Culture of faeces and urine

Fig. 21.1 Investigation of a patient with suspected enteric fever.

A An early diagnosis with prompt and aggressive treatment instituted in hospital is important in avoiding the complications that account for fatalities. These include:

- toxaemia with hepatic, renal and bone marrow dysfunction
- gastrointestinal perforation (single or multiple) and haemorrhage
- metastatic infection such as osteomyelitis, endocarditis
- persistent infection resulting in relapse or chronic carriage (see Box 21.1).

Q What is the treatment of enteric fever?

A Antimicrobial chemotherapy is essential as this is a systemic condition with life-threatening complications. The agent chosen should be active against the infecting strain as confirmed by sensitivity testing. Chloramphenicol has traditionally been the agent of choice, as most isolates are sensitive, but ciprofloxacin is increasingly being used

B21.1 Epidemiology and spread of enteric fever

Spread

The bacterium enters the body via the mouth and humans are the only reservoir. Person-to-person spread possible with poor standards of hygiene, but less likely than with other GI pathogens, e.g. *Shigella*

Chronic carrier

Arises from inadequate treatment. Bacterium may persist in the gallbladder

Water-borne

Important source in underdeveloped world and spread occurs where sewage contaminates drinking water supplies

Food-borne

Food washed or prepared with contaminated water
Food handler with poor standards of hygiene who is a chronic carrier

because it is as effective and does not have the bone marrow side-effects of chloramphenicol. It should, however, be used with caution in children, as it can adversely affect growing cartilage and bone. Alternative antibiotics include ampicillin and co-trimoxazole, which are less effective. Management must also include treatment of complications, such as fluid replacement for dehydration, blood transfusion following haemorrhage, surgery for perforation, and organ support if required.

Belinda is admitted to hospital, initially for observation and investigation. Blood and faeces cultures taken on admission grow *S. typhi*, sensitive to ampicillin, chloramphenicol and ciprofloxacin. She is started on ciprofloxacin intravenously, which is subsequently changed to oral administration. Investigations to exclude typhoid fever in her husband and children are negative. Before discharge she remarks in conversation that she helps her brother a couple of days a week in a sandwich bar.

Q Why was ciprofloxacin preferred to ampicillin?

A Ciprofloxacin and chloramphenicol achieve relatively high intracellular concentrations and this, together with good penetration into the intestinal mucosa, probably explains the superior efficacy of these agents compared to ampicillin or co-trimoxazole, despite their being sensitive *in vitro*.

Q How can enteric fever be prevented?

A Prevention in the undeveloped world is achieved by the separation of drinking water supplies from sewage, and greater attention to the preparation of food. Travellers from the developed world to endemic areas should be careful about what they eat, especially when eating out (see Case 19). A whole-cell heat-killed vaccine consisting of *S. typhi*

is available which should be given as a primary course of two doses 4–6 weeks apart. Recently an oral typhoid vaccine has been produced consisting of a live attenuated strain which appears to be as efficacious as the parenteral vaccine. Vaccination is recommended for travellers to countries where hygiene is poor, that is, Africa, Asia, Central and South America etc., and for laboratory workers handling specimens which may contain the typhoid bacillus. Vaccination is not recommended for contacts, carriers, or as part of the management of an outbreak.

Q What are the characteristics of enteric *S. typhi* and *S. paratyphi* and non-enteric salmonellae?

A Both enteric and non-enteric salmonellae share many similar features which distinguish them from other members of the Enterobacteriaceae, and which are important in distinguishing them from other bacteria in the laboratory (see Box 21.2).

The non-enteric salmonellae are animal in origin and are a major cause of food poisoning (see Case 17). They may be contracted from poultry (chickens, turkeys), cows, pigs and, to a lesser extent, birds and domestic pets. Infection is usually by ingestion of contaminated food such as eggs (*S. enteritidis*) or meat (*S. typhimurium*) and the symptoms are similar to those of other causes of food poisoning. Unlike infection caused by the enteric salmonellae, most cases are self-limiting, sporadic, and do not require antimicrobial chemotherapy. The incidence is highest in the period from July to November in the UK. Cross-infection may occur occasionally in institutions if hygiene standards are poor. Some species, such as *S. virchow* and *S. cholerasuis*, may be more virulent and are associated with bacteraemia, meningitis and osteomyelitis. When this occurs aggressive antimicrobial chemotherapy is required.

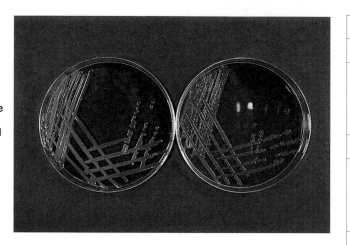

Fig. 21.2
E. coli (lactose fermenter) on left, compared with salmonella species (non-lactose fermenter) on right on MacConkey agar.

Summary: Enteric fever

Presentation

Pyrexial illness with non-specific gastrointestinal symptoms in a traveller returned from an endemic area. Physical examination often unremarkable

Diagnosis

Culture of blood and faeces for *S. typhi* or *S. paratyphi*. Urine and bone marrow may also be positive. Serology often not diagnostic, especially if vaccinated in the past

Management

Careful attention to food hygiene and pre-exposure vaccination when travelling will prevent acquisition. Chloramphenicol or ciprofloxacin are the antibiotics of choice

B21.1 Genus *Salmonella*

- Lactose-negative coliforms, of which there are >200 species
- Ferment glucose and mannitol, which distinguishes them from other non-lactose fermenters in stool specimens
- Kauffmann–White scheme classifies salmonellae to species on the basis of somatic (cell wall), flagellar and capsular antigens

Q What measures may be taken to minimize the incidence of salmonella food poisoning?

A At a national level steps have been taken to minimize the incidence of salmonellosis among poultry and cattle by improving animal husbandry and the slaughter of infected poultry flocks. Avoiding the use of raw eggs in cooking, adequate defrosting and cooking of poultry, and good standards of hygiene in the home, with particular attention to hand washing, are essential.

Q The patient described above was a food-handler, i.e. prepared food in a restaurant or retail outlet. What precautions need to be taken to prevent spread in this setting?

A Six consecutive negative specimens of faeces are required before it is considered safe for her to go back to work, because of the serious consequences of prolonged carriage with subsequent transmission to the general public.

Q How do these precautions differ in a food-handler who has contracted salmonella food poisoning?

A A food-handler who has contracted non-enteric salmonellosis such as food poisoning may return to work when symptoms have resolved if he or she can be relied upon to practise good personal hygiene, even if the faeces are still positive. Clearance specimens (negative faeces) are therefore not necessary, but if good personal hygiene cannot be guaranteed negative specimens usually are required.

CASE 22
Anorexia, malaise and nausea in Eddie, 25 years old

Eddie, a 25-year-old man, presents with a 5-day history of anorexia, malaise, fever and nausea. He has been persuaded to see his GP by his friends, who have told him his eyes have become yellow (Fig. 22.1), and he has also noticed some abdominal discomfort on the right-hand side. On closer questioning he admits to smoking 15 cigarettes a day, but has not been able to face one since he began to feel ill. He has noticed that over the past couple of days his urine has become very dark, which he attributes to not having taken in much fluid. He has not noticed any change in the colour or consistency of his stools. Prior to this illness he has been fit and healthy, with no past medical history of note. He is not on any regular medication.

Q What is the likely diagnosis?

A Eddie is clearly jaundiced. Although there are a large number of causes of jaundice, the non-specific prodromal illness with fever is highly suggestive of an acute infective – most probably viral – hepatitis. Other possibilities include acute alcoholic hepatitis and drug-induced hepatitis, either of which may mimic acute viral hepatitis. Many patients with acute hepatitis

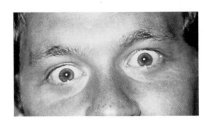

Fig. 22.1 Eddie's eyes.

give a history of tobacco and alcohol intolerance. The right upper quadrant pain is due to enlargement of the liver, stretching the sensitive liver capsule. Occasional patients, especially those with hepatitis B virus infection, may give a history of a rash and/or a polyarthritis prior to the onset of jaundice, features which arise from immune complex formation between virus and antibody.

Q What are the possible causative agents of acute infective hepatitis?

A A large number of infectious agents can cause acute hepatitis, including hepatitis A, B, C, D and E viruses, Epstein–Barr virus, cytomegalovirus, yellow fever virus and leptospira.

Q What further clinical details should be elicited from Eddie in order to pinpoint the most likely cause of his hepatitis?

A The answer to this question depends on an understanding of the risk factors that expose an individual to infection with each of the different agents, which in turn necessitates knowledge of their routes of spread. This information is outlined in Table 22.1. In simple terms, it is useful to remember the following summary of the hepatitis A–E viruses:

- Enteric spread: HAV, HEV
- Parenteral spread: HBV, HCV, HDV (also known as delta virus)

Note that HCV and HEV were formerly known as non-A non-B (NANB) viruses, prior to their identification in 1989 (HCV) and 1991 (HEV). The disease caused by these viruses was referred to as NANB hepatitis (NANBH).

Table 22.1 Routes of spread and risk groups for hepatitis viruses

Hepatitis A virus (HAV)

Routes of spread
 Faecal–oral
Risk groups
 Those who eat/drink contaminated food, e.g. shellfish and water
 Travellers to areas of high endemicity with low hygiene standards
 Carers or contacts of cases of acute HAV infection

Hepatitis B virus (HBV)

Routes of spread
 Vertical, i.e. mother to baby
 Sexual
 Contact with blood or blood products
Risk groups
 Newborns of carrier mothers
 Members of ethnic groups with high carriage rates
 Sexually promiscuous, both hetero-sexual and male homosexuals
 Intravenous drug abusers who share needles
 Patients receiving or exposed to blood or blood products, e.g. haemophiliacs, haemodialysis patients, blood transfusion recipients
 Health-care workers exposed to blood or blood products

Hepatitis C virus (HCV)

Routes of spread
 Contact with blood or blood products
 Natural route of transmission unknown
 Sexual transmission very inefficient compared to HBV
Risk groups
 Intravenous drug abusers who share needles
 Patients and health-care workers receiving or exposed to blood or blood products, as per HBV above

Hepatitis D virus (HDV)

Routes of spread
 Can only infect simultaneously with HBV, or patients who are already HBV infected, therefore routes as for HBV
Risk groups
 As for HBV. In the UK most HDV-infected patients are intravenous drug abusers

Hepatitis E virus (HEV)

Routes of spread
 Faecal–oral
Risk groups
 HEV is not endemic in the UK, therefore HEV infections are only likely in travellers to areas where HEV is endemic, e.g. Russia, India, South America

Yellow fever virus

Routes of spread
 Mosquito bites
Risk groups
 Travellers to countries where yellow fever infection exists, i.e. Africa, S. America

Note: EBV, CMV and leptospirosis infections are dealt with in Cases 9, 50 and 53 respectively

Eddie is not on any form of medication and his alcohol intake amounts to an average of 3–4 pints of beer per week. He gives no history of travel abroad in the last 6 months. He does not eat shell-fish. He has not been in contact with anyone else who is jaundiced. He denies ever having used intravenous drugs, and has never received a blood transfusion. He works for an estate agency. When questioned about his sexual partners he reveals that he is a prac-tising homosexual, and he acquired a new regular partner about 4 months ago. On examination he is jaundiced, his liver is tender and palpable 2 cm below the intercostal margin, but he has no stigmata of chronic liver disease and there are no other clinical signs.

Q How should Eddie be investi-gated further?

A The most likely diagnosis is now acute HBV infection, most probably acquired from his new sexual part-ner, although HAV infection from an unknown source is also a possi-bility. Apart from the standard in-vestigations of full blood count and liver function tests, blood should also be sent to the microbiology laboratory with a provisional diag-nosis of acute hepatitis, and asking for diagnostic assays to exclude HAV and HBV infection. All samples from Eddie should be clearly marked as 'Risk of infection' to alert porters and laboratory staff to the potential dangers of handling such material and to ensure safe transport. Note that the diagnosis of both HAV and HBV infection relies on the detection of the viruses or of antibodies to the viruses using serological techniques; neither virus can be grown in routine tissue culture, so it is *not* useful to send a faecal sample to the laboratory.

The following preliminary report is received from the micro-biology laboratory: hepatitis A IgG detected; hepatitis A IgM result to follow.

Q What are the significant differ-ences between IgM and IgG anti-bodies?

A IgM antibodies are only present for a short period following infec-tion, whereas IgG antibodies persist for many years, if not for life. Thus the presence of virus-specific IgM in a serum sample is a definitive indi-cation that the patient has recently been infected with that virus, where-as the presence of virus-specific IgG only indicates that the patient has been infected with that virus at some unspecified time during his or her life (see also Figure 55.2, in Case 55). One other important dif-ference, not relevant in this par-ticular case, is that IgM, being a large pentameric molecule, is un-able to cross the placenta, whereas IgG can.

Q How can the above results be interpreted?

A The HAV serology provided by the laboratory at this stage is not particularly helpful. The IgG anti-HAV indicates that the patient has at some stage been infected with HAV, but whether his acute illness is due to recent infection will only be revealed by the IgM anti-HAV result.

Q What diagnostic assays are available for characterizing HBV infection?

A A schematic diagram of HBV is shown in Figure 22.2. Various com-ponent parts (i.e. antigens) of the virus can be detected in the lab-oratory. Similarly, antibodies to these antigens can also be detected. The antigen–antibody systems can be summarized as follows:

Antigen		Antibody
Hepatitis B core antigen	HBcAg	Anti-HBc
Hepatitis B e antigen	HBeAg	Anti-HBe
Hepatitis B surface antigen	HBsAg	Anti-HBs

'e' is short for 'extractable'. eAg is in fact a breakdown product of cAg.

Q What assay will the laboratory perform to test for HBV infection?

A An assay for the presence of HBsAg. HBV is different from many other viruses in that virus, or anti-gens derived from it, can be detected in the bloodstream during infection.

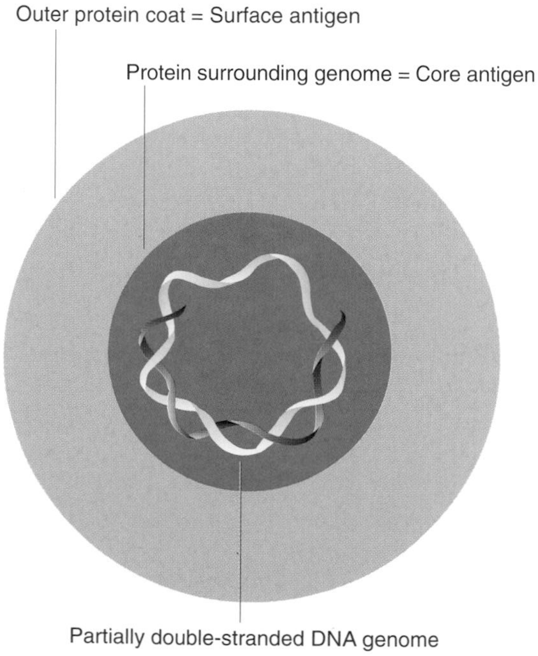

Outer protein coat = Surface antigen

Protein surrounding genome = Core antigen

Partially double-stranded DNA genome

Fig. 22.2 Diagram of HBV.

When HBV replicates within hepatocytes excess surface protein spills over into the blood, and this antigen (HBsAg) can be detected by the very sensitive assays available in the laboratory. This is therefore the primary screening assay for the diagnosis of HBV infection. A positive result would indicate that the patient is infected with HBV.

Q How would the laboratory confirm that infection with HBV was recent?

A As explained above, the best serological marker of recent infection is the presence of IgM class antibodies to the virus. In the case of HBV, the standard diagnostic assay is to look for the presence of IgM against the HBV core antigen. The significance and usefulness of the other markers of HBV infection are discussed below.

A further report from the laboratory reads: Hepatitis A IgM – NEGATIVE; no evidence of recent hepatitis A virus infection; HBsAg – POSITIVE; IgM anti-HBc – POSITIVE; indicates recent infection with hepatitis B virus.

Q What are the possible consequences of acute HBV infection?

A These are shown in diagrammatic form in Figure 22.3. The high mortality associated with acute fulminant hepatitis, together with the propensity for HBV infection to become chronic and the consequent risk that this will ultimately lead to cirrhosis and liver cell cancer, are the reasons why HBV is such a feared infection. The risk of chronic carriage is not related to the severity of the acute infection but to the age at acute infection: 10% of otherwise immunocompetent children or adults will become chronic carriers following acute infection, whereas over 95% of neonates become carriers. Patients who are immunosuppressed are also at greater risk of becoming chronic carriers, e.g. HIV-infected patients, transplant recipients.

Q What steps should be taken in the further management of Eddie?

A

1. He should be observed carefully during the acute stage of the illness. If there is any indication of fulminant hepatitis (e.g. impairment of conscious level, liver flap), he should be referred to hospital for specialist care.

2. He, and all those responsible for caring for him, should be aware that he is an infection risk. His blood and body fluids will contain HBV. Care should be taken to avoid needlestick accidents (this is standard practice whether or not a patient has HBV infection). He should be advised not to share razors or toothbrushes as the amount of blood present on these may be sufficient to transmit infection.

3. After Eddie has recovered from his acute illness he should be followed up to determine whether he is one of the 10% of patients who become chronic carriers. Chronic carriage is defined as the persistence of HBsAg for longer than 6 months.

4. Eddie's sexual partner should also be tested for HBsAg. If positive, he should also be followed to determine whether he is a chronic carrier or not. If negative, he should be offered appropriate prophylaxis (see below).

5. Both Eddie and his partner should be counselled about HIV infection (see Case 30).

Eddie recovers from his episode of jaundice, although it takes him 4 months before he feels his normal self again. Follow-up testing demonstrates the disappearance of HBsAg from his serum after 12 weeks, and the appearance of anti-HBs after 16 weeks, confirming elimination of the virus. His partner gives a history of jaundice 1 year previously, and on testing of serum samples taken 6 months apart is shown to be HBsAg positive, confirming that he is a chronic carrier. The laboratory report also indicates that his serum is HBeAg positive.

Q What is the purpose of testing for HBeAg and anti-HBe?

A eAg is a breakdown product of core antigen and is a surrogate marker of the extent of HBV replication occurring in the liver. The 'e' status of all carriers should be determined. The interpretation of the results is:

- HBeAg positive; anti-HBe negative
  extensive HBV replication occurring in the liver, with spillover into serum
  serum extremely infectious, e.g. via needlestick injury
  increased risk of long-term liver damage

- HBeAg negative; anti-HBe positive
  low-level viral replication in liver
  serum very much less infectious, e.g. transfusion of unit of blood needed to transmit infection

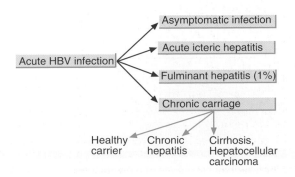

**Fig. 22.3
Consequences
of acute HBV
infection.**

Acute HBV infection → Asymptomatic infection

Acute icteric hepatitis

Fulminant hepatitis (1%)

Chronic carriage → Healthy carrier → Chronic hepatitis → Cirrhosis, Hepatocellular carcinoma

reduced risk of long-term liver damage
- HBeAg negative; anti-HBe negative
  in process of seroconverting to eAg (i.e. will become anti-HBe positive)
  regard as for HBeAg-positive individuals until anti-HBe is detectable

Note that HBeAg and anti-HBe are only *surrogate* markers of what is going on in the liver of HBsAg carriers. A more exact measure is the presence and quantity of HBV DNA in serum, but assays for this are not available in most routine diagnostic laboratories.

Figure 22.4 shows in diagrammatic form the serological results obtained from various categories of patients infected with HBV.

Further investigation of Eddie's partner reveals moderately deranged liver function tests, with a raised alanine aminotransferase. A liver biopsy reveals chronic active hepatitis.

Q Is there anything further that should be done for him?

A Yes. He is a candidate for α-interferon therapy. This immuno-modulatory agent works by enhancing the elimination of HBV-infected hepatocytes by the host's own immune system. Patients who respond to IFN become HBeAg negative, and then anti-HBe positive. Loss of HBsAg and complete elimination of the virus may take some years. However, seroconversion from eAg to anti-HBe positivity is a successful clinical endpoint, as the risk of progressive hepatitis is now much reduced and the patient is very much less infectious. Not all patients respond to IFN. Response rates are reduced in carriers who have been infected since birth, and in immuno-suppressed patients (e.g., HIV infected).

Q Is HBV infection preventable?

A Yes, by both passive and active immunization.

- Passive immunization:
  hyperimmune hepatitis B immuno-globulin (i.e. contains high-titre anti-HBs)
  for newborns of carrier mothers
  for non-responders to vaccine who suffer exposure, e.g. needlestick injury
- Active immunization:
  hepatitis B vaccine – recombinant HBsAg (i.e. a subunit vaccine)
  no risk of inadvertent transmission of HBV
  3 i.m. injections at 0,1 and 6 months
  check anti-HBs levels 4–6 weeks after end of course
  non-responders (up to 10% of recipients) are not protected

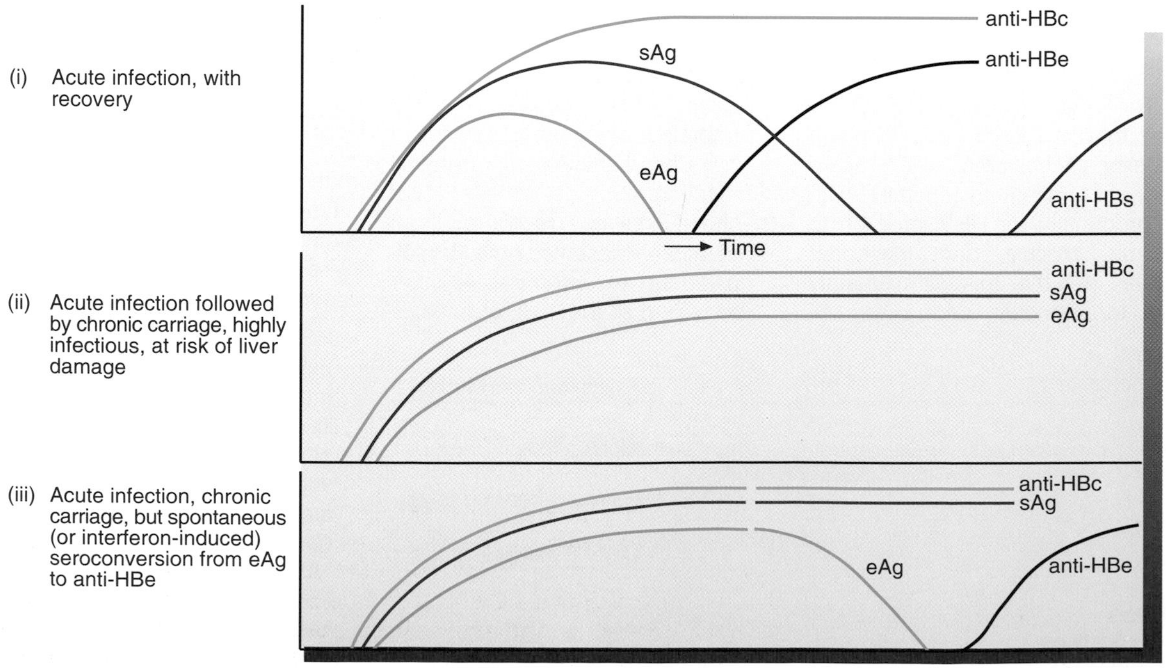

(i) Acute infection, with recovery

(ii) Acute infection followed by chronic carriage, highly infectious, at risk of liver damage

(iii) Acute infection, chronic carriage, but spontaneous (or interferon-induced) seroconversion from eAg to anti-HBe

Fig. 22.4 The serological results obtained from various categories of patients infected with HBV.

for newborns of carrier mothers
for all others at risk of HBV infection (see Table 22.1).
booster doses currently recommended after 5 years

Note: newborns of carrier mothers should be given both passive and active prophylaxis (i.e. anti-HBs in one thigh, course of vaccine begun in other thigh immediately after birth). This regimen gives over 90% success in interrupting vertical transmission

Table 22.2 summarizes the relevant information relating to hepatitis viruses A, C, D and E.

Summary: Viral hepatitis
Presentation
Non-specific prodrome, fever, malaise, nausea, alcohol and nicotine intolerance, followed by jaundice
Causative agents
Hepatitis viruses A–E, occasionally EBV, CMV
Diagnosis
Serology –IgM anti-HAV, HBsAg, anti-HCV
Spread
Faecal–oral route (HAV, HEV); vertical, sexual, blood contact (HBV, HCV, HDV)
Complications
Fulminant hepatitis; chronic hepatitis leading to cirrhosis and liver-cell cancer (HBV and HCV only)
Treatment
Supportive; interferon (chronic HBV and HCV); liver transplantation (fulminant hepatitis, end-stage chronic hepatitis)
Prevention
Reduction in risk activities, e.g. not sharing needles, practising safe sex; vaccination (against HAV, HBV) for selected at-risk groups; screening of blood supply (HBV, HCV)

Table 22.2 Salient features of the hepatitis viruses A, C, D and E

Hepatitis A virus

Incubation period 2–6 weeks
Diagnosis – the presence of IgM anti-HAV
Outcome – asymptomatic seroconversion
    acute hepatitis
    fulminant hepatitis, but risk much lower than for HBV
    recovery is associated with clearance of virus, i.e. no chronic carrier state, no risk of chronic liver disease
Immunization – passive: administration of normal human immunoglobulin
    active: killed whole virus vaccine
Indications for immunization
    frequent travellers; sewage workers; possibly health-care workers and workers looking after small children, e.g. in child-care centres, nurseries

Hepatitis C virus

Incubation period not known; 4–12 weeks if transmitted by blood transfusion
Diagnosis – anti-HCV positivity indicates infection; detection of HCV RNA in serum by polymerase chain reaction assay indicates chronic carriage
Outcome – asymptomatic seroconversion
    acute hepatitis
    fulminant hepatitis (less common than with HBV)
    chronic carriage with risk of chronic hepatitis, cirrhosis, hepatocellular carcinoma
Prevention – screening of blood supply to prevent post-transfusion acquisition

Hepatitis D virus (defective virus, requires HBsAg for its surface coat)

Diagnosis – detection of δ antigen, anti-δ antibodies
Outcome – acute hepatitis
    fulminant hepatitis (increased risk in coinfections of HBV and HDV)
    chronic carriage (increases risk of progressive liver disease in HBV carrier)
Prevention – as for HBV. Anti-HBs will prevent HDV infection

Hepatitis E virus

Diagnosis – assays not widely available at present. Diagnosis by exclusion
Outcome – as for HAV, except increased mortality in pregnant women (10%), pathogenesis unexplained
Prevention – no passive or active prophylaxis available

CASE 23
Upper abdominal pain in Gareth, a 46-year-old sheep farmer

Gareth, a 46-year-old sheep farmer, complains of upper abdominal pain of increasing severity which has been present for about 1 month. Nausea, anorexia and a general lassitude have recently affected his work. On examination Gareth is apyrexial and anicteric, with a pulse rate of 80/min. In the right upper abdominal quadrant there is a smooth and well circumscribed mass, which appears to be hepatic in origin.

Q What specific investigations are likely to be useful in determining the cause of this hepatic mass?

A The differential diagnosis includes neoplasia (primary hepatic, although relatively rare, and secondary), haemangioma, gallbladder disease or an abscess. Ultrasound, which is usually available and is non-invasive, should outline the nature of the mass and indicate whether it is cystic, solid or fluid filled. CT or MRI scans may be required to confirm this.

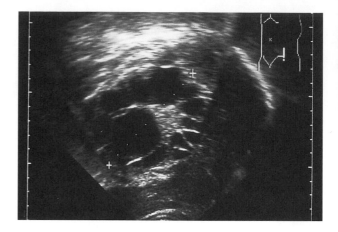

Fig. 23.1 Ultrasound of R lobe of liver.

Ultrasound showed a double-walled cystic lesion in the right lobe of the liver (see Figure 23.1). The full blood count revealed an eosinophil count of $1.2 \times 10^9/l$ $(0.04-0.4) \times 10^9/l$.

Q What is the likely diagnosis?

A The appearance of this mass and the background history of sheep farming (herbivorous animals), together with a peripheral eosinophilia, is compatible with hydatid disease caused by the tapeworm *Echinococcus granulosus* (see Fig. 23.2).

Q The radiologist who performed the ultrasound examination offers to aspirate the contents of this cyst to confirm the diagnosis. The attending physician refuses. Why?

A Rupture of the cyst and spillage of the contents is a possible complication of this procedure, and were this to happen severe systemic symptoms such as rigors and high fever might ensue. Serological investigation for antibodies to *E. granulosus* using enzyme immunoassay (often only available in reference centres) should confirm the diagnosis. The Casoni skin sensitivity test rarely adds further to the diagnosis.

Q Is surgical removal required?

A Unless the cyst is very large such that there are pressure effects or the patient is unresponsive to chemotherapy, surgical removal is not indicated. Most patients respond to abendazole, an imidazole agent, or praziquantal, but these should be continued for 6 weeks.

Q What other microbes cause liver abscesses?

A Most liver abscesses are pyogenic and caused by bacteria such as *Streptococcus milleri* (see Case 3), *Staphylococcus aureus, Bac-*

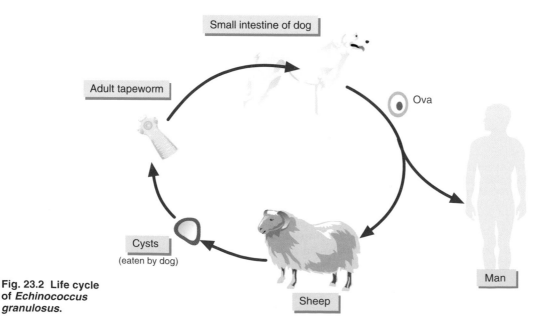

Small intestine of dog

Adult tapeworm

Ova

Cysts
(eaten by dog)

Sheep

Man

Fig. 23.2 Life cycle of *Echinococcus granulosus*.

teroides spp. and coliforms such as *Escherichia coli* originating from the large bowel (see Case 20). Fungal infections of the liver may also involve the spleen, and are usually found only in the severely immunocompromised, such as bone marrow transplant patients. *Entamoeba histolytica* liver involvement following amoebic colitis may occur in patients or travellers from endemic areas (see Box 23.1).

B23.1 Amoebic liver abscess
Clinical features
Younger age group than pyogenic abscesses Diarrhoea or colitis in 30–40% Point tenderness may be present
Investigations
Eosinophilia in 80% Amoebae may be seen in biopsy of edge of abscess; rarely seen in aspirated fluid Rise in antibodies
Treatment
Metronidazole, with perhaps diloxanide furoate

Summary: Hydatid disease
Presentation
Abdominal mass/liver abscess Occupation may be relevant
Diagnosis
Ultrasound but not aspiration Serology
Management
Abendazole, surgery occasionally

CASE 24
Continuous non-bloody diarrhoea in Paul, a 35-year-old aid worker

Paul, a 35-year-old male aid worker who has spent the previous 6 months working in a refugee camp, becomes ill during a 12-hour flight from Lima, Peru, to London. He complains of almost continuous non-bloody diarrhoea for the preceding 18–24 hours, nausea and severe fatigue. On arrival in the airport health centre he is apyrexial, dehydrated, drowsy and has postural hypotension.

Q What additional information would be helpful in coming to a provisional diagnosis?

A The presence of abdominal pain and the passage of blood per rectum would suggest a colitis or enteritis due to *Salmonella, Campylobacter* or *Shigella* (dysentery). A history of similar symptoms from fellow passengers or aircraft crew might indicate an outbreak of toxin-mediated food poisoning caused by *Staphylococcus aureus, Bacillus cereus* or *Clostridium perfringens*, and a food history point to the source and likely cause (see Case 17). Further information from the patient is required concerning the nature of his work in the refugee camp, the social conditions there and whether colleagues have had similar symptoms.

Further questioning of Paul indicates that there has been minimal if any abdominal pain, and that he is now passing liquid stools every 30–40 minutes. Before he left Lima he had been engaged for the last 2 weeks in fieldwork in the foothills of the Andes, where conditions had been primitive and water in short supply.

Q What is the likely diagnosis?

A The profuse watery diarrhoea without abdominal pain leading to marked dehydration is consistent with cholera (aetiological agent *Vibrio cholerae*). Cholera has been endemic in many parts of Asia for some years, and is spread along trade and travel routes rather than

B24.1 *Vibrio cholerae*
• Motile Gram-negative curved bacillus • Requires specific media but grows luxuriantly in alkaline medium, which is used to isolate it from stool specimens • Causes diarrhoea by the production of an enterotoxin, whereas other *Vibrio* spp. such as *V. parahaemolyticus* are invasive • Classic biotype replaced by El Tor in the 1960s and different serotypes, e.g. *Ogawa, Inaba* distinguished by somatic (O) antigens

by human carriage. Since 1991 there has been an epidemic in Peru involving over a million people. Risk factors include drinking untreated or unboiled water and attendance at social events where food washed in untreated water may be consumed. This outbreak is due to *V. cholerae* 01, serotype *Inaba* (see Box 24.1).

Q How does *V. cholerae* induce diarrhoea?

A The bacterium does not gain access to the bloodstream and never enters any tissue of the body. It replicates only in small intestine following attachment where it finds suitable conditions. There it elaborates an enterotoxin which acts by stimulating adenylate cyclase (see Figure 24.1), not unlike some of the toxins elaborated by *Escherichia coli* or *Salmonella*. The toxin's effects on water and electrolyte metabolism results in an alkaline

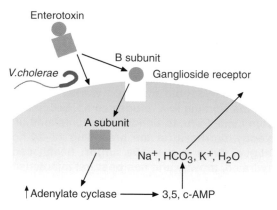

Fig. 24.1
Mechanism of action of cholera enterotoxin.

Summary: Cholera
Presentation
Continuous watery diarrhoea in a resident of an endemic or epidemic area or a returned traveller
Diagnosis
Culture of faeces on selective media (should be requested as not routine) Urea and electrolytes to assess degree of dehydration
Management
Fluid replacement (e.g. saline with glucose and potassium); antibiotics (i.e. tetracyclines) sometimes necessary

environment, which in turn provides ideal growth conditions for the bacterium.

Q What is the management of cholera?

A Fluid replacement is the key to effective management and in severe cases this should be by the parenteral route. Lactated Ringer's solution or saline with added glucose and potassium may be used, with regular assessment of electrolytes, blood glucose and acid balance. Antibiotics are believed to shorten the diarrhoea. Tetracyclines are the agents of choice, with co-trimoxazole, chloramphenicol and quinolones as alternatives.

Q How may cholera be prevented?

A Improved sanitation, especially the separation of sewage from drinking water, reduces endemic disease. Untreated water and con-taminated food (e.g. shellfish) or food washed in water should be avoided. Cholera, whether micro-biologically confirmed or otherwise, should be notified and stool speci-mens forwarded to the laboratory accompanied by appropriate travel and or other details, as culture for cholera is not routine. A phenol- and heat-inactivated parenteral vaccine is available but is only 50% protective and effective for 3 months only. It is indicated for travellers to endemic areas but is not useful for the control of out-breaks. An orally administered killed whole-cell vaccine combined with a B-subunit peptide is currently being evaluated and shows promise as an alternative.

CASE 25
Colicky abdominal pain and diarrhoea in Winston, a 68-year-old man with chronic leukaemia

Winston is a 68-year-old man who is admitted to hospital complaining of nausea and vomiting, colicky abdominal pain and diarrhoea for a number of days. Winston has not been abroad recently, but up to his retirement 3 years previously he worked for the United Nations, trav-elling back and forth to southeast Asia. He lives with his wife, Edith, who is well. He suffered a myocardial infarction 8 years previously and chronic lymphatic leukaemia was diagnosed 4 years ago, but he has since remained well on no medication. His physical examination is unremarkable.

Q What microbiological investi-gations should be instigated?

A Stool samples for culture should be sent to the microbiology lab-oratory for the diagnosis of gastro-enteritis caused by *Campylobacter, Shigella, Salmonella* etc., and for microscopy to detect ova and parasites. Blood cultures should also be taken because his chronic leukaemia renders him immuno-suppressed. If any food is incrimi-nated this should also be analysed. Consideration should be given to non-infectious causes such as diver-ticulitis, inflammatory bowel disease and bowel neoplasia, and appro-priate investigations undertaken, e.g. ultrasound, colonoscopy, especially if the symptoms do not settle.

Forty-eight hours after admission Winston develops a temperature of 39.5°C and rigors, and becomes cold, clammy and hypotensive. He is immediately transferred to the intensive therapy unit (ITU) for resusci-tation. Blood cultures sub-sequently grow *Escherichia coli*. Urine culture is sterile. The laboratory also reports seeing larvae in the second sample of faeces submitted.

Q What might these larvae be?

A Rhabditiform larvae of *Strongyloides stercoralis* were seen following concentration of faeces. This is a roundworm which is endemic in the tropics but may be seen in temperate climates in institutions, where continuous self-infection may occur. Alternatively it may be diagnosed in patients who have spent some time in the tropics (the organism is acquired from soil and is endemic in indigenous populations) even some years previously, as in the case described here. In the immunosuppressed patient (e.g. those with leukaemia, lymphoma or on corticosteroids) there may be an interval of some years between the original infestation and presentation. The diagnosis is usually made by seeing larvae in the stool or by detecting a rise in antibodies by enzyme immunoassay (only available in reference laboratories).

Q Is there a connection between the strongyloidiasis and the Gram-negative bacteraemia?

A Acute presentation as described here may also be accompanied by bacteraemia induced by gastrointestinal upset in the immunosuppressed host, and this may be fatal.

Q How is strongyloidiasis contracted and what are the common clinical presentations?

A Filariform larvae penetrate the skin, especially the soles of the feet, enter the bloodstream, migrate to the lungs and eventually settle in the small intestine where they mature. This sequence takes about 2–3 weeks. The larvae may remain in the intestine for some years, and where personal standards of hygiene are poor, repeated autoinfection may occur. Patients with strongyloidiasis may present with:

- asymptomatic infestation (diagnosed on screening)
- nausea, vomiting, diarrhoea, abdominal pain

- a malabsorption-type syndrome
- creeping skin eruptions occurring over many years
- pneumonitis with eosinophilia
- infestation accompanied by bacteraemia.

Winston is successfully resuscitated in the ITU with intravenous fluids but does not require ventilation. The bacteraemia is treated with intravenous cefotaxime (see Case 44). Winston is also started on thiabendazole, which is given for 3 days to treat the strongyloidiasis, and follow-up stool samples are clear of larvae.

Q What is the commonest roundworm infestation in the UK?

A *Ascaris lumbricoides* is probably the commonest worm (helminth) encountered in temperate climates (see Box 25.1) and infestation is usually seen in children 3–8 years of age, who present with failure to thrive, bowel obstruction or eosinophilia accompanied by respiratory symptoms. Piperazine is the treatment of choice.

B25.1 Other helminths (worms) and the diseases they cause	
Nematodes (roundworms)	**Diseases**
Ascaris lumbricoides	Intestinal obstruction
Onchocerca volvulus	River blindness (onchocerciasis)
Wuchereria bancrofti	Elephantiasis
Enterobius vermicularis (thread or pinworm)	Perianal irritation
Toxocara canis	Asthma, epilepsy, ocular lesions
Cestodes (tapeworms)	
Taenia solium (pig)	Epilepsy from cysticercosis may occur
Echinococcus granulosus (dogs)	Hydatid disease with cysts (see Case 23)
Trematodes (flukes)	
Schistosoma spp.	Cystitis (bilharzia, see Case 31), GI bleeding
Fasciola hepatica	Cholangitis, cholecystitis

Summary: Strongyloidiasis
Presentation
Usually acquired in tropics, with symptoms of diarrhoea and abdominal pain. Occasionally overwhelming infection
Diagnosis
Larvae seen in faeces under microscopy, eosinophilia in blood count and rise in antibodies
Treatment
Thiabendazole

CASE 26
Gillian, a 23-year-old receptionist with frequency, dysuria and haematuria

Gillian, a 23-year-old receptionist, has a 2-day history of frequency, dysuria and slight haematuria. She also complains of suprapubic pain but there is no vaginal discharge. Three weeks previously her GP had prescribed ampicillin for 5 days for a similar episode, and the symptoms had gradually resolved. There is no relevant previous history and physical examination is unremarkable.

Q What is the likely diagnosis and why?

A The symptoms as described above in a young woman are very suggestive of urinary tract infection, and cystitis in particular. A urethritis or cervicitis due to *Neisseria gonorrhoea* or other sexually transmitted diseases would be characterized more by dysuria during the early part of micturition, and a discharge (see Case 28). Enquiries about changes in sexual habits or partners, however, should always be made with this type of presentation.

Q What are the possible complications of this infection?

A Symptoms such as frequency, dysuria and haematuria are indicative of lower renal tract involvement. Infection of the kidney or renal pelvis is more likely to be accompanied by fever, vomiting, rigors, and perhaps abdominal or flank pain. Loin or renal angle tenderness is typical of pyelonephritis, which may be accompanied by bacteraemia.

Gillian's family doctor obtains a midstream urine specimen (MSU), which is cloudy, and sends it to the local Public Health Laboratory (microbiology laboratory) for microscopy and culture before starting her on trimethoprim for 5 days. The microscopy report on the urine is as follows: >100 white cells/mm³; <10 red cells/mm³; moderate numbers of epithelial cells seen (see Fig. 26.1).

A

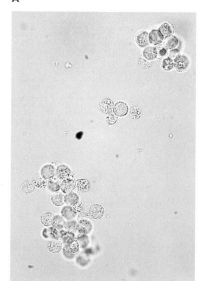

B

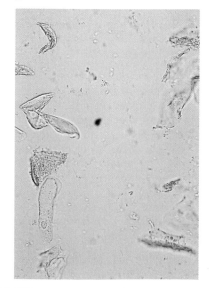

Fig. 26.1 Microscopy of (A) infected urine with numerous 'pus' cells; (B) contaminated urine with squamous epithelial cells.

Q What is the interpretation of the above microscopy report?

A Normally, urine has <5 white or pus cells/mm^3 and a count of 10–30/mm^3 may indicate early or partly treated infection. Large numbers of pus cells (>100/mm^3) are diagnostic of infected urine, although this may not occur if the patient is incapable of mounting a normal inflammatory response, as with neutropenia. The epithelial cells represent possible vulval or vaginal contamination, and consequently culture may grow more than one organism or insignificant numbers of harmless skin flora. A Gram stain is rarely indicated for urine specimens as it does not add to the above or indicate the most appropriate therapy.

Q What pathogens most frequently cause urinary tract infection?

A Gram-negative bacilli such as *Escherichia coli* are most commonly implicated, as outlined in Table 26.1.

Culture of the urine grew a pure growth of >10^5/ml of *Staphylococcus saprophyticus*, which on sensitivity testing was resistant to ampicillin, nitrofurantoin, cephradine and nalidixic acid, but sensitive to trimethoprim (see Table 26.2). The patient's symptoms completely resolved after 2–3 days of the 5-day course of trimethoprim, and a follow-up urine sample taken after the course was sterile.

Q Could the isolation of a *Staphylococcus* here not represent skin contamination as indicated by the microscopy?

A No. The presence in pure growth of a recognized urinary pathogen, *S. saprophyticus*, is diagnostic here. *S. saprophyticus* is a coagulase-negative staphylococcus which is distinguished in the laboratory by intrinsic resistance to novobiocin, a rarely used antibiotic. It is second in importance to *Escherichia coli* as a cause of cystitis in young women

Table 26.1 Aetiology of urinary tract infection (UTI)

Organism	Frequency %	Comment
Escherichia coli	>50	Commonest cause by far
Proteus spp.	10–15	Often associated with renal stones
Klebsiella spp.	10	May be hospital- or catheter-associated
Enterococci	8–10	Usually low-grade pathogens
S. saprophyticus	5–8	Confined to young women
S. epidermidis/aureus	2–6	Hospital acquired, associated with urinary catheters or bacteraemia (*S. aureus*)
Pseudomonas aeruginosa	4	Recurrent UTI or underlying pathology

Table 26.2 Commonly prescribed oral antibiotics to treat UTI

Antibiotic	Comment
Ampicillin	Most hospital and up to 50% of community isolates resistant
Trimethoprim*	Very useful agent to treat UTI in hospital and the community
Nalidixic acid	Early quinolone, urinary antiseptic. Poor against staphylococci and streptococci. Less frequently used now
Nitrofurantoin*	Useful agent and a urinary antiseptic. Inactive against *Proteus*
Co-amoxyclav	Effective against many ampicillin-resistant isolates
Cephalexin ⎫ Cephradine ⎭	As for co-amoxyclav
Fosfomycin	Recently introduced to the UK but widely used throughout Europe; single dose usually effective
Ciprofloxacin	Second-line agent to treat complicated UTIs or more resistant organisms
Norfloxacin*	

*Preferred agents for antimicrobial prophylaxis before instrumentation or lithotripsy, recurrent infections or those associated with coitus.

(see Table 26.1). It is almost exclusively confined to women during the reproductive years, and there appears to be a seasonal peak incidence in late summer and early autumn. Like most urinary pathogens it is acquired from the rectum, and although not sexually acquired *per se* is associated with recent sexual intercourse or menstruation. Like many coagulase-negative staphylococci, such as *S. epidermidis*, *S. saprophyticus* is often resistant to β-lactam agents such as ampicillin and cephradine (Table 26.2).

Q Does Gillian warrant further investigation?

A No. Although urinary tract infection may occur as a result of underlying disease of the genitourinary tract, it is not uncommon in females and the recent episode described here probably represents relapse of an earlier infection, partially treated with ampicillin. High concentrations of many antibiotics are achieved in the urine as this is the route of excretion, and although the *S. saprophyticus* was resistant to ampicillin *in vitro* some inhibition of growth is likely to have occurred; this, together with increased oral fluid intake leading to a dilution effect, ensured a temporary resolution in symptoms. The presentation and outcome described do

B26.1 Indications for radiological investigations

Adults (IVU or US)	First infection in men Recurrent infection or persistent symptoms Frank or persistent haematuria Unexpected pathogen Suspected renal abscess (US)
Children (US)	All children require ultrasound investigation
	<u><2 years</u>: if normal, cystoscopy and scintigraphy; if abnormal, IVU, micturating cystourethrography <u>2–10 years</u>: if normal, no further investigations; if abnormal, IVU and micturating cystourethrography (IVU: intravenous urography; US: ultrasound)

B26.2 Urethral syndrome

Definition

Symptoms of dysuria and frequency in women during the reproductive years, without significant bacteriuria ($>10^5$/ml).

Possible causes

Less common urinary pathogens, e.g. *Chlamydia*, *Neisseria gonorrhoea*, *Gardnerella vaginalis*, herpes simplex.
Conventional bacteria but with counts as low as 10^2/ml.
Fastidious bacteria such as lactobacilli, diphtheroids.
Non-infective, e.g. psychological factors, trauma from intercourse

suggest complicated UTI, and consequently none of the factors necessary to merit further investigation are met (see Box 26.1).

Q Do the symptoms and the microbiology results fulfil the criteria for the 'urethral syndrome'?

A No. This patient had a significant bacteriuria with a well recognized cause of urinary infection and there is nothing especially unusual about this episode. The features of the 'urethral syndrome' are outlined in Box 26.2.

Summary: Urinary tract infection

Presentation

Frequency, dysuria and haematuria indicate lower tract infection. Fever, vomiting, rigors and flank pain are more suggestive of upper renal tract involvement

Diagnosis

An MSU should reveal pyuria and a bacterial colony count of $>10^5$/ml. Lower counts may be seen in partly treated infection or less common causes, as seen in the urethral syndrome

Management

Increased fluid intake and an oral antibiotic or urinary antiseptic such as trimethoprim or nitrofurantoin. Ultrasound or intravenous pyelogram should be considered in children, men, and following recurrent episodes in women

CASE 27
Joan's cloudy bag

A 55-year-old woman, Joan, has chronic renal failure secondary to pyelonephritis and is on continuous ambulatory peritoneal dialysis (CAPD). She has noticed that the bag containing the dialysate has become cloudy in the past few days. She has also experienced some mild abdominal discomfort, but she is apyrexial. She has no other abdominal or gastrointestinal symptoms.

Q What is the likely diagnosis?

A The dialysate bag is normally clear, but a cloudy bag in a patient on CAPD with or without abdominal symptoms is characteristic of CAPD peritonitis. CAPD has been widely used since the mid-1980s as a form of renal replacement, and is based upon hyperosmolar ultrafiltration across the peritoneal membrane. This is achieved by insertion of a Tenckhoff catheter (see Figure 27.1), which is permanent and allows the continuous instillation of 1–2 l of

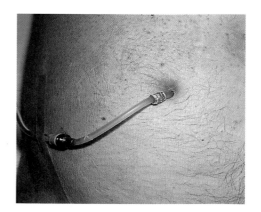

Fig. 27.1 Tenckhoff catheter inserted into the abdomen.

dialysis fluid for 4–8 hours. Compared with haemodialysis it is more economical, does not require vascular access, entails fewer electrolyte restrictions, is less likely to be associated with elevated blood pressure and ensures greater mobility for the patient.

Q How frequent is CAPD peritonitis and how does it arise?

A The rate of infection is around 1–1.5 episodes per patient per year, which is about half of what it was during the early years. This is a relatively low incidence, considering that there is permanent access to the peritoneal cavity and that this sealed system is broken about 1500 times a year. Infection may arise from the exit site, the tunnel through which the catheter passes (see Figure 27.2), the peritoneum itself or via the haematogenous route. The latter two sources are relatively infrequent.

Q How may the diagnosis be confirmed?

A A sample of fluid should be sent to the laboratory for microscopy and culture or, if this cannot be done immediately, the fluid should be refrigerated. A cloudy bag usually contains >100 pus cells/mm^3, predominantly polymorph neutrophils. The Gram stain is relatively insensitive in detecting microorganisms and consequently culture is essential to confirm an aetiological diagnosis. Samples of fluid are incubated aerobically and anaerobically after centrifugation and enrichment to maximize the yield from culture.

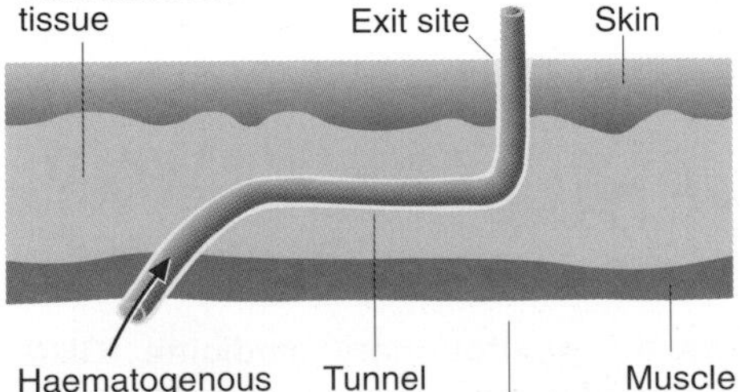

Pending the results of culture and sensitivity testing, her renal physician prescribes intraperitoneal cefuroxime and vancomycin (administered in the dialysis fluid) for Joan, and follow-up is arranged. In the peritoneal fluid 250 white cells/mm^3 are seen and *Staphylococcus epidermidis* (the most common aetiological agent), sensitive to vancomycin but resistant to cefuroxime, is isolated. The cefuroxime is discontinued and over the next few days the bag becomes less cloudy and her symptoms resolve.

Q What local factors contribute to staphylococcal peritonitis?

A Considerably fewer bacteria are required to cause CAPD than surgical peritonitis. The presence of the catheter results in the formation of a biofilm on the external surface, composed of extracellular slime which protects organisms from the body's host defences such as mononuclear cells and inhibits penetration by antibiotics. The low pH and relatively high osmolarity of CAPD fluid will also suppress the activity of these cells in the dialysate.

Q What is the success rate for the treatment of CAPD peritonitis with first-line antimicrobial agents?

A The conventional approach to the management of uncomplicated CAPD peritonitis before the results of culture are available is usually intraperitoneal vancomycin plus an aminoglycoside, but if symptoms are more severe a loading dose of an intravenous antibiotic is administered. This approach is successful in approximately 80% of cases. Antibiotic treatment should be modified following antimicrobial sensitivity

results, and it is possible to subsequently administer the aminoglycoside to alternate bags rather than each bag.

Occasionally it is necessary to remove the Tenckhoff catheter if infection persists or relapses, if there is an associated tunnel infection, or if infection is caused by fungi or *Pseudomonas*, both of which are difficult to eradicate. The newer quinolone antibiotics have been used recently because they may be administered orally and achieve excellent intraperitoneal levels.

Six months later, after making a full recovery from the first episode, Joan becomes seriously ill with vomiting, severe abdominal pain and a cloudy dialysate. This time she is admitted to hospital and *Escherichia coli* and *Bacteroides fragilis* are isolated from her dialysis fluid.

Q What is the significance of these two organisms compared with *S. epidermidis*?

A Skin organisms such as *S. epidermidis* are most frequently

Subcutaneous tissue | Exit site | Skin

Haematogenous route of infection (occasionally) | Tunnel | Peritoneal cavity | Muscle

Fig. 27.2 Anatomy and source of infection of CAPD.

Table 27.1 Organisms most frequently implicated in CAPD peritonitis

Organism	Frequency (%)	Comment
Coagulase −ve staphylococci	45	*S. epidermidis* in 80%
Staphylococcus aureus	15	Associated with tunnel infections
Streptococci	12	Include enterococci
Escherichia coli	8	Consider bowel perforation
Other coliforms	5	Consider bowel perforation
Pseudomonas aeruginosa	4	Tunnel infection and abscesses
Diphtheroids	2	Relapse common
Fungi	2	*Candida albicans* most frequent
Miscellaneous	7	

implicated in CAPD peritonitis (see Table 27.1). Coliforms and other gut flora are less common, but when they occur they often reflect intra-abdominal pathology, such as a perforated viscus. Consequently, investigation and management should be as for surgical peritonitis (see Case 20) and include abdominal X-rays, ultrasound, surgical consultation, and possibly a laparotomy.

Following investigation, diverticulitis with localized abscess formation is diagnosed which requires removal of the catheter, surgical resection and drainage. Following a course of intravenous cefotaxime and metronidazole Joan makes a full recovery, but because of distortion to the peritoneum arising from the surgical peritonitis she is unable to go back on peritoneal dialysis and is haemodialysed instead.

Q What measures may be taken to minimize CAPD infection?

A Strategies to prevent infection very much depend on the patient and the attention that he or she gives to the procedure of changing bags. It also involves:

- insertion of the Tenckhoff catheter by an experienced surgical team who carry out the procedure regularly
- training of patients in the cleaning and dressing of the exit site and the application of occlusive dressings. Patient motivation is all-important
- eradication of nasal carriage with mupirocin where *S. aureus* infection recurs
- development of improved catheter materials which inhibit the adhesion of bacteria and the formation of biofilms, and the incorporation of antimicrobial agents in the catheter
- there may be a place in some cases for the use of filters, routine alcohol rinses or prophylactic antibiotics.

Q Where else are coagulase-negative staphylococci, especially *S. epidermidis*, important as pathogens?

A These skin bacteria are likely to cause infection whenever foreign bodies are inserted into the bloodstream or a body cavity. These include intravascular catheters (peripheral, arterial and central), prosthetic joints (see Box 27.1) etc. The ubiquitous distribution of these bacteria, their resistance to multiple antibiotics, the production of extracellular slime resulting in biofilm

B27.1 Important infections caused by coagulase-negative staphylococci
Bacteraemia
common organism (see Case 44)
Endocarditis
5% of native and 40% of prosthetic valve infection
CSF shunt
50% of infections. Diphtheroids increasing in importance
Prosthetic joint
30% of infections, usually introduced at time of surgery
Vascular grafts
60% of infections, e.g. aortofemoral
UTI
S. saprophyticus in young women (see Case 26)

formation, and problems with typing which hampers our understanding of their epidemiology, make the prevention and treatment of infection especially difficult.

Q What are the risk factors for intravascular catheter infections?

A These include:

- inexperience or poor technique by the operator
- insertion of central rather than peripheral catheters
- insertion during an emergency, e.g. cardiac arrest
- duration of catheterization, especially if longer than 3–4 days.

Many intravascular devices become infected during insertion, but infection may also arise from contaminated infusates (rare now but implicated previously in outbreaks of *Citrobacter* spp. bacteraemia) and contamination of hubs or giving-set junctions.

Summary: CAPD peritonitis
Presentation
Cloudy bag or dialysate. Frank abdominal pain less a feature than with surgical peritonitis
Diagnosis
>100 pus cells/mm^3 and bacteria grown from fluid after centrifugation or enrichment. *S. epidermidis* the commonest cause
Management
Intraperitoneal antibiotics. Removal of catheter rarely required

CASE 28
Elizabeth, a 28-year-old prostitute, attends the clinic for a check-up

Elizabeth, 28 years old, attends the genitourinary medicine (GUM) clinic for a check-up. She has recently started work in a 'massage parlour' and it is the policy of the owner to ensure that all girls attend for regular assessment. She has no relevant past medical history and

is not on any regular medication, apart from the oral contraceptive pill. Her last menstruation was 2 weeks ago. She has noticed a whitish vaginal discharge, not very profuse, over the past couple of days, but no other symptoms related to the genitourinary tract, in particular no dysuria or vaginal irritation. On examination the vaginal walls do not look inflamed, although there is a small amount of purulent material visible. When a speculum is passed a mucopurulent discharge is seen coming from the cervix.

Q What is the provisional diagnosis?

A Elizabeth has a mucopurulent cervicitis. The vaginal discharge has presumably arisen from the cervix. The absence of vaginal irritation or signs of vaginal wall inflammation support this hypothesis.

Q What organisms may cause this condition?

A Mucopurulent cervicitis may arise from infection with *Neisseria gonorrhoeae* (see Box 28.1) or *Chlamydia trachomatis* strains D–K (see below). Herpes simplex virus may also infect the cervix, resulting in a profuse mucopurulent discharge, especially during a primary attack of genital herpes (see Case 29), but the absence of visible ulceration makes this diagnosis less likely.

B28.1 *Neisseria gonorrhoeae*

- Gram-negative intracellular diplococcus
- Males: usually symptomatic, with involvement of urethra (profuse purulent discharge + dysuria; anus and rectum, pharynx (from oral sex), prostate, epididymis and testes may also be involved
- Females: often asymptomatic, with involvement of endocervix, urethra, rectum, pharynx. May cause pelvic inflammatory disease (see below)
- Bacteraemia may occur (more common in females), with involvement of skin and joints
- Diagnosis by smear and culture
- Antibiotic treatment: depends on knowledge of local resistance patterns, as penicillin resistance is no longer uncommon and not always due to β-lactamase production. Examples include a single high dose of amoxicillin plus probenecid; single dose of a quinolone (e.g. ciprofloxacin)

Q What investigations should be performed?

A A cervical smear should be Gram stained. The presence of poly-morphs on a smear supports the clinical diagnosis of cervicitis. Gonococci may be seen as intra-cellular Gram-negative diplococci. A swab for culture for *N. gonorrhoeae* should preferably be plated out on appropriate media in the GU clinic (the organism is fragile and may not survive prolonged storage prior to plating out). A further cervical swab, together with a urethral swab for chlamydia diagnosis, should also be taken.

Q How will the laboratory attempt to confirm infection with *C. trachomatis*?

A Although chlamydia are classified as bacteria, they do not grow on inanimate media. Thus, isolation is attempted in cell culture, where the replicating organisms produce large inclusion bodies, the presence of which can be demonstrated by appropriate staining. Such cell culture is time consuming and labour intensive, and many laboratories have switched to more rapid diag-nostic techniques such as antigen detection by ELISA or by staining with fluorescently labelled monoclonal antichlamydia antibodies. These latter techniques may not be as sensitive as cell culture.

Q Should you offer Elizabeth any other tests?

A All new female patients attend-ing a GUM clinic, regardless of sexual proclivity, should be offered:

- serological screening for syphilis (see Box 28.2)

B28.2 Syphilis

- **Causative agent** *Treponema pallidum*, a spirochaete
- **Stages of disease**
  Primary: painless, indurated ulcer ('hard' chancre), usually in genital area
  Secondary: 6–8 weeks later, fever, headache, widespread rash, generalized lymphadenopathy, +/- mucosal mouth ulcers and wart-like lesions (condylomata lata) in moist warm sites
  Latent: may then ensue and last several years
  Tertiary: includes granulomatous lesions (gummata) at various sites (e.g. skin, bones, joints)
  Quaternary: involves the cardiovascular (e.g. aortic aneurysm) and central nervous systems (tabes dorsalis, general paralysis of the insane)
  Congenital syphilis: in offspring of infected mothers
- **Diagnosis** Serology includes non-specific screening tests based on cardiolipin or reagin (e.g. WR, VDRL, RPR), and confirmation with specific treponemal tests (e.g. TPHA, FTA). Dark-ground microscopy may demonstrate organism in exudate from chancre, mucous ulcers, condylomata lata, but not in later stages of disease
- **Treatment** High-dose penicillin, with appropriate serological follow-up to confirm cure

---

- cervical smear for cytology if due or clinically indicated
- cervical smear and culture for *N. gonorrhoeae* and *C. trachomatis*
- vaginal smear, culture or wet prep as clinically indicated (see below)
- throat and/or rectal cultures for *N. gonorrhoeae*, dependent on sexual history
- urinalysis.

Q What investigations are routine for new male patients attending the GUM clinic?

A New male patients should be offered:

- syphilis screening
- microscopy and urinalysis of initial voided urine
- urethral smear and culture for

N. gonorrhoeae and *C. trachomatis* if symptomatic or at high risk for these infections.

For patients of either sex HIV serology may be offered if appropriate after pretest counselling and consent (see Case 30). Similarly, those at risk of HBV infection should be offered HBV serology, and if negative for both HBsAg and anti-HBc (see Case 22), a course of vaccination.

Patients such as Elizabeth, who are at continued risk of acquiring sexually transmitted diseases, will require screening at regular intervals for all of the above.

Q What treatment would you offer Elizabeth at this stage?

A If the cervical smear is positive for Gram-negative diplococci you should treat her for gonorrhoea (see Box 28.1) and also for a presumptive chlamydial infection (e.g. with a 7-day course of tetracycline, or erythromycin if pregnant), as the two infections can often coexist. If the smear is negative you should treat the presumptive chlamydial infection only.

Q What are the other principles of management of a patient with a sexually transmitted disease?

A

1. Contact tracing: Treating the patient with antibiotics is only half the battle. In simple terms, 'it takes two to tango'! Identification and tracing of all contacts of patients with an STD is a vital function of the clinic. Contacts should be advised to attend the clinic in person, when appropriate counselling, testing and treatment can be offered.
2. Prevention of infection: The most effective method is the use of barrier methods of contraception (i.e. condoms and diaphragm), the use of which should be encouraged.
3. Education: It is important that any patient with an STD should

appreciate that they are potentially infectious, and they should therefore abstain from sexual intercourse until their infection has been appropriately treated.

Elizabeth's cervical smear, examined in the clinic, shows many polymorphs but no organisms are seen. A 1-week course of doxycycline is prescribed, and Elizabeth is counselled about the risks of spreading her infection and advised to abstain from sexual intercourse for 7 days. She is asked to return to the clinic in 2 weeks' time. The cervical swab from Elizabeth is reported as 'Chlamydia culture POSITIVE'. At her return visit to the clinic, speculum examination reveals a normal cervix.

Q Are any further investigations warranted?

A Yes. A 'test-of-cure' cervical culture for chlamydia should be performed.

Q What clinical syndromes are associated with genital *C. trachomatis* infection?

A

- Non-specific urethritis (NSU, see Box 28.3)

B28.3 Non-specific urethritis (NSU)

- Previously known as non-gonococcal urethritis (NGU), commonest STD in UK
- Urethral symptoms (dysuria, mucopurulent discharge) usually only in males
- Causative organisms include *C. trachomatis* (30–60%), certain strains of ureaplasma and mycoplasma, and possibly *Trichomonas vaginalis*
- May coexist with gonococcal urethritis
- In asymptomatic patients, presence of polymorphs in urethral smear or initial voided urine may indicate urethritis
- Treatment: a tetracycline or erythromycin. Relapse may occur

---

- Prostatitis or epididymitis
- Mucopurulent cervicitis (this case)
- Pelvic inflammatory disease (see Box 28.4)
- Reiter's syndrome (triad of arthritis, conjunctivitis, NSU, usually in HLA B27-positive individual)
- FitzHugh–Curtis syndrome (right upper quadrant pain due to perihepatitis). High titres of antibodies to *C. trachomatis* may be diagnostic
- Trachoma inclusion conjunctivitis (infection of neonate acquired on passage through infected birth canal; see Case 56)
- Infertility (in females, may not be a history of symptomatic infection).

Elizabeth returns to the clinic at regular intervals for routine checks. At one such visit she complains of a thin smelly vaginal discharge.

Q What are the common causes of a vaginal discharge?

A Candidosis, trichomoniasis and 'bacterial vaginosis' (see Boxes 28.5–28.7).

B28.4 Pelvic inflammatory disease (PID)

- **Presentation**: Lower abdominal pain and tenderness (+/- peritonism), dyspareunia, pelvic pain and tenderness (+/- mass *per vaginam*), mucopurulent cervicitis and fever
- **Differential diagnosis**: Appendicitis, ectopic pregnancy, tuboovarian abscess
- **Causative organisms**: *N. gonorrhoeae*, *C. trachomatis*, coliforms and streptococci, anaerobes
- **Management**: Varies from outpatient antibiotics to cover chlamydia and anaerobes (e.g. a tetracycline, and metronidazole) to urgent admission to hospital for laparotomy and drainage. Partner should be investigated and treated accordingly

B28.5 Vaginal candidosis

- Causative agent *Candida albicans* (a yeast). May be part of normal flora of gastrointestinal tract and thus not necessarily a sexually transmitted disease
- Predisposing factors include diabetes mellitus, oral contraceptives, pregnancy, broad-spectrum antibiotics, steroid therapy
- Presents with profuse white vaginal discharge and vaginal itching. Diffuse erythema extending to vulva seen on examination
- Diagnosis by vaginal smear (budding yeasts and pseudomycelium seen) and/or swab of exudate cultured on Sabouraud's medium
- Treatment with topical clotrimazole, miconazole or oral fluconazole or itraconazole
- Attacks may recur. Consider treatment of sexual partner if he is symptomatic

B28.6 Trichomoniasis

- Causative agent *Trichomonas vaginalis*, a protozoan
- Presents with thin yellowish discharge with an offensive smell, +/- irritation, dysuria. Punctate erythema and abundant discharge seen on examination
- Diagnosis by microscopy of vaginal wet preparation. Difficult to culture
- Treatment with metronidazole or tinidazole for both patient and partner

B28.7 Bacterial vaginosis (also known as non-specific vaginitis)

- Causative agents a heterogeneous mix of anaerobes, *Gardnerella vaginalis*, mycoplasmas
- Presents with scanty but offensive-smelling discharge
- Diagnosis: vaginal pH >5 (normal <4.5), positive amine test, vaginal smear shows 'clue' cells – epithelial cells coated with Gram-variable bacteria, and absence of lactobacilli
- Treatment with metronidazole

Summary: Sexually transmitted diseases
Presentation
May be asymptomatic (especially in females); vaginal, cervical or penile discharge; frequency and dysuria; pelvic pain, dyspareunia; genital ulceration
Diagnosis
Urethral and cervical smears, vaginal, urethral, cervical swabs for appropriate culture, vaginal wet prep, serology, urinalysis
Management
Antibiotic therapy where appropriate; contact tracing; education and encouragement of safe sex practices; regular screening of the sexually promiscuous (e.g. prostitutes)

CASE 29
Sharon, a 24-year-old personnel manager with a blistering genital rash

Sharon, a 24-year-old personnel manager, attends the genitourinary medicine (GUM) clinic in great distress. She has developed several painful blisters in and around her vagina over the past 72 hours. She complains that passing urine is excruciatingly painful, and she is also finding it difficult to walk. On examination Sharon is febrile (38°C) and looks generally unwell. Painful inguinal lymphadenopathy is noted bilaterally. The appearance of the external genitalia is shown in Figure 29.1. A mucopurulent cervical discharge is seen on speculum examination, and there are ulcers visible on the cervix.

Q What is the diagnosis?

A Sharon has an extensive blistering rash. Ulcers can be seen where the roofs of the blisters have been eroded. These lesions are typical of herpes simplex virus (HSV) infection. The systemic manifes-tations (fever, malaise), bilateral lymphadenopathy, and widespread distribution of the lesions, including spread on to the adjacent skin of the thigh, are typical of a primary attack (classification of HSV infections is discussed in Case 2).

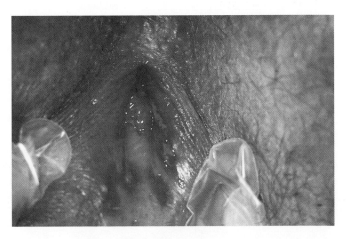

Fig. 29.1 Extensive genital ulceration.

Q How can this diagnosis be confirmed?

A By sending vesicle fluid or a swab of an ulcer base for virus isolation. HSV grows readily in cell culture in 24–48 hours. Electron microscopy of vesicle fluid will demonstrate the presence of herpes virus particles.

Q What complications may arise from an attack of primary genital herpes?

A These are listed below:

• Lesions near to urethra/urethral meatus may lead to acute urinary retention
• Sacral nerve root involvement may also lead to urinary and/or faecal retention
• Spread to meninges, leading to meningitis
• Local extension to cervix (cervicitis), uterus and Fallopian tubes, leading to pelvic inflammatory disease (rare).

Q How should this patient be managed?

A Primary genital herpes is a clear indication for acyclovir therapy – without treatment, this severe debilitating illness may continue for 2–3 weeks. Although oral therapy on an outpatient basis may suffice for many patients, the extent of Sharon's attack warrants admission to hospital.

B29.1 Epidemiology of HSV-2 infection

• Seroepidemiological studies indicate that 15–30% of the adult population has evidence of HSV-2 infection
• Less than 25% of anti-HSV-2-positive individuals give a history of symptomatic genital herpes
• Asymptomatic shedding from anti-HSV-2-positive individuals without a positive history is usually of low titre and transient (e.g. 24 hours only). Recent evidence suggests a transmission rate of 10% per year to uninfected partners

---

Sharon is admitted to hospital and intravenous acyclovir therapy initiated. Within 48 hours her fever subsides, she feels much better, and no new lesions have appeared. However, her husband of 5 years, Jason, wants to know how his wife acquired her infection. Although Sharon steadfastly denies it, Jason believes that she must be having an extramarital affair, as he himself has never had genital herpes. Sharon has previously been questioned about this, and the doctors are convinced she is telling the truth.

Q How, then, might Sharon have acquired the infection?

A There are two possibilities. First, Jason may suffer from cold sores, i.e. recurrent orolabial herpes. These lesions contain high titres of infectious virus, which can be passed to the genital area of a sexual partner either by orogenital sex or by direct inoculation via contaminated fingers. Although orolabial herpes is usually due to infection with HSV-1, and genital herpes due to HSV-2, both viruses can infect at either site, and primary genital infection with HSV-1 is clinically indistinguishable from that due to HSV-2.

Secondly, despite the absence of previous symptoms, Jason may nevertheless have acquired genital herpes, possibly many years ago, with an asymptomatic primary infection. Virus will have spread to his sacral ganglia, where for the most part it will exist in a latent state but may reactivate from time to time. Such recurrent attacks, although subclinical, will give rise to infectious virus on his external genitalia.

Genital HSV infection is an emotionally charged subject, and the emergence of disease in one partner of an apparently monogamous couple, such as described here, inevitably raises suspicions. Jason may not take kindly to being told that he does, after all, have HSV infection, and may also find the sugestion that he has passed this on to his partner after 5 years of monogamy faintly ludicrous. It may be as well to reiterate the salient data on which this conclusion is based (see Box 29.1).

Jason and Sharon accept these explanations, and after 72 hours of intravenous therapy Sharon is discharged with a further 7 days of oral acyclovir. On her return to the clinic 2 weeks later, although physically well she bursts into tears, and after much coaxing explains that she is afraid her life will be blighted by painful recurrent attacks of genital herpes.

Q What are the risks of recurrent disease?

A Having acquired the virus she will indeed carry it for the rest of her life (prompt acyclovir therapy does *not* prevent HSV latency). She may suffer recurrences, but it is impossible to predict their frequency, which may vary from none to one every 3–4 weeks, even in immunocompetent individuals. The basis for this variability in the virus–host relationship is not understood.

Q Are recurrent attacks likely to be as severe as the primary attack?

A No. Recurrences are less severe; systemic manifestations are rare; the number of lesions will be dramatically less; the lesions will be localized (usually unilateral, no spread to adjacent skin, cervical lesions in 5% cases only); the average time to healing is 6–7 days.

Despite reassurances about the milder nature of recurrent disease, Sharon is still worried in case she falls into the category of having very frequent recurrences.

Q Is there any intervention that can improve the lot of such individuals with frequent recurrences?

A Yes, prophylactic acyclovir therapy. Continous low-dose therapy for months at a time dramatically reduces the frequency of attacks. Breakthrough attacks may occur, but are usually mild and infrequent. Unfortunately, attacks return on cessation of therapy, at the same frequency as before. Many patients in the USA have now been on such regimens for a number of years, without ill effects.

Q Is there a potential drawback to such a strategy?

A An initial worry was that continuous therapy would lead to the emergence of acyclovir-resistant mutants. Although such mutants have been described, most are of reduced pathogenic potential and therefore not a clinical problem. The one setting where fully virulent mutants may emerge is in immunosuppressed patients (e.g. those with HIV infection).

Sharon's final anxiety concerns the effect her genital herpes may have should she become pregnant, but she can be reassured on that point (see Case 58).

Q Many patients attending GUM clinics have much less florid disease than Sharon e.g. solitary ulcers. What is the differential diagnosis of solitary genital ulceration?

A The common causes of ulceration confined to the genital area are genital herpes, chemical burns from disinfectants, trauma (including excoriation of marked acute candidal vulvitis), pyogenic infection and fixed drug eruption. Other causes include:

- syphilis (primary chancre, see Case 28)
- chancroid, granuloma inguinale and lymphogranuloma venereum (see Boxes 29.2–29.4) are seen almost exclusively among travellers
- genital ulceration as part of systemic diseases such as Behçet's disease, or erythema multiforme (HSV infection may act as a trigger for the latter)

Any of these conditions may closely mimic one another, although intact vesicles are almost exclusive to HSV infection. Single lesions, which may appear trivial to the patient (e.g. 1 mm in diameter) are often due to genital herpes and should not be ignored.

Q How can it be proved that a solitary ulcer is due to HSV?

A By taking a swab of the ulcer base for virus isolation. If a more rapid diagnosis is required, direct immunofluorescence can be performed by staining cells from the ulcer base with appropriately labelled monoclonal antibodies. Isolation of virus from such a lesion is absolute proof of cause and effect. Another potential benefit of virus isolation is that it is possible to type the virus to determine whether it is HSV-1 or HSV-2, by staining with appropriate monoclonal antibodies.

B29.2 Chancroid

- Causative organism *Haemophilus ducreyi*
- 'Soft chancre' – single or multiple papules on the genitalia, which ulcerate
- Lack of induration distinct from 'hard chancre' of syphilis
- Inguinal adenopathy prominent, may break down to form an abscess or discharging sinus in groin
- Diagnosis – Gram-negative bacilli in smears
- Treatment is with tetracycline

B29.3 Granuloma inguinale

- Causative organism *Donovania granulomatis*
- Papules on genitalia or groins. Subsequently ulcerate and become secondarily infected
- Diagnosis – biopsy appearance of Donovan bodies (intracellular bacilli) in macrophages
- Treatment is with tetracycline

Q Is virus typing clinically useful?

A Most laboratories do not type HSV. However, typing may be useful in tracing routes of spread of infection, e.g. in suspected child sexual abuse, where the child may have acquired genital herpes by direct inoculation of virus from his or her own orolabial source (likely to be type 1) rather than from the genital area of the abuser (likely to be type 2). Typing of virus also has some limited prognostic value: genital type 2 infection is more likely to recur than genital type 1 infection, whereas the reverse is true of orolabial infection.

B29.4 Lymphogranuloma venereum

- Causative organism *Chlamydia trachomatis*, strains L 1–3
- Small genital ulcer, may go unnoticed
- Presentation with painful enlarged inguinal nodes, leading to multiple abscesses which may rupture
- Diagnosis – serology or intradermal skin test with Frei's LGV antigen
- Treatment is with tetracycline

Summary: Genital herpes simplex

Presentation

Primary – extensive painful genital ulceration, inguinal adenopathy, fever. *Recurrence* – asymptomatic; if lesions, then few in number, localized, not indurated; no adenopathy or systemic response

Diagnosis

Clinical; swab in viral transport medium for virus isolation; demonstration of virus in vesicle fluid/ulcer base by electron microscopy, antigen detection

Management

Acyclovir for primary attack and prophylaxis if frequent or severe recurrences; barrier methods of contraception to prevent spread

CASE 30
Jane, 27, requests an AIDS test

Jane, a 27-year-old accountant previously fit and well, arrives at the surgery in a state of great agitation. Immediately after sitting down she asks for an 'AIDS test'. It quickly becomes clear that Jane is worried that she may be infected with the human immunodeficiency virus (HIV). Before ordering an appropriate diagnostic test it must be ascertained whether Jane has any risk factors for acquisition of HIV infection.

Q What are the routes of transmission of HIV?

A There are three possible means of HIV spread:

- Sexual
- Vertical (i.e. mother to baby)
- Exposure to infected blood or blood products, e.g. transfusion of blood, administration of factor VIII, sharing of needles between injecting drug users, and needlestick injuries.

There is no evidence to suggest that HIV can be transmitted via droplet spread or by insects.

It transpires that Jane has just returned from a holiday abroad with friends. During this trip she had unprotected sexual intercourse with a casual acquaintance, whom she has just learnt is an injecting drug user. Intercourse took place on one occasion only, this being 5 days ago. On direct questioning Jane denies any other risk factors for HIV infection. Apart from her understandable anxiety, she has no other symptoms and examination reveals no abnormalities.

Q What is the basis of the standard laboratory test for HIV infection?

A Laboratory diagnosis of HIV infection is made by demonstrating the presence of antibodies to the virus in patients' sera, not by detection of the virus or viral antigens. Note that there is no such thing as an 'AIDS test'.

Q Jane is obviously distraught. Are you able to confirm whether or not she has contracted HIV infection?

A Unfortunately, the answer is no. There is a time lag (known as the 'window period') between infection with HIV and the production of antibodies. This varies, but the vast majority of HIV-infected patients will be antibody positive by 3 months after infection. A test on Jane's serum now would be negative, but you could not exclude the possibility of HIV infection until a sample taken 3 months after exposure is also shown to be negative.

This dilemma is explained to Jane, and she is asked to return in 3 months' time for an anti-HIV test. In fact she returns 2 weeks later, complaining of a sore throat and non-specific malaise. On examination there is a fine macular rash on her trunk and moderate cervical and axillary lymphadenopathy.

Q What is the differential diagnosis, and what investigations should be ordered?

A Jane now has a glandular fever-like illness. Although the commonest cause of this syndrome is acute Epstein–Barr virus infection (see Case 9) there is also the possibility that this may be due to acute HIV infection. This syndrome, referred to as 'HIV seroconverting illness', occurs 1–6 weeks after exposure to HIV in 40–70% of patients.

A full blood count and film would be useful, as well as diagnostic tests for EBV infection. However, a negative anti-HIV test at this stage would again not rule out this diagnosis, as HIV seroconverting illness can occur before the presence of detectable antibodies.

All specimens sent to the laboratory should be clearly indicated as 'high risk'. If Jane is suffering from acute HIV infection her blood will be infectious, and it is important that laboratory staff are aware of this.

Q What is the risk of transmission of infection via a needlestick incident involving blood from a known anti-HIV-positive patient?

A The transmission rate after inoculation of known infected blood via percutaneous injury is 0.3%. Transmission following splashing of HIV-infected material on to mucous membranes has been described, but the risk is likely to be considerably less than that for percutaneous injury. There are no reports of HIV infection following splashing on to intact skin.

A full blood count from Jane reveals a moderate lymphocytosis, with atypical mononuclear cells seen. The monospot is negative. At Jane's insistence an anti-HIV test is requested, the result of which is negative. Jane makes an uneventful recovery from her illness, and returns 4 weeks later for a repeat anti-HIV test. The result of this test is positive.

Q Is there anything further to be done before accepting the diagnosis of HIV infection?

A Yes: because of the seriousness of the diagnosis a repeat anti-HIV test should be ordered. Even though the patient has a defined risk exposure, and her illness 4 weeks previously is entirely consistent with an acute HIV infection, the diagnosis should *always* be confirmed by sending a repeat serum sample for testing. In any laboratory there is the possibility of error (e.g. mislabelling of tubes, inserting the wrong sample in the test, assigning a result to the wrong patient), and there are well-documented instances where such errors have led to the erroneous labelling of a patient as being anti-HIV positive.

Q What is the risk of acquisition of HIV infection through unprotected intercourse with a known HIV-positive partner?

A It is difficult to quote a precise risk, although it is considerably less than for some other sexually transmitted diseases (e.g. gonorrhoea, syphilis). Factors which affect the likelihood of transmission include the stage of HIV infection in the donor (progression of HIV infection to AIDS is associated with higher titres of virus in peripheral blood and genital secretions), and the presence of genital ulceration in either partner. Although it will be no comfort to her, Jane may consider herself very unlucky to have aquired infection after a single sexual exposure.

After much anguish, Jane eventually comes to terms with her diagnosis and is able to resume her normal life.

Q What is Jane's prognosis?

A HIV infection is a necessary, but not sufficient, cause of the acquired immunodeficiency syndrome (AIDS). HIV-infected individuals may exhibit a range of clinical consequences, from asymptomatic infection through to the severe debilitating immunodeficiency state known as AIDS. The mean incubation period between

Table 30.1 CDC classification of HIV infection

Group I Acute infection
Group II Asymptomatic infection
Group III Persistent generalized lymphadenopathy
Group IV (AIDS) Other diseases
  Subgroup A Constitutional disease
  Subgroup B Neurological disease
  Subgroup C Secondary infectious diseases
    Category C-1 Specified secondary infectious diseases listed in the CDC surveillance definition for AIDS (Explained in Case 48, see Appendix 4)
    Category C-2 Other specified secondary infectious diseases
  Subgroup D Secondary malignancies
  Subgroup E Other conditions

infection with HIV and the development of AIDS is 8–10 years, but this estimate has been revised upwards as the HIV epidemic has progressed. In recognition of the different stages of HIV infection, and in order to facilitate comparison of patient groups in different studies, the Centres for Disease Control in Atlanta, USA, have devised a classification system for HIV infection (Table 30.1). Jane has progressed through group I, and is now within group II. There is no evidence to suggest that the prognosis of those patients (like Jane) who suffer an acute HIV illness is any different from those who do not.

Q How should the progression of Jane's HIV infection be monitored?

A At present, cofactors which enhance the progression of HIV infection through to AIDS have not been unequivocally identified, and there is therefore no way of predicting how quickly an individual patient will progress. There are, however, ways of monitoring the progression of disease by measuring a number of so-called 'surrogate markers', such as the absolute number of circulating CD4-positive lymphocytes, the target cells of HIV infection. Declining numbers of CD4 cells is a poor prognostic indicator. Many management decisions are made on the basis of the CD4 count, e.g. when to start prophylaxis against opportunistic infection, particularly *Pneumocystis carinii* (see Case 48). Another surrogate marker is the p24 antigen. This is a component of HIV which appears in peripheral blood late in the course of infection. Its presence is therefore a poor prognostic indicator.

Q To which family of viruses does HIV belong?

A The retroviruses.

Q Why are retroviruses so called?

A Retroviruses have an RNA genome, but can convert this into a DNA copy by virtue of the virally

encoded enzyme reverse transcriptase. One of the central tenets of molecular biology is that genetic information flows unidirectionally from DNA to RNA to protein. Thus, the apparent 'backward' step of making RNA into DNA led to the adoption of the term 'retroviruses' to describe this family of viruses. Eukaryotic cells do not have a reverse transcriptase, and thus this enzyme is an ideal target for antiretroviral drugs.

Q Should Jane be offered any antiretroviral therapy?

A Currently the only effective antiviral agents in widespread use are reverse transcriptase inhibitors, of which azidothymidine (AZT) is the best known. There is considerable controversy surrounding the optimal use of this drug. Early trials demonstrated that AZT treatment of patients with AIDS resulted in improved survival. However, although AZT therapy in the earlier stages of HIV infection may delay the onset of AIDS, this benefit is short-lived and survival is not prolonged. This paradoxical finding may be related to the earlier emergence of AZT-resistant mutants in these patients, rendering the drug ineffective.

Jane asks about the possibility of passing her infection to her children, should she have any.

Q What information can you give her about the risk of vertical transmission?

A The risk varies according to the status of the mother. Overall, transmission occurs in approximately 15% of pregnancies in HIV-positive women, but risk factors which enhance this are maternal p24 antigenaemia and a CD4 count of less than 700/μl. Transmission can be transplacental (*in utero*) or occur perinatally or postnatally (via breast milk). Caesarian section may reduce the risk of vertical transmission, as may maternal AZT therapy during pregnancy. In countries where there

CASE 30

is an adequate alternative, HIV-infected mothers are advised not to breastfeed.

Q What problems are there in diagnosing HIV infection in the offspring of carrier mothers?

A Diagnosis of HIV infection in a neonate is complicated by the passage of maternal antibodies across the placenta. Thus the presence of anti-HIV at or near birth in the neonate is not evidence of infection. Serological diagnosis of infection can only be made routinely by demonstrating the persistence of anti-HIV antibodies after 18 months of age. Alternative means of diagnosis include HIV culture from, or detection of viral genome in, neonatal blood, but these techniques are only available in research laboratories. Much interest is now focused on the use of indirect diagnostic indicators such as hyper-gammaglobulinaemia or β_2-microglobulin levels as predictors of neonatal infection.

The diagnosis and management of AIDS are discussed in detail in Case 48.

Summary: HIV infection
Routes of infection
Vertical (mother-to-baby); sexual; blood and blood products
Diagnosis
Detection of anti-HIV; may take 3 months to appear after contact
Stages of infection
CDC classification recognizes acute infection (glandular fever-like illness); asymptomatic carriage; progressive generalized lymphadenopathy (PGL); acquired immunodeficiency syndrome (AIDS)

CASE 31
Suprapubic pain and haematuria in Gavin, a 35-year-old sales executive

Gavin, a 35-year-old sales director, presents to his GP with suprapubic pain when passing urine, which contains blood. He has no past history of these symptoms or of urethral discharge and has no relevant previous medical history. Gavin is on no medications and his wife, Hannah, and his four children, are well.

Q What is this condition and what may cause it?

A Gavin has haematuria (frank blood *per urethram*) and, with the presence of pain, probably has haemorrhagic cystitis, which is usually characterized by obvious blood on micturition. The possible causes of this are:

- bladder carcinoma – diagnosed on cystoscopy and histology
- cyclophosphamide – a chemotherapeutic agent which results in severe ulceration and may lead to bladder contraction
- irradiation – following treatment for bladder carcinoma
- cystitis – uncommon in uncomplicated cases but may occur as part of 'honeymoon cystitis' in females following sexual intercourse (see Case 26)
- Reiter's disease – abnormal host response to a number of infecting agents, such as chlamydia (see Case 28), salmonella, shigella, yersinia (see Case 64) etc. Characterized by urethritis, arthritis, uveitis and, occasionally, skin lesions. Hyperacute cystitis with haematuria is occasionally part of the presenting illness

CASE 31

- schistosomiasis – a helminth infection (see Case 25) due to a trematode (fluke) seen in travellers to the developing world, and seen endemically there also
- adenoviruses and polyomaviruses – occasionally (see Case 39 for adenovirus infections).

It transpires that Gavin had been to Egypt as part of an export sales drive for his company some weeks ago. During the visit he had taken a pleasure trip down the Nile and had bathed in the river. Culture of his urine is negative for bacterial pathogens.

Q What is a possible diagnosis given the history, and how might it be confirmed?

A Schistosomiasis due to *Schistosoma haematobium* is very possible in the light of recent travel to Egypt and the history of bathing. Peripheral blood eosinophilia may also point to a parasitic cause. A diagnosis may be confirmed by microscopic examination of concentrated or filtered urine for ova. Alternative approaches include bladder biopsy to demonstrate granulomata, examination of faeces for ova and parasites, or a rectal biopsy when gastrointestinal symptoms are prominent, and finally, serology, which is only available through reference laboratories.

Microscopy shows over 100 pus cells/mm³ and ova of *Schistosoma haematobium* (see Figure 31.1) with the characteristic terminal spine. Gavin is prescribed one dose of praziquantal (an effective antischistosomal agent), his symptoms resolve and a follow-up urine sample is clear.

Q How is schistosomiasis acquired?

A There are a number of species responsible for a variety of clinical syndromes (see Box 31.1). Humans are the principal host, with the snail as the intermediate host. Eggs are

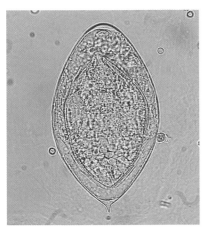

Fig. 31.1 Ovum of *S. haematobium* in urine.

excreted in the urine or faeces, hatch in fresh water and are taken up by the snail, in which cercariae (fork-tails) develop. These are subsequently released into the fresh water habitat from which people become infected via the skin.

Q What complications may ensue from untreated or undiagnosed urinary schistosomiasis?

A These arise mainly in the indigenous population, where facilities for diagnosis and treatment may be inadequate. Complications include:

- secondary bacterial infection and renal stones
- bladder granulomata and papillomata
- ureteric blockage with hydronephrosis
- bladder carcinoma.

Q How may schistosomiasis be prevented?

A Irrigation and water conservation schemes in developing countries make control increasingly difficult, as snails are disseminated. Measures to control the snail population will reduce the risk of infection. Other measures include:

- introduction of modern sewage disposal facilities
- measures to encourage people not to urinate in fresh water (difficult in the developing world)
- avoidance of bathing or walking barefoot in fresh water by visitors to endemic areas
- research on immune response, leading to the development of a vaccine.

Summary: Schistosomiasis
Presentation
Haematuria or diarrhoea and dysentery in the returned traveller
Diagnosis
Clinical suspicion and examination of urine, faeces or biopsy material for ova
Treatment
One dose of praziquantal. Surgery occasionally required for complications

B31.1 Species, geographical distribution and clinical syndromes caused by schistosomia
<ul><li>*S. haematobium* (Egypt, Middle East, Africa)</li><li>*S. mansoni* (Middle East, Africa, Latin America, West Indies)</li><li>*S. japonicum* (Far East)</li><li>Also *S. intercalatum, S. mekongi*</li></ul>
<ul><li>Purpuric papular skin rash – 'swimmers itch' (*S. mansoni, S. haematobium*)</li><li>Cystitis (*S. haematobium*)</li><li>Katayama fever, a serum sickness-like syndrome with fever, eosinophilia, lymphadenopathy and splenomegaly</li><li>Cor pulmonale, infiltration of lungs leading to obstruction of blood flow (*S. japonicum*)</li><li>Liver fibrosis, liver failure due to vascular obstruction</li><li>Chronic schistosomiasis, diarrhoea, dysentery, immune-mediated disease</li></ul>

CASE 32
Mark, a 42-year-old solicitor, has a lump on his penis

Mark, a 42-year-old solicitor, comes to the genitourinary medicine clinic complaining of a small painless lump on his penis. He is concerned that he might have developed genital herpes. He is unmarried, having split from his long-term girlfriend a year ago. He has had four casual sexual partners since then. He has no urethral discharge, no dysuria, and there are no other symptoms related to the genitourinary tract. His past medical history is unremarkable, although he does suffer from occasional cold sores. He is on no regular medication. Examination is normal apart from the physical sign shown in Figure 32.1. There is no inguinal adenopathy.

Q What is the diagnosis?

A The appearance is that of a wart. The absence of vesicles or ulcers clearly distinguishes this from genital HSV infection.

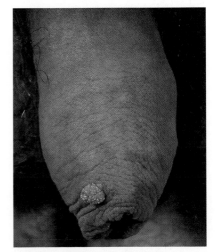

Fig. 32.1 Mark's penis.

Q Name the infectious agent responsible.

A Human papillomavirus (HPV), sometimes referred to as wart virus.

Q How are papillomaviruses classified?

A Papillomaviruses contain a double-stranded DNA genome and belong to the Papovavirus family. The term papova is derived from papilloma–polyoma–vacuolar, which indicates that this family contains three distinct genera of viruses. They are classified into types, of which there are over 60 that infect humans, on the basis of the degree of DNA sequence homology of the viral genome.

Q At what anatomical sites may HPV infection occur?

A HPVs infect and replicate in squamous epithelium on both keratinized and mucosal surfaces. Infections are extremely common. Clinical presentation may be:

1. Cutaneous:
   * usually the hands (verruca vulgaris) and feet (verruca plantaris, or plantar wart), but may occur elsewhere, e.g. the face
   * most frequent in childhood and early adolescence
   * due to types 1–4
2. Mucosal:
   * single papillomas may occur in the mouth, at any age, and rarely recur after surgical excision
   * multiple papillomas associated with HPV types 6 and 11 are the commonest benign epithelial tumours of the larynx, are more frequent in children than adults, and frequently recur after surgical excision
3. Anogenital:
   * an increasingly common sexually transmitted disease
   * benign warts (condylomata acuminata) may occur on the penis, vulva, urethra, cervix and perianal areas, due to types HPV 6 or 11
   * malignant transformation in the cervix associated with HPV types 16 and 18 (and others).

Q How should Mark be treated?

A Warts may regress spontaneously, although this is unpredictable and may take many months. Treatment of genital warts is in general unsatisfactory. Many lesions will recur, and this should be clearly explained to Mark before treatment is undertaken. The treatment options available for removal of small numbers of lesions are:

* podophyllin or podophyllotoxin: must be applied carefully as normal skin may be severely burned; should be washed off after 4 hours
* cryotherapy, e.g. with a slurry of cardice (solid CO_2) and acetone. May be painful!
* interferon therapy: injected either intramuscularly or intralesionally; still under evaluation
* surgery: persistent or extensive warts, or urethral warts or warts extending to the anal canal, may be surgically excised.

After appropriate discussion Mark agrees to cryotherapy of his wart. He returns to the clinic 2 weeks later and there are now no visible lesions. However, he has brought his current girlfriend with him, who is anxious that she may be at risk of cervical cancer.

Q What is the evidence linking cervical HPV infection with cancer of the cervix?

A There are a number of lines of evidence suggesting that infection with certain HPV types (e.g. 16, 18) is an important cofactor for the development of cervical malignancy:

* The epidemiology of carcinoma of the cervix strongly resembles that of a sexually transmitted disease
* Papillomaviruses are known to be oncogenic in animals
* A rare autosomal disease, epidermodysplasia verruciformis, is associated with multiple skin warts and the development of squamous-cell carcinoma, the malignant cells of which contain HPV (usually type 5)
* 80–90% of cervical carcinomas contain HPV 16 or 18 DNA. In most cases this DNA is integrated into the host chromosomes.

Q How may HPV infection of the cervix be diagnosed?

A Evaluation of women with HPV lesions of the cervix is largely dependent on the detection of cytologic abnormalities in cervical smears, and on colposcopic examination and biopsy of suspicious lesions. Some authorities have suggested that screening women for the presence of HPV 16 DNA using the polymerase chain reaction is more sensitive in detecting premalignant and malignant lesions of the cervix than is cytology. However, at present this is a controversial subject, and women with genital warts, and female partners of males with genital warts, should be advised to have regular cervical smears.

Summary: Genital warts
Presentation
Painless warts in genital area
Diagnosis
Clinical; HPV type can be determined by biopsy and genome analysis
Complications
HPV 16 and 18 are associated with cervical carcinoma
Treatment
None; topical podophyllin; cryotherapy; interferon; surgery

CASE 33
Howard, a 10-year-old boy with scaly skin lesions

Howard, a 10-year-old boy, is referred to the dermatology outpatients because of skin lesions on his arm which have been present for 3–4 months. He has never previously been seriously ill, is on no medications and there is no family history of eczema or any other skin disorder. On examination he is seen to be a fit and active child, and the lesions are scaly, with raised margins (see Figure 33.1).

Q What is the diagnosis?

A These lesions are typical of tinea or dermatophytosis, which is most commonly seen during childhood. They are caused by filamentous fungi which invade the stratum corneum. Three genera are responsible: *Trichophyton*, *Microsporum* and *Epidermophyton* (contains only one species, *E. floccosum*). Tinea is infectious.

Q What other questions might Howard or his parents be asked?

A Howard should be asked whether his brothers, sisters or playmates have similar marks on the skin and whether there is a cat or dog at home, as some of the fungi are acquired from animals or on a farm.

A history of a similar condition in other members of the family may reflect common exposure or increased genetic susceptibility, which may be mediated by differences in T-lymphocyte response.

Q Where else on the body might you look for tinea infections?

A Tinea infections may be found all over the body and are traditionally classified according to the anatomical location. Examples include:

- tinea pedis (feet): infects the interdigital spaces (also known as 'athlete's foot'), which may result in itching leading to blisters and secondary bacterial infections. Most commonly caused by

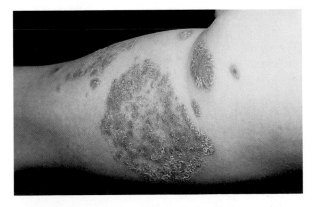

Fig. 33.1 Scaly lesion on Howard's arm.

B33.1 Classification of dermatophyte infections according to source		
Zoophilic	Acquired from animals such as cats, dogs, rodents, cattle	*M. canis*, *T. mentagrophytes* (rats), *T. verrucosum* (cattle)
Geophilic	Acquired from soil: more important in the tropics	*M. gypseum*
Anthrophilic	Acquired from siblings, playmates, school friends via desquamated skin scales etc.	*T. rubrum* (commonest), *E. floccosum*

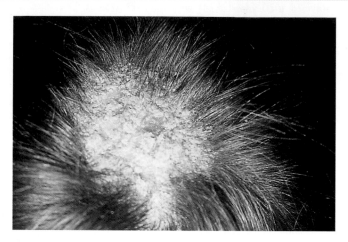

Fig. 33.2 Tinea capitis due to _M. audouinii_.

T. rubrum, _T. mentagrophytes_ (_interdigitale_)

- tinea cruris (groin): may present in genitourinary medicine clinics
- tinea corporis (body): classically referred to as 'ringworm', and may affect the arms, trunk and legs. Most commonly caused by _T. rubrum_
- tinae capitis (head): infection of the scalp and hair. Characterized by scaling of the scalp, severe dandruff and broken hairs. Rare in adults (see Figure 33.2)
- onychomycosis: infection of the nailbeds, resulting in unsightly fingers and toes.

Q How may a diagnosis of tinea be confirmed?

A The classic appearance of the scaly lesions is diagnostic of 'ringworm' and frequently investigations are not conducted or warranted. Investigations will confirm the diagnosis and may indicate a possible source, such as a domestic animal (see Box 33.1). Investigations include:

- ultraviolet light illumination of scalp (Wood's light): _Microsporum_ infections fluoresce green. Not applicable, however, for other genera or other body sites
- microscopy: fungal elements may be seen following digestion of skin scales, nail clippings or hairs in 10–20% potassium hydroxide. _Swabs are unsuitable_. Skin scales

should be obtained from the _edge_ and not the centre of the lesion

- culture: scales, hair or nail clippings may be cultured for fungi on Sabouraud agar containing antibiotics and cycloheximide to suppress other flora. This may take up to 3 weeks, however.

A clinical diagnosis of tinea corporis was made, which was confirmed by the presence of fungal elements on microscopy and the isolation from skin scales of _T. rubrum_. Howard was prescribed a topical antifungal agent and when he was seen again at the outpatients 1 month later the lesions were almost gone.

Q What options are there for the treatment of tinea infections?

A There are a limited number of drugs available (see Table 33.1). The mainstay of treatment is still a

topical azole preparation, or griseofulvin taken orally. Skin infections require 2–4 weeks whereas those affecting nails and hair may require 3–9 months of therapy.

Q What other non-bacterial infections or infestations of the skin may present with a rash or itching?

A These include:

- superficial candida: may affect skin, nail or feet
- pityriasis versicolor: caused by the yeast _Malassezia furfur_ and is characterized by hypo- or hyper-pigmented macules, which are not usually itchy. Very difficult to grow _in vitro_ and diagnosis is made clinically and with microscopy
- scabies: caused by the insect _Sarcoptes scabiei_ and is found worldwide, especially in immigrants and the homeless. Affects the clefts between the fingers, the hands, forearms and genital area. Pruritus is characteristic. Scabies is quite infectious and may be acquired by close contact, such as during sexual intercourse, by a family member or even by a health-care worker during the care of an infested patient. Treatment with agents such as permethrin must be applied to the whole body and not just the affected area, bedclothes and clothing should be changed and washed, and all members of the household plus close contacts also treated

Table 33.1 Commonly used agents to treat dermatophyte infections	
Whitfield's ointment	Consists of salicylic and benzoic acid. Inexpensive but very messy. Has largely been replaced by azoles
Azoles	Include clotrimazole (topical), miconazole (topical), ketoconazole (oral, a major advance in the treatment of nail infections) and, more recently, itraconazole
Griseofulvin	Administered orally and preferentially deposited in newly formed keratin, therefore ideal for nail and hair infections
Terbinafine	Allylamine agent administered orally. Still relatively new but appears to be as effective as griseofulvin over a shorter period

- lice: different types may infest the head, body or pubic area (also known as crab louse). Common among vagrants and children
- viruses: a variety of viral illness may manifest with a skin rash or itchy lesions. These include herpes simplex (see Cases 2, 29 and 58), enteroviruses (see Case 35), measles (see Case 37), rubella (see Case 55) and parvovirus (see Case 62).

Summary: Tinea
Presentation
Scaling skin infections with a less inflamed centre. May also infect nails and hair. Contagious and may be acquired from domestic or farm animals
Diagnosis
Clinical presentation often diagnostic. Skin scales, nail scrapings or hairs should be sent to the laboratory for microscopy and culture. Dermatophytes rarely ever isolated from swabs
Treatment
A topical azole for 2–4 weeks (skin infection) and oral griseofulvin or terbinafine for 3–9 months (nail or hair infections)

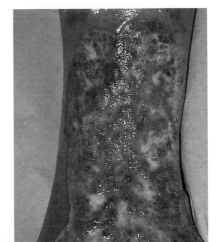

Fig. 34.1 Leg ulcer with surrounding discoloration of skin.

CASE 34
Hannah, a 67-year-old widow with a leg ulcer

Hannah, a 67-year-old overweight widow, comes to the surgery because of a leg ulcer (see Figure 34.1). Two weeks ago a swab was taken from the ulcer for culture and oral amoxycillin prescribed for 10 days. The result of the swab is as follows:

- **Heavy growth of *Escherichia coli* isolated**
- **Moderate growth of *Proteus mirabilis* isolated**
- **Moderate growth of *Enterococcus faecalis* isolated**
- **Scanty growth of *Bacteroides* spp. isolated after 48 hours.**

Hannah tells you that the ulcer has been increasing in size but there is little or no pain.

On examination she is mildly hypertensive and has bilateral varicose veins. Examination of the leg reveals an ulcer with discoloration of the surrounding skin and some oedema. Arterial pulses are strong and there is no tenderness, pus, erythema, cellulitis or lymphangitis.

Q What kind of ulcer does Hannah have?

A The position of the ulcer, the presence of strong arterial pulses, the induration, oedema and trophic changes as manifest by discoloration of the surrounding skin caused by haemosiderin deposition, the presence of varicose veins and the absence of pain are all highly suggestive of a venous ulcer caused by inadequate superficial and deep venous drainage of the lower limb. Approximately 20% of elderly adults develop varicose or venous ulcers, but they are five times more common in females.

Q Is it surprising that the laboratory has not included the result of a Gram stain in the report?

A Most bacteriology laboratories do not routinely carry out Gram films on superficial swabs because the large number of mixed bacteria on the skin, especially in the ulcer base, often obscures the presence of pathogens which may be detected following culture.

Q Which of the bacteria from the swab are likely to be clinically significant?

A It is highly unlikely that any of the bacteria are of pathogenic significance. Microbes recovered from the skin may be subdivided into two populations:

- Normal resident flora, present on intact skin or in hair follicles. These include staphylococci (occasionally *Staphylococcus aureus*), micrococci, diphtheroids and propionibacteria
- Transient flora, removed by washing with soap or disinfectants such as chlorhexidine and originating from the general environment, contact with other individuals or other parts of the body (e.g. the anus). Such flora are limited by the dryness of the

normal skin and the secretion of inhibitory fatty acids, but often flourish in moist conditions or where there is a break in skin integrity. Transient flora include *S. aureus*, streptococci, enterococci (see Box 34.1), coliforms such as *E. coli* and *Proteus* (see Box 34.2) spp., *Pseudomonas aeruginosa* and even *Candida* spp.

Q Should sensitivities to antibiotics have been included in the report?

A No. The reporting of antibiotic sensitivities would be misleading, as these organisms are unlikely to be pathogens here. Indeed, it would have been helpful if the report had included a comment to this effect!

B34.1 Enterococci (faecal streptococci)

- May be haemolytic or non-haemolytic and some belong to Lancefield group D. Include *Enterococcus faecalis*, *E. faecium*
- Part of the normal upper respiratory and gastrointestinal flora. Cause urinary infection (see Case 26), bacteraemia and endocarditis (see Case 44), and intraabdominal infection (see Case 20). Increasingly important as hospital pathogens
- Unlike other streptococci, resistant to most penicillins (except ampicillin, usually) and the cephalosporins

---

B34.2 *Proteus* spp.

- Oxidase-negative Gram-negative bacilli, e.g. *Proteus mirabilis*, *P. vulgaris*
  Grow well on most laboratory media but have a tendency to swarm.
  Urease production is characteristic
- Part of the normal gastrointestinal flora but may cause urinary infection (see Case 26) and bacteraemia (see Case 44). Commonly colonize moist or broken skin, e.g. ulcers, otitis externa (see Case 7)
- Most isolates are sensitive to the penicillins and cephalosporins

---

Q Is this an infected ulcer?

A The absence of pain, erythema, pus, cellulitis or systemic symptoms such as fever suggest that this is not an infected ulcer and that the bacteria isolated from the swab are colonizing the area of broken skin.

Q How may infected leg ulcers be classified?

A Most are secondarily infected rather than primary (where infection causes the ulcer):

1. Primary:
   - Ecthyma gangrenosum, caused by *Pseudomonas aeruginosa*, usually in the immunosuppressed patient, and may be accompanied by bacteraemia
   - Syphilis, with a hard chancre usually on the external genitalia (see Case 28)
   - Tuberculosis, often in the form of lupus vulgaris, or associated with BCG administered subcutaneously to immunosuppressed patients
   - Anthrax, caused by infection with *Bacillus anthracis* due to contact with infected animals, hides or other animal products. Generally occurs in farmers, vets, tanning workers etc. Presents as a pimple leading to a pustule surrounded by inflammation (malignant pustule), with the centre becoming necrotic
   - Parasitic, e.g. cutaneous leishmaniasis (see Case 52)
   - Anaerobic, e.g. *Bacteroides* spp. causing perianal ulcers with undermining of the edge and necrosis.

2. Secondary:
   Associated with pressure sores, varicose veins or arterial disease (e.g. peripheral vascular disease) and diabetes mellitus. Commonly colonized by Gram-negative bacilli (coliforms, *Pseudomonas*) but infections are usually caused by Gram-positive cocci (*S. aureus*, streptococci) and anaerobes.

Q What investigations should routinely be carried out in patients with leg ulcers?

A When the ulcer is secondary to venous or arterial disease, with little or no evidence of local or systemic infection, no laboratory investigations are required. If there is erythema or cellulitis a swab should be taken to diagnose staphylococcal or streptococcal infection, and if the patient is systemically unwell they should be admitted to hospital to exclude accompanying bacteraemia.

Where the ulcer is thought to be primary, dark-ground microscopy or serology (to exclude syphilis) and Ziehl–Neelsen stain and culture (to exclude tuberculosis, see Case 49) may be necessary, but these should be arranged in advance with a microbiology laboratory or advice sought from other specialist services, e.g. the genitourinary medicine department. A biopsy of the ulcer for histology as well as microscopy and culture, should also be considered to diagnose some of the above conditions and to rule out malignancy.

Hannah's antibiotic is discontinued and she is advised about diet to lose weight, which is felt to be exacerbating the problem. She is also encouraged to exercise the leg, such as by ankle flexing to improve venous function. Following hydrocolloid dressings and compression bandages organized at the surgery, and with the assistance of the community nurse, her leg ulcer improves over the next 4 weeks. Her blood pressure returns to normal when she loses weight over the next 2 months.

Q Was oral amoxycillin the most appropriate antibiotic?

A No. As discussed earlier, an antibiotic was not indicated unless the ulcer looked infected, but in any case amoxicillin is not the agent of choice here.

Q Why is amoxicillin inappropriate here?

A Amoxycillin is active against aerobic and anaerobic streptococci, but most strains of *S. aureus* produce β-lactamase and hence will be resistant to penicillin and ampicillin (equivalent in its antibacterial activity to amoxycillin). Flucloxacillin alone, or in combination with amoxycillin, would be more appropriate pending the results of sensitivity testing. Alternatively, co-amoxiclav, which will cover both pathogens and is active against β-lactamase-producing isolates of *Bacteroides fragilis*, would also be appropriate.

Summary: Leg ulcers
Presentation
Breaks in the skin associated with venous or arterial disease in most cases
Diagnosis
Clinical. Microbiological investigations usually not necessary unless the ulcer looks infected (i.e. presence of swelling, erythema, tenderness etc.) or a less common aetiology suspected
Management
Correction of the underlying disease, e.g. varicose veins, weight loss or surgery with dressings/bandages and occasionally antibiotics

---

CASE 35
Victoria, 4 years old, with painful mouth ulcers

For the past 2 days 4-year-old Victoria has complained of a painful mouth and sore throat, and has been unable to eat properly. Her past medical history is unremarkable and she has received the standard childhood vaccinations (DPT, polio, HiB and MMR). Two weeks ago she started attending a playgroup, and her mother reports that a number of children at the playgroup have suffered a similar illness. On examination she has a fever of 38.5°C, and a number of vesicles and ulcers can be seen on the palate, tonsils and tongue.

Q What is the differential diagnosis?

A The three commonest causes of painful oral ulceration in a young child are primary orolabial herpes, herpangina, and hand, foot and mouth disease. The first of these is illustrated in Figure 35.1 and the characteristic features are given in Box 35.1.

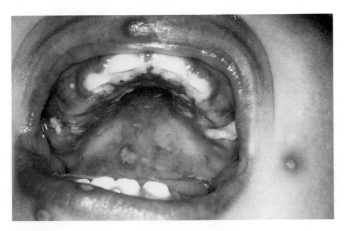

B35.1 Orolabial herpes

Causative agent – Herpes simplex virus (HSV) type 1 or 2
Age – Primary infection is usually in children, but can be seen in older individuals
Clinical features – Primary disease:

- extensive gingivostomatitis
- spread to adjacent skin (see Figure 35.1)
- systemic upset, with fever and cervical adenopathy
- 2–3 weeks before cessation of new lesion formation

Secondary disease (i.e. recurrent cold sores):
- due to reactivation of latent virus in trigeminal ganglion
- much milder disease, e.g. few lesions, unilateral
- no systemic reaction
- resolution in 5–7 days

Complications

- Self-inoculation of virus to other sites, e.g. eyes, genitals
- Secondary bacterial infection, e.g. staphylococci, streptococci
- Patients with eczema – *eczema herpeticum* – extensive contiguous spread of infection. Can arise from primary and/or secondary infection. Access to bloodstream through damaged skin may lead to infection of internal organs, e.g. hepatitis, pneumonitis
- Immunodeficient patients – viraemic spread may occur, with internal organ involvement. Suffer more frequent and extensive recurrences.

Treatment – Acyclovir (see Appendix 3).
Indications for use are:

- Primary disease – will reduce time to cessation of new lesion formation, and time to healing to 7–10 days
- Reactivations – in patients at risk of eczema herpeticum
               – in immuno-deficient patients

(Note: not usually worthwhile for recurrences in other patients, as clinical benefit is marginal)

Fig. 35.1 Orolabial herpes simplex.

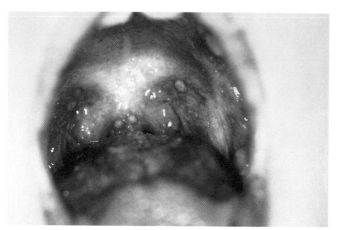
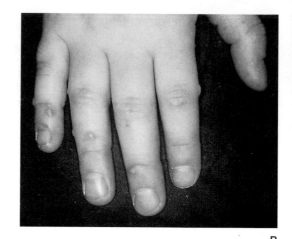

Fig. 35.2 (A) Mouth lesions; **(B)** Hand lesions.   **A**   **B**

More careful examination of Victoria shows that she has a few vesicles on her fingers (Fig. 35.2) and on her feet.

Q What is the causative agent of her illness?

A The diagnosis is now one of hand, foot and mouth disease. It is not uncommon for outbreaks of this to occur in child-care settings. This is a manifestation of infection with a Coxsackie virus, usually a Coxsackie A strain.

Q To which genus of viruses do the Coxsackie viruses belong, and what are the other members of this genus?

A The enteroviruses (see Box 35.2). There are a large number of enteroviruses that infect humans, and the somewhat *ad-hoc* nomenclature makes then rather confusing. Coxsackie is the name of a town in the USA where an outbreak of polio-like paralytic disease was caused by a hitherto unidentified virus, hence the origin of the name Coxsackie viruses. Echo stands for Entero Cytopathic Human Orphan, and arises from the isolation of viruses from faeces which produced a cytopathic effect in tissue culture, but which were not initially associated with disease. More recently discovered entero-viruses are now simply given the prefix EV and a number. The value of remembering that all these viruses are enteroviruses lies in the fact that this gives an indication of their mode of spread: they enter through the mouth and are excreted in the faeces. Hence viral culture of a throat swab and faeces are appropriate for the investigation of possible enteroviral infection.

Q What other diseases are associated with infection with enteroviruses?

A These viruses give rise to a wide range of clinical syndromes, outlined in Table 35.1. Entero-viruses are an important cause of morbidity and mortality, and appear in the differential diagnosis of a number of the case histories presented in this text. They have not, however, been proven to cause disease of the gastrointestinal tract.

In addition, there are a number of important diseases where enteroviral infection has been suggested to play an aetiological role, including polymyositis and dermatomyositis, the chronic fatigue syndrome, dilated cardiomyopathy and diabetes mellitus. However, the links between enterovirus infection and these diseases have not yet been conclusively proven.

There is no specific antiviral therapy available at present for treating enteroviral infections.

Q How may enteroviral infections be prevented?

A Polio virus vaccines (see Box 35.3) are effective in preventing infection with the three types of

---

B35.2 The enteroviruses

- Polioviruses (types 1, 2, and 3)
- Coxsackie A viruses (23 types)
- Coxsackie B viruses (types B1–B6)
- Echoviruses (31 types)
- Enteroviruses types 68–71

B35.3 Polio virus vaccines

- Component of routine childhood vaccination schedule
- Two types:
1. Live attenuated (Sabin)

    - Given orally, therefore provides mucosal immunity
    - May revert to virulence, resulting in vaccine-associated poliomyelitis

2. Killed (Salk)

    - Given by i.m. injection, therefore less effective in inducing mucosal immunity and hence herd immunity
    - No risk of reversion to virulence
    - Vaccine of choice in immunosuppressed individuals

Table 35.1 Consequences of enterovirus infections

General
Asymptomatic infection
The commonest sequela of infection
Infection in the newborn
Neonatal enteroviral infection can be life-threatening, owing to the multisystem nature of the infection in this patient group (e.g. myocarditis, hepatitis, encephalitis). Outbreaks may occur in neonatal units
Skin and mucous membranes
Fever and exanthem
Non-specific illness, often in the summer months
Herpangina
Usually Coxsackie A viruses. Discrete small vesicles on the posterior pharynx, palate, tonsils, tongue
Hand, foot and mouth disease
Coxsackie A or B viruses. Intraoral lesions are ulcerative, the lesions on hands and feet usually vesicular.
Conjunctivitis
Coxsackie A 24 and EV 70 associated with epidemics of acute haemorrhagic conjunctivitis in Africa, the Americas and the Far East (see Case 39)
Musculoskeletal system
Pleurodynia (Bornholm disease or epidemic myalgia)
Usually Coxsackie B viruses. Chest pain may mimic myocardial infarction
Central nervous system
Poliomyelitis
This is a syndrome of flaccid paralysis resulting from motor neuron damage, usually due to polioviruses but rarely other enteroviruses
Meningitis
The enteroviruses are one of the two commonest causes of aseptic meningitis, the other being mumps virus
Encephalitis
May represent spread of infection from the meninges or, rarely, occur in the absence of meningitis
Respiratory system
Upper RTI
e.g. common-cold-like illness, pharyngitis
Lower RTI
e.g. bronchiolitis or pneumonia, usually in young children
Cardiovascular system
Acute myo- and pericarditis
Coxsackie B viruses

polio virus, but do not provide cross-protection against infection with the other members of the genus. There are two types of vaccine available. Both are effective and both have been adopted as prophylaxis by different countries. The WHO has the objective of worldwide elimination of poliomyelitis by the year 2000. This might just be achieved.

Summary: Enteroviruses
Genus consists of polio-, Coxsackie A- and B-, echoviruses
Presentation
Wide range of clinical manifestations, including meningitis, myocarditis, poliomyelitis, rashes, upper and lower respiratory tract infections; do not cause diarrhoea
Diagnosis
Viral culture of throat swab, faeces, CSF; serology
Management
No specific therapy; polio is preventable by vaccination

CASE 36
Jamie, a 5-year-old with a troublesome graze

Jamie, a 5-year-old child, is seen in the Accident and Emergency department. Four days previously he was playing with his two sisters when he fell and sustained a graze over his left elbow. This was dressed and looked after by his mother, who is now concerned that the wound is infected, and she claims that Jamie now cries whenever she or anybody else goes near it. In the past Jamie has been a healthy child and has received all his vaccinations to date, including tetanus and haemophilus. On examination Jamie is apyrexial but a little irritable, and screams when the casualty officer approaches his elbow. There is a small area of erythema with some tenderness surrounding the graze, but there is no pus, lymphangitis or lymphadenopathy. Movement of the elbow is not restricted.

Q What is the diagnosis and the likely aetiology?

A Jamie has cellulitis, as evidenced by the erythema and tenderness, which is most probably caused by a β-haemolytic streptococcus or possibly *Staphylococcus aureus* (see Case 51) acquired following the injury.

Q How are streptococci classified?

A Streptococci are Gram-positive cocci which appear in chains under microscopy but unlike staphylococci are catalase negative. Streptococci

are found as part of the normal flora of the upper respiratory, gastro-intestinal and lower genital tracts. Classification is based upon the ability of many streptococci to produce exotoxins, i.e. haemolysins, capable of breaking down red blood cells. Streptococcal haemolysis (see Table 36.1) may be:

- α: partial haemolysis with a surrounding area of green coloration
- β: clear zone of haemolysis (often, can read through the agar plate!)
- γ: no haemolysis

Table 36.1 Guide to streptococci (excluding anaerobes) and their clinical importance

Group	Haemolysis	Examples	Infections
α or viridans streptococci	α	S. mutans, S.mitior, S. sanguis	Bacteraemia, infective endocarditis (see Case 46)
		S. pneumoniae	Pneumonia (see Case 12)
β streptococci	β	S. pyogenes	Superficial and deep infection, including bacteraemia
γ streptococci	None	S. salivarius	? dental disease
Enterococci	α or β or γ	E. faecalis	UTIs, endocarditis

Q How are the β-haemolytic streptococci subdivided?

A These streptococci are divided on the basis of the Lancefield groups, which reflect differences in carbohydrate antigens of the cell. This grouping can be carried out on isolates in the diagnostic laboratory with appropriate antisera by pre-cipitation or latex agglutination. Within the different groups there may be one or more species:

Group   Species
A   S. pyogenes: may be sub-divided according to Griffith types (M, T, R), based upon surface protein antigens
B   S. agalactiae: causes in-fection in the mother and neonate during the post-partum period (see Case 54)
C   S. equi and S. equisimilis: very similar to group A but probably less virulent
D   include the enterococci such as E. faecalis, E. faecium (see Case 34)
F   S. anginosus (previously known as S. milleri): part of the normal gastrointestinal flora but may cause liver, lung and brain abscess (see Case 3)
G   very similar to A and C

Q How do group A streptococci cause disease?

A Group A streptococci are capable of producing an array of extra-cellular enzymes and toxins (many also produced by other β-haemolytic streptococci) which are considered to be potent virulence determinants. They include:

- haemolysins
- erythrogenic toxins: production mediated by lysogenization by bacteriophages and responsible for the rash in scarlet fever; also implicated in streptococcal toxic shock syndrome (see Case 40)
- streptolysins O and S: induce lysis in red blood cells (haemolysis) and are cytotoxic to other cells, such as neutrophils
- streptokinase: converts plasmin-ogen to plasmin; now used in the emergency treatment of ischaemic thrombotic heart disease
- deoxyribonuclease: at least four of these are known
- hyaluronidase: partly responsible for spread of infection in cellulitis and erysipelas.

The severity of disease may also be related to underlying disease such as diabetes mellitus, but severe in-fections may also occur in the young, fit and healthy population.

Q Which streptococci cause cellulitis?

A Groups A, C and G. Group A causes the most severe or life-threatening form.

Q What is the antibiotic of choice to treat cellulitis caused by β-haemolytic streptococci?

A Benzylpenicillin as all group A streptococci are still very sensitive to penicillin. It is also the treatment of choice for infections caused by groups B, C and G. Treatment should be continued for at least 10–14 days, as there is initially often a slow response. Where oral therapy is appropriate (i.e. in the absence of systemic infection) it may be substituted by amoxycillin/ampicillin. Alternatives include erythromycin, a cephalosporin or clindamycin, especially in the penicillin-allergic patient.

Q Are the enterococci sensitive to penicillin?

A No. The enterococci are penicillin resistant but are less resistant to ampicillin/amoxycillin, and this is the treatment of choice for enterococcal urinary tract infection. Systemic enterococcal infection requires a combination of a penicillin and an aminoglycoside, or a glycopeptide such as vancomycin or teicoplanin.

Jamie is discharged from the Accident and Emergency depart-ment on a course of amoxycillin for 10 days. Three days later when he is reviewed, the area of cellulitis has decreased and is less tender. A report from the microbiology laboratory indicates that a group A streptococcus, sensitive to penicillin, has been isolated from a swab taken from the wound site.

Q What other infections are caused by group A streptococci?

A These include:

- tonsillitis: less common than viruses
- quinsy: peritonsillar abscess which requires drainage
- impetigo: common in childhood and associated with overcrowding; also caused by groups C and G β-haemolytic streptococci and S. aureus
- erysipelas: more superficial than cellulitis

- scarlet fever
- bacteraemia: often with multiple organ failure and a high mortality, even in young patients (see Case 44)
- necrotizing fasciitis: often associated with other pathogens, such as *S. aureus*, coliforms and anaerobes.

Q What other measures should be taken in cases of group A infection admitted to hospital?

A This bacterium is highly infectious and spreads by direct contact or by the airborne route (e.g. tonsillitis). Patients with tonsillitis, cellulitis or wound infection who require admission to hospital should be isolated in a single room where at all possible, until 48 hours of antibiotic treatment have elapsed. Plastic aprons and gloves are necessary for patient contact and hand-washing is essential.

Q What other bacteria cause wound infection?

A The bacteria that most commonly cause wound infection are:

- *S. aureus*, responsible for 50–60% (see Case 51)
- groups A, C and G β-haemolytic streptococci
- aerobic Gram-negative bacilli, e.g. *Escherichia coli*, *Klebsiella aerogenes* etc. but colonization with these bacteria is more common than infection (see Case 34)
- anaerobes, e.g. *Clostridium perfringens*, *Bacteroides fragilis*.
- less commonly enterococci, *Pseudomonas aeruginosa* and *S. epidermidis* (difficult to distinguish from normal skin flora). These are usually hospital acquired and occur in debilitated patients or following complicated procedures
- dog bites may lead to wound infection due to less common Gram-negative bacilli, e.g. *Capnocytophaga canimorsus* and *Pasteurella multocida*, which can

---

B36.1 Classification of surgical wounds
Clean
No break in any viscus or hollow organ, e.g. inguinal hernia, infection rate of <2%
Contaminated
Involves incision into the gastrointestinal or respiratory tract, with possible spillage but no pus, e.g. cholecystectomy, infection rate of 10–40%
Infected
Surgery where there is infected tissue or a collection of pus, e.g. incision and drainage of peritoneal abscess, infection rate of >50%

---

occasionally result in systemic infection such as bacteraemia.

Q What are the risk factors for contracting post-surgical wound infection?

A Specific factors which influence the risk of contracting infection following surgery include the type of surgery and the anatomical location (see Box 36.1), whether a drain is left *in situ* where there is residual infected material, the experience and expertise of the surgical team, the patient's age, underlying disease such as diabetes mellitus, and finally, whether antibiotic prophylaxis was used (see Case 20).

Three weeks later Jamie is seen in the paediatric outpatients department because his parents have noticed a low-grade fever, generalized weakness, some swelling around the face in particular, and blood while passing urine over the last week. The graze and the surrounding area of cellulitis have healed, and there is no longer any tenderness.

Q What possible diagnosis must be considered now?

A Post-streptococcal glomerulonephritis, despite treatment and resolution of the infection. Glomerulonephritis may be confirmed by the detection of red blood cell casts in the urine and elevated serum urea and creatinine. This condition is due to a cross-reaction between certain streptococcus antigens and those of the host, e.g. on the basement membrane of the glomerulus, leading to deposition of immune complexes and infiltration with polymorphonuclear and eosinophil leukocytes within the glomerulus, as seen on renal biopsy. Complement activation leads to depressed C_3 of the complement cascade. Certain Griffith types of group A streptococci are associated with glomerulonephritis, and these include M12 (post-tonsillitis) and M49, M55 and M57 (post impetigo).

Q Name another important post-streptococcal disease.

A Rheumatic fever (see Box 36.2) where the pathogenesis is similar.

Q Are there any laboratory tests apart from culture which might indicate recent group A streptococcal infection?

A A number of serological tests are available in most diagnostic or

---

B36.2 Rheumatic fever
Clinical features
Fever, arthralgia, nodules, skin rash (erythema marginatum) 1–5 weeks after a streptococcal infection. Only 15–20% are culture +ve for group A streptococci from throat or other site, e.g. wound
Diagnosis
High probability if two *major* criteria (carditis, polyarthritis, chorea, erythema marginatum, subcutaneous nodules) or 1 *major* and 2 *minor* criteria (previous history of rheumatic fever, arthralgia, fever, elevated ESR or CRP, abnormal ECG) with laboratory evidence of recent streptococcal infection

reference laboratories which may indicate recent or previous infection. These include antistreptolysin O titre or ASOT (normal value <250), anti-DNAse B titre (normal value <320) and antihyaluronidase (normal value <300). One or more of these is usually considerably elevated in cases of rheumatic fever or post-streptococcal glomerulonephritis.

Summary: β-haemolytic streptococci

Presentation

A variety of superficial (wound infection, tonsillitis, erysipelas, impetigo) and systemic (bacteraemia with multiple organ failure) infections. Immune-mediated complications may ensue

Diagnosis

Culture of appropriate specimens, e.g. throat or wound swab, blood etc. Serology useful especially in immune-mediated disease

Management

Penicillin is the antibiotic of choice for treatment of infection

CASE 37
Simon, 4 years old, develops a rash

Simon, 4 years old, has developed a rash in the last 24 hours. He has been unwell for the past 3 days, with a fever, a runny nose and an unproductive cough. His GP yesterday prescribed amoxycillin. Simon was vaccinated against diphtheria/pertussis/tetanus, HiB and polio as an infant. Until this illness he has been fit and well, with no history of allergy, and on no regular medication. On examination in addition to the rash (see Fig. 37.1) he is generally miserable and febrile (39.2°C), with a respiratory rate of 30/min. There is no lymphadenopathy or evidence of lower respiratory tract disease.

Q What is the differential diagnosis?

A The salient clinical features of a prodromal illness with fever, cough, coryza and conjunctivitis, followed by a rash starting on the face in an unvaccinated child are highly suggestive of measles (Box 37.1). A further diagnostic clue is that children with measles are usually very miserable. Alternative diagnoses include:

- rubella: prodromal illness is not a feature and posterior cervical adenopathy is usually more marked
- upper respiratory tract infection with an allergic reaction to ampicillin
- roseola infantum (see Box 37.2).

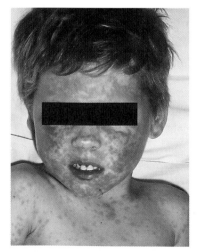

Fig. 37.1 Simon's rash — day 1.

B37.1 Clinical course of uncomplicated measles infection

Transmission – droplet spread of respiratory secretions
Entry – through upper respiratory tract or conjunctiva
Incubation period – 10–14 days; leucopenia develops as virus replicates in lymphoid tissue
Prodromal illness – 2–4 days, as described above
Rash – develops over 2–3 days, then fades
Infectious period – from prodromal stage and for 4 days after onset of rash

Q How can the diagnosis be confirmed?

A By noting the presence of Koplik's spots on Simon's buccal mucosa. These small greyish-white lesions (see Figure 37.2) are present during the prodromal stage but fade once the rash appears. Virus isolation from the throat and serology may also help.

An acute measles virus infection is diagnosed and the antibiotic stopped. Over the next few days Simon's rash spreads to his trunk and limbs and then begins to fade, leaving a brownish discoloration. His respiratory symptoms improve and his fever subsides. However, on day 6 after the onset of the rash, Simon complains of a headache, becomes increasingly irritable, and his fever returns.

Q What complication may now be developing?

B37.2 Roseola infantum (exanthem subitum, 6th disease)

Causative agent – primary infection with human herpes virus types 6 or 7 (HHV6, HHV7)
Age – 6 months to 2 years old
Clinical features – 3–4 days pyrexia without localizing signs, with morbilliform rash appearing as fever subsides

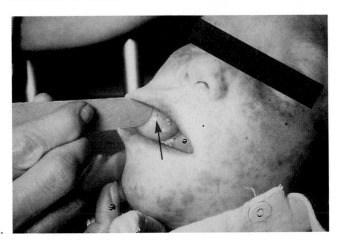

**Fig. 37.2
Koplik's spots.**

A Acute measles postinfectious encephalitis. Features of this serious complication include recrudescence of fever, headache, seizures, cerebellar ataxia and declining levels of consciousness, within 8–10 days of the onset of measles, in 1 per 1000–5000 cases of measles. Histology of affected brain shows demyelination and perivascular cuffing.

Q What is meant by the term 'postinfectious'?

A This refers to the pathogenetic mechanism underlying the disease. Neither whole virus or viral antigens can be detected in affected brain tissue. The damage is therefore believed to arise from an aberrant immune response to the virus, hence the term 'postinfectious'. Postinfectious encephalitis may also be seen after varicella-zoster and influenza virus infections.

Q What is the prognosis of acute measles postinfectious encephalitis?

A Poor. There is no specific treatment and corticosteroids have not been shown to be of value. Fifteen per cent of cases are fatal and up to 40% of survivors suffer long-term neurological sequelae.

Q What are the other complications of measles infection?

A Most complications arise from secondary infection of the necrotic epithelial surfaces of the respiratory tract, and include:

- bronchitis/bronchopneumonia
- bronchiectasis
- otitis media
- purulent conjunctivitis
- laryngotracheitis.

Central nervous system complications include:

- acute measles postinfectious encephalitis (see above)
- subacute sclerosing panencephalitis (SSPE, see below).

Another serious complication, fortunately rare, is:

- giant-cell pneumonia, a severe protracted illness, often fatal, with characteristic giant cells seen on histology. Due to the direct spread of virus to the lower respiratory tract. Occurs usually in patients with underlying disease, e.g. leukaemia.

Q How does SSPE differ from acute measles postinfectious encephalitis?

A The pathogenesis and clinical presentations of these two complications are quite distinct. The salient features of SSPE are shown in Box 37.3.

Q How does the epidemiology of measles differ in the developing world?

A The peak incidence of measles infection occurs at less than 2 years of age. Measles is still a major cause of death with mortality approaching 5–15%. WHO estimates there may be up to 1 million deaths per year arising from measles infection worldwide. Factors contributing to this heavy toll are the immuno-suppressive effects of measles, due to infection and death of lymphoid cells, in a population that may already have reduced immuno-competence arising from malnutrition. Infection is therefore often complicated by life-threatening bacterial pneumonia (including tuberculosis) and severe diarrhoea.

Q Is measles preventable?

A Yes, by means of a live attenuated vaccine. This is now incorporated into the MMR (measles–mumps–rubella) vaccine that should be given to all children at age 12–18 months. Measles is *not* a trivial illness, and infection carries a significant risk of serious morbidity and mortality. Measles is highly infectious, and there have been outbreaks of disease in populations with respectable levels of vaccine coverage. Every effort should therefore be made to ensure and maintain high levels of vaccination.

Vaccination at 15 months of age in developing countries, however, may be too late to prevent much measles-associated mortality, which occurs in younger children, while vaccination at 9 months is not as

CASE 37

effective in inducing protective immunity. This paradox has yet to be satisfactorily resolved.

Q What are the contraindications to measles vaccination?

A Genuine contraindications are few:

- Acute febrile illness on presentation for immunization, which should be deferred
- Untreated malignant disease or altered immunity
- Allergy to neomycin or kanamycin (these antibiotics are present in the vaccine)
- Vaccine should not be given within 3 weeks of receipt of another live vaccine, or within 3 months of an injection of immunoglobulin
- Allergy to egg, but only if this is manifested by an anaphylactic reaction.

Summary: Measles
Presentation
Prodrome of upper respiratory tract symptoms, fever and rash in an ill child
Diagnosis
Clinical (rash, Koplik's spots); serology; virus isolation
Complications
Secondary bacterial infections; acute postinfectious encephalomyelitis; subacute sclerosing panencephalitis; giant-cell pneumonia
Management
No antiviral therapy; preventable by vaccination

CASE 38

Emma, 8 years old, also develops a rash

Eight-year-old Emma has developed a generalized itchy rash, which first appeared 2 days ago on her face, as discrete red spots. These spots developed into small vesicles and spread over her trunk, with a few lesions also appearing on her limbs. She has no other symptoms. There is no relevant past medical history, and she has not taken any drugs recently. On examination, Emma has a temperature of 37.9°C, and the rash appears as shown in Figure 38.1.

CASE 38

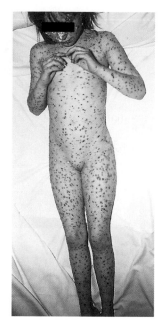

Fig. 38.1 Emma's rash.

Table 38.1 Clinical features of chicken-pox
Incubation period 13–17 days
Rash usually appears first on the trunk, then spreads to involve face, scalp and limbs
Lesion evolves from macule to papule to vesicle in a few hours, to crust in 4 days
Usually several lesions in the mouth; pharynx and conjunctiva may also be involved
Cropping occurs over several days, so that lesions of differing ages may be present
Some generalized lymphadenopathy may occur
The rash is itchy in some, but not all, patients

Q What is the diagnosis?

A The florid vesicular rash is characteristic of chicken-pox, i.e. the manifestation of primary infection with varicella-zoster virus (VZV). In the early stages, or if the rash is less profuse, other possibilities would include herpes simplex virus infection or a drug reaction. The diagnosis is essentially a clinical one – the features of the chicken-pox rash are given in Table 38.1. If necessary, the diagnosis can be confirmed by isolation of the virus from vesicle fluid, or by demonstrating a rise in antibody titre in serum samples taken a few days apart.

Table 38.2 Complications of chicken-pox
Secondary bacterial infection of vesicles
Scarring – increased risk if lesions traumatized or infected
Varicella pneumonia
usually in adults 2–3 days after onset of rash
chest X-ray shows diffuse patchy nodular infiltration
may also occur in neonates
Encephalitis
uncommon. Usually 7–10 days after onset
CSF normal or increase in cells and protein
cerebellar syndrome most often seen. Hemiplegia also described recovery usually complete, but sequelae and fatalities may occur
Haemorrhagic varicella
rare. Usually associated with thrombocytopenia
bleeding from mucous membranes, into lesions and into unaffected skin
often fatal

Q What are the possible complications of chicken-pox?

A These are listed in Table 38.2.

Q Which patient groups develop chicken-pox pneumonia?

A Pulmonary involvement arises as a result of haematogenous spread of the virus. Thus, patients who are immunosuppressed (or immuno-immature, i.e. neonates), especially those with reduced cell-mediated immunity, are at considerable risk of developing pneumonia as they are less able to prevent the spread of virus in the bloodstream. Pneumonia is also more common in adults than in children, and there is evidence to suggest that pregnant women are more susceptible than non-pregnant women (see Case 57). The incidence of pneumonia in immunocompetent adults is 1–5%, although X-ray changes indicating involvement of the lungs are more frequent (e.g. 10–15%).

Q What pathogenetic mechanisms may account for the encephalitis which may follow chicken-pox?

A As discussed in Case 37, possible mechanisms of brain damage in viral encephalitis include direct spread of the virus into the brain itself, and immune system-mediated damage due to an aberrant immune response to the virus cross-reacting with brain antigens (postinfectious encephalitis). The pathogenesis of varicella encephalitis is not known with certainty, but the timing, coincident with the development of a measurable immune response, suggests that this is a postinfectious encephalitis rather than the result of direct virus infection of the brain.

Despite Emma's florid rash, she feels well in herself and is keen to go back to school.

Q When should she be allowed to do so?

A Chicken-pox is highly infectious, as patients excrete virus in droplets from the pharynx. In addition, the vesicles contain high titres of infectious virus. Emma will have been infectious for a couple of days prior to the development of her rash, and will remain so until her last crop of vesicles have crusted over. She should not be allowed back to school until no new lesions have appeared for 2 days, provided the existing lesions have crusted.

By chance, the very next patient to enter the surgery has a rash, very similar in appearance to Emma's, but localized to an area of skin on his back and chest (see Figure 38.2). He is Mr Carter, a 48-year-old hospital administrator, previously fit and well, who first noticed pain on his back and chest a week ago. This was followed by an odd sensation when he touched the area of skin involved, and, 3 days ago, by the emergence of several red spots. He has no other symptoms. In his social history he says he has been under considerable stress recently in his job, and 2 weeks ago his mother died.

Q What is the diagnosis?

A The vesicular appearance and dermatomal distribution of the rash are typical of herpes zoster, or shingles, involving a thoracic nerve root. This represents reactivation of latent VZV from within a dorsal root ganglion. The characteristic clinical features of an attack of shingles are listed in Table 38.3.

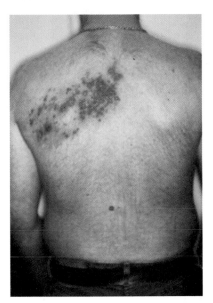

Fig. 38.2 Mr Carter's rash.

Table 38.3 Clinical features of herpes zoster

Malaise and pyrexia
Pain and tenderness over 2–3 adjacent roots precedes the eruption by a few days
Rash – groups of small, irregular, tense vesicles on an erythematous and oedematous area of skin appear in crops
Lesions evolve to pustules to scabs in 5–10 days
Regional lymph nodes may be enlarged and tender
Commonest sites: thoracic, cervical and cranial nerve V(a), in that order, but any segments may be involved

---

Q What is the relationship, if any, between this rash and that of Emma?

A VZV, like all the human herpes viruses (see Case 2, Box 2.1), exhibits the phenomenon of *latency*, whereby primary infection is followed by lifelong carriage of the virus, which can then be reactivated at some later stage, resulting in a secondary, or recurrent, infection. The site of latency for VZV is within the nerve cell body, or ganglion. As primary VZV infection is a generalized phenomenon, latent virus may be found in multiple dorsal root ganglia around the body. Following reactivation from within a ganglion, virus tracks down the axon to the skin supplied by that particular nerve, resulting in the characteristic dermatomal distribution of zoster.

Q What are the risk factors for the development of herpes zoster?

A

- Increasing age, presumably reflecting declining immunity to VZV – >20% of individuals over the age of 80 will give a history of zoster

- Trauma (including surgery) to an area of the body may be followed by zoster appearing in that area some days later
- Stress
- Immunodeficiency or -suppression – results in increased frequency of reactivation of all herpes viruses. Bloodstream spread may result in a generalized zoster rash and life-threatening involvement of internal organs, e.g. lungs and liver, in this patient group.

Q What are the possible complications of herpes zoster?

A These depend to some extent on which nerve is involved, and are listed in Table 38.4.

Analgesics are prescribed and Mr Carter is told that the shingles is likely to last for a few days only. However, over the next 3 weeks his rash shows no sign of resolving, and in fact becomes more extensive.

Q What should be considered now?

A In the immunocompetent host VZV reactivation is a self-limiting disease. The continued appearance of new lesions in any patient raises the possibility of an underlying immunodeficiency disorder. A severe attack of zoster can be the presenting feature of a number of diseases, all of which have in common an element of immune dysfunction – see Table 38.5. Mr Carter should be investigated accordingly.

After further investigation, Mr Carter was in fact diagnosed as having chronic lymphocytic leukaemia.

Q What options are available for the management and prevention of VZV infection?

A The mainstay of therapy is acyclovir, or the recently developed derivatives thereof (famciclovir, valaciclovir). A higher dose is necessary to inhibit VZV compared to HSV replication, and in life-threatening VZV disease it is necessary to administer the drug intravenously. Indications for such therapy include chicken-pox pneumonia, chicken-pox or herpes zoster in an immunocompromised patient, and severe ophthalmic zoster. The value of treating uncomplicated chicken-pox or herpes zoster with acyclovir is unresolved. There is a high-dose oral preparation of acyclovir, licensed in the UK for the treatment of herpes zoster in the elderly (>65 years old). Although this undoubtedly reduces the time to healing, to cessation of new lesion formation, and the pain of the acute attack, its effect on the incidence of postherpetic neuralgia is controversial.

There is a live attenuated VZV vaccine (the Oka strain), which has been shown to prevent the serious complications of primary VZV infection when given to children in remission from leukaemia. It is currently available in the UK only on a named-patient basis for such children.

Table 38.4 Complications of herpes zoster

Postherpetic neuralgia
  pain in the rash-affected area for more than 3 months after the rash itself has resolved
  can be debilitating and result in clinical depression
  likelihood of occurrence increases with increasing age
Motor nerve involvement
  e.g. C4 zoster + wasting of deltoid muscle
  seventh cranial nerve, leading to facial palsy
Ocular involvement
  with cranial nerve V(a), leading to keratitis
Dissemination, with internal organ involvement
  in the immunodeficient or -suppressed
Autonomic nerve involvement
  e.g. retention of urine in sacral zoster
Neurological (rare)
  zoster encephalitis, transverse myelitis

Table 38.5 Predisposing factors for severe herpes zoster

HIV infection
Malignancy, especially of the reticuloendothelial system, e.g.
  chronic lymphocytic leukaemia, multiple myeloma,
  Hodgkin's and non-Hodgkin's lymphomas
Immunosuppression for transplant recipients
Chemotherapy
High-dose steroid therapy
Radiotherapy

Summary: Chicken-pox
Presentation
Generalized vesicular rash, usually in a child
Diagnosis
Clinical; if any doubt, demonstrate virus in vesicle fluid by electron microscopy, culture, antigen detection
Complications
Pneumonia; postinfectious encephalitis; internal organ involvement in the immunosuppressed
Treatment
Acyclovir – for immunosuppressed patients, pneumonia
Complications of reactivation
Postherpetic neuralgia, ocular involvement, motor nerve involvement, dissemination

CASE 39
Steven, a 42-year-old accountant, with a red, painful eye

Steven, a 42-year-old accountant, has a routine eye check-up by his local optometrist, who notes that his intraocular pressure is on the high side and suggests he should seek ophthalmological advice. Steven therefore presents to Eye Casualty, where he is fully examined, but tonometry is normal. He is reassured and discharged. One week later he notices a gritty sensation, initially in his left eye, and pain when looking into bright light. He develops a watery discharge from both eyes, which become puffy and red (see Figure 39.1), so he returns to Eye Casualty. Examination of the left eye reveals oedema of both conjunctivae and eyelids, and a subconjunctival haemorrhage, and punctate epithelial lesions are seen following fluorescein staining. Similar but less marked changes are seen in the right eye. Bilateral enlarged preauricular lymph nodes are also noted.

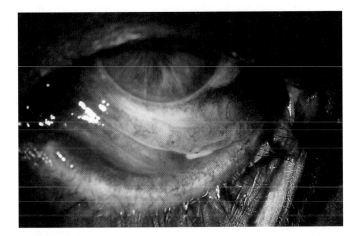

Fig. 39.1 Steven's left eye.

Q What is the likely diagnosis?

A The inflamed conjunctivae, together with the corneal lesions, indicate a keratoconjunctivitis. The acute onset is highly suggestive of an infectious aetiology. Viral infections of the eye are common, and the absence of visible pus also makes bacterial infection less likely in this particular case.

Q How would you manage this patient?

A An eye swab should be taken, broken off into viral transport medium and sent to the laboratory. Steven should be given topical chloramphenicol ointment to prevent secondary bacterial infection. He should also be instructed about scrupulous hand-washing to prevent the accidental spread of infection. The presence of corneal lesions means that referral to an ophthalmologist is mandatory. Treatment of the acute episode may include a cycloplegic agent (e.g. cyclopentolate) to relax the ciliary body and iris, which will relieve his pain.

Q What is the likely outcome of Steven's infection?

A His symptoms should improve over the next 7–14 days. However, as the conjunctivitis resolves epithelial opacities, which may impair vision, may become prominent. Steven will require long-term outpatient follow-up, as these lesions may take months or years to disappear.

Q What are the common infectious causes of conjunctivitis?

CASE 39

A

1. Viruses

   - Adenoviruses, the most likely infection in this case. The cornea may also be involved (keratitis)
   - Herpes simplex virus – see Box 39.1; HSV keratitis is the commonest infectious cause of corneal blindness in the UK
   - Varicella-zoster virus – involvement of the ophthalmic division of the trigeminal nerve is common in herpes zoster (see Case 38)
   - Enteroviruses (see Case 35) particularly Coxsackie virus A24 and enterovirus 70, associated with epidemics of acute haemorrhagic conjunctivitis in Africa, the Americas and the Far East
   - Measles. Conjunctivitis is a common manifestation during the prodrome (See Case 37)

2. Bacteria. Involvement of the cornea is unusual in bacterial infection unless secondary to virus infection, trauma, or in association with contact lens use

   - *S. aureus* – gives rise to 'sticky eye' in neonates
   - *H. influenzae*
   - *Str. pneumoniae*
   - *Chlamydia trachomatis* – causes conjunctivitis and trachoma (see Case 56)

B39.1 Eye involvement with herpes simplex virus

- Primary conjunctivitis may arise by self-inoculation from an orolabial source
- May cause blepharitis, conjunctivitis, keratitis
- Reactivated infections may give rise to superficial (dendritic) corneal ulcers
- Complications include keratitis, disciform ulceration, permanent scarring, iridocyclitis
- Management includes topical acyclovir; steroids contraindicated in early infections; complications require expert ophthalmological care

- *N. gonorrhoeae* – causes ophthalmia neonatorum (see Case 56)
- *Ps. aeruginosa* – opportunist infection, e.g. after trauma.

3. Other

- Fungi, e.g. Candida – in immunosuppressed patients
- Acanthamoeba – severe keratitis associated with contaminated contact lenses
- Worms – *Onchocerca volvulus*, giving rise to river blindness.

Ten days after Steven's second visit to Eye Casualty, the laboratory issues a preliminary report of the eye swab stating 'Adenovirus isolated – type to follow'. Two weeks later a further report is issued: 'Adenovirus type 8 isolated'.

Q How might Steven have acquired his adenovirus infection?

A The incubation period of adenoviral keratoconjunctivitis is of the order of 7 days. Steven visited Eye Casualty 7 days before the onset of his illness. The worry here is that the infection may have been nosocomially acquired, i.e. the adenovirus was introduced into Steven's eye during his first visit to Eye Casualty.

Q How do nosocomial outbreaks of adenoviral keratoconjunctivitis occur?

A Adenoviruses are difficult to remove by disinfection – the absence of a lipid envelope and the presence of a tight-knit protein capsid renders such viruses stable to most of the commonly used disinfectants. Thus, unless appropriate agents (chloramine T or 1% sodium hypochlorite) are used for disinfection, virus may be passed from patient to patient via contaminated instruments, e.g. tonometers. The skin of staff handling these instruments may also become contaminated. Staff may therefore inadvertently spread virus to otherwise sterile instruments, and thence into patients' eyes. A further route

of spread arises if multidose vials are used, e.g. to administer local anaesthetic or fluorescein dye to the eye, again allowing patient-to-patient spread of virus. All of the above routes of spread are highly efficient, as virus is inoculated directly into the recipients' eyes.

Q How might the hospital infection control team investigate a nosocomial outbreak of adenovirus eye infection?

A The first task is to gather evidence that such an outbreak has occurred. A continuous record of adenovirus isolates and typing results from eye swabs should be maintained, so that any increase in isolation rates, or the emergence of new or unusual serotypes, can be identified quickly. The dates of the eye swabs should be carefully noted, and whether those particular patients were attending Eye Casualty for the first time (in which case their infections were community acquired) or were reattenders. During a nosocomial outbreak most patients will fall into the latter category, suggesting that the virus was acquired from their first visit.

Q What are the principles of management of a nosocomial outbreak?

A These consist of reviewing and tightening up infection control policies within the unit. The importance of basic precautions, such as rigorous hand-washing by all staff between patients, must be emphasized. Disinfection protocols must be checked to ensure efficacy. All multidose vials should be abandoned – the increased costs of single-dose vials will be more than offset by the reduction in infections. Infected patients should also be educated about the possibility of spread to household and other casual contacts.

Q How are adenoviruses classified?

A Classification of adenoviruses is a complex subject. Suffice to say that over 40 serotypes of adeno-

viruses, grouped into six subgenera (A–F), may infect humans. Subgenus F contains serotypes 40 and 41, which behave somewhat differently from the other adenoviruses (see below).

Q What diseases do adenoviruses cause?

A Adenoviruses give rise to a number of distinct clinical syndromes:

1. Upper respiratory tract infection (see Case 8)

- Usually in young children, adenoviruses 1–7 give rise to pharyngitis, tonsillitis, adenoidal enlargement, conjunctivitis, nasal congestion, cough

2. Lower respiratory tract infection

- Laryngotracheobronchitis, bronchiolitis, pneumonia
- Account for 10% of pneumonia in children
- Outbreaks may occur in young adults crowded together, e.g. military recruits.

3. Infections of the eye

- Pharyngoconjunctival fever describes one particular syndrome
- Follicular conjunctivitis may appear as a separate entity
- Epidemic keratoconjunctivitis, as described in this case. Type 8 is the commonest cause.

4. Gastroenteritis

- Mainly in young children (see Case 18). May or may not be associated with respiratory symptoms. Associated particularly with types 40 and 41, which are thus referred to as enteric adenoviruses.

5. Rare syndromes

- Acute haemorrhagic cystitis – dysuria and haematuria (see Case 31)
- Meningitis, encephalitis
- Hepatitis in the immunosuppressed, e.g. bone marrow recipients.

Q What techniques are available for the laboratory diagnosis of adenovirus infections?

A These encompass the more common approaches to viral diagnosis, including:

- virus culture. May take up to 3 weeks to grow in laboratory tissue culture. Enteric adenoviruses do not grow in routine cell culture lines
- electron microscopy. Enteric adenoviruses are excreted in large amounts in stool, and can be visualized under EM
- antigen detection. Cells from a nasopharyngeal aspirate, for example, can be stained with monoclonal anti-adenovirus antibodies, the binding of which can be detected by immunofluorescence (see Case 15)
- serology. A rising titre of antibodies may be detected in a pair of acute (i.e. taken at presentation) and convalescent (i.e. taken 7–10 days later) sera.

Q What specific antiviral therapy is available for serious adenovirus infections?

A No agent has undergone clinical trials, but there are anecdotal reports of the successful use of tribavirin in the treatment of life-threatening adenoviral infections.

Summary: Viral kerato-conjunctivitis
Presentation
Painful red eye
Causes
Adenoviruses (may be nosocomial and result in corneal opacities); Herpes simplex virus (may recur, leading to corneal blindness)
Diagnosis
Viral culture of eye swab
Treatment
Requires ophthalmological expertise; topical acyclovir for HSV

must, however, be considered during the months of July and August, even in Britain! The following should also be considered:

- Menigococcaemia: the absence of meningism does not exclude this but the skin rash is not typical of this condition, which is usually characterized by a purpuric rash (see Case 1)
- Gram-negative infection: a high fever, gastrointestinal symptoms (loose bowel motions) and low blood pressure may indicate endotoxic shock (see Case 44) and must always be considered. A rash does not usually occur with this condition, however
- Gram-positive infection: staphylococcal and streptococcal bacteraemia or certain toxin-mediated diseases may give rise to a high fever, a rash and other features, e.g. depression of myocardial muscle function
- Leptospirosis: the absence of a history of contact with rats or jaundice should not exclude infection caused by *Leptospira interrogans*, especially in the presence of conjunctivitis (see Case 50). Again the rash is atypical
- Viral illness: adenoviruses (see Case 39) and enteroviruses (see Case 35) may occasionally present like this in children, but are less common in adults and are usually characterized by a maculo-papular rash
- Stevens–Johnson syndrome: a widespread erythematous rash accompanied by painful erosive lesions in the mouth and palate are features of this condition, which may be caused by drugs (e.g. sulphonamides, barbiturates) or herpes simplex infections (see Cases 29 and 58)
- Kawasaki syndrome: an erythematous rash of the hands and feet, a strawberry tongue, conjunctivitis and lymphadenopathy are diagnostic of this condition, which is usually seen during

CASE 40
Extensive rash, headache, fever and myalgia in Avril, a 20-year-old woman

It is the middle of July; 20-year-old Avril has been brought to hospital by her boyfriend and two flatmates. The history from her friends is that up to a couple of days ago she had been fit and healthy, and had even enjoyed a day out by the sea in the sun the previous day. Avril initially complained of feeling hot, a frontal headache, loose bowel motions and muscle aches and pains, for which she had taken some paracetamol. As far as is known she has never been seriously ill before or required admission to hospital, and is on no medications. There has been a steady deterioration in her condition over the last 24 hours, and this morning she is confused and clearly quite ill. On examination Avril has a temperature of 40°C, a pulse rate of 120/min and a blood pressure of 90/60 mmHg. There is a widespread erythematous rash over the trunk, mild conjunctivitis and inflamed mucous membranes of the mouth, but there is no meningism.

Q What is the differential diagnosis?

A The combination of confusion, a high fever and hypotension suggests

a serious systemic infection. The presence of the rash might suggest sunstroke, but hypotension would be unusual unless severe. This

childhood. The aetiology is uncertain, but death may occur due to arrhythmias arising from cardiac involvement

- Rickettsial disease: many tick-borne diseases which are geographically defined, such as Rocky Mountain Spotted Fever, caused by *Rickettsia rickettsii*, may cause a systemic illness with a widespread rash, which is, however, usually macular.

Further questioning of Avril's female friends reveals that she had started her menses the previous day. A tampon is discovered on vaginal examination, which when removed reveals a red and inflamed vaginal mucosa. Initial investigations reveal a leukocytosis of $18 \times 10^9/l$, thrombocytopenia ($60 \times 10^9/l$), abnormal liver function tests and elevated urea (24 mmol/l) and creatinine (198 μmol/l).

Q What microbiological investigations should be done?

A At least two sets of blood cultures should be taken to exclude bacteraemia, and other specimens essential for culture include urine (to exclude a urinary tract infection with bacteraemia), faeces (to exclude *Salmonella* or *Campylobacter* infection) and a high vaginal swab, not forgetting the tampon (to exclude toxic shock syndrome, TSS). Acute serum should also be taken for virological studies (a convalescent serum also when available) and, where appropriate, to exclude rickettsial disease.

Q How should this case be managed initially?

A Irrespective of the aetiology, certain general principles apply. Intravascular fluid replacement in the form of saline or colloids is essential, and this should go some way towards normalizing the blood pressure. Organ support in an intensive care unit may be required, especially if the patient is hypoxic

and requires ventilation or if there is myocardial dysfunction necessitating inotropic support. A broad-spectrum antibiotic to cover both Gram-negative and Gram-positive bacteria, e.g. cefotaxime, should be administered intravenously. An appropriate alternative would be a combination of penicillin, flucloxacillin and gentamicin. Renal support in the form of haemofiltration or dialysis and parenteral nutrition may be required if initial attempts at resuscitation are unsuccessful.

Avril is transferred to the intensive care unit that evening for observation and a Swan–Ganz catheter is inserted to observe closely her haemodynamic status. Intravascular fluid replacement with colloid is started and intravenous cefotaxime commenced, but ventilation is not required. The next day her temperature is down to 38.5°C, serum creatinine is 140 μmol/l and she has become more lucid.

Q What is the most likely diagnosis?

A The combination of a high fever, an extensive skin rash, hypotension, other organ involvement and the finding of an inflamed vaginal mucosa with a tampon suggests the toxic shock syndrome (see Box 40.1).

Q What pathogen is likely to have been responsible?

A *Staphylococcus aureus* is the most likely cause of toxic shock syndrome, although group A β-haemolytic streptococci (see Case 36) may also cause a similar syndrome. These bacteria both have the ability to produce an array of extracellular enzymes and toxins. Both toxic shock syndrome toxin (TSST-1) and enterotoxins produced by *S. aureus* are implicated in toxic shock syndrome, and many of the isolates recovered from TSS cases belong to phage group 1 when typed using bacteriophages (viruses

that induce lysis, often according to well-recognized patterns).

***Staphylococcus aureus*, resistant to penicillin but sensitive to flucloxacillin, is isolated from the vaginal swab and the tampon. On subsequent referral to a reference laboratory the isolate is TSST-1 positive. Blood cultures are sterile, examination of faeces reveals no pathogens and serological investigations are negative. The cefotaxime is changed to flucloxacillin and over the next couple of days there is a marked improvement in Avril's condition. She is transferred to a medical ward on day 3, and subsequently widespread skin desquamation becomes evident, especially on the palms of the hands and the soles of the feet (see Figure 40.1).**

Q What factors are important in the pathogenesis of the toxic shock syndrome?

A When the toxic shock syndrome was first described in the late 1970s, it was believed to be confined to menstruating women from whom *S. aureus* was isolated, usually from the vagina or a tampon. It is

---

B40.1 Diagnostic features of the toxic shock syndrome

- Temperature of >38.9°C
- Hypotension and/or decreased urinary output
- Widespread rash, usually erythematous with desquamation later
- Involvement of three or more organ systems, including gastrointestinal tract (e.g. diarrhoea), kidneys (elevated creatinine), mucuous membranes (red, inflamed), respiratory tract (e.g. hypoxia), liver (abnormal function tests), blood (e.g. thrombocytopenia) and central nervous system (e.g. confusion)
- Negative serology for Rocky Mountain Spotted Fever (where appropriate), leptospirosis, adenovirus infection etc.

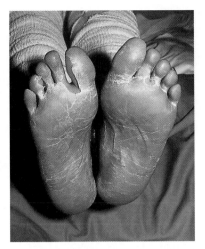

Fig. 40.1 Desquamation of the feet in toxic shock syndrome.

now recognized, however, that this is just one form of the disease, and non-menstruating cases e.g. following skin infection, may outnumber those associated with the menses in females. The relevant pathogenic factors appear to be:

- *Staphylococcus aureus*, usually from phage group I, capable of producing TSST-1 or one of the enterotoxins. Streptococcal toxic shock has also been described associated with the erythrogenic or pyrogenic toxins (see Case 36). These toxins are now considered to be superantigens (antigens which react non-specifically with T lymphocytes, leading to their activation and the release of cytokines which is overwhelming and inappropriate). Bacteraemia is unusual as this is a toxaemic state.
- tampons. First reports were associated with the use of certain makes of tampon in 70–80% of cases. It is believed that these tampons, which were hyper-absorbable, facilitated the local growth of *S. aureus* and the expression of TSST-1. This may have been due to the presence locally of an aerobic environment or magnesium binding by the tampons. In non-menstruating

cases similar factors may be important, but it is not clear how they arise.

- antibodies to TSST-1. More than 85% of patients with toxic shock due to *S. aureus* have low titres of antibodies to TSST-1 compared with healthy controls, 88% of whom have high titres. Healthy controls probably acquire antibodies through asymptomatic contact with toxin-producing strains. Patients who develop toxic shock and fail to mount a serological response are also at greater risk of relapse.

Q What other conditions associated with *S. aureus* are toxin mediated?

A Both staphylococcal food poisoning/gastroenteritis and the scalded skin syndrome are due to the production of specific toxins rather than systemic or localized infection. The main features of these conditions are:

- gastroenteritis, due to preformed enterotoxins in food. There are seven enterotoxins, the most commonly implicated ones being enterotoxins A and B. These induce a self-limiting disease charac-

terized by a short incubation period, vomiting and diarrhoea (see Case 17)

- scalded skin syndrome, caused by epidermolytic toxins which induce skin desquamation, most commonly seen during childhood. Histologically there is cleavage of the middle layers of the epidermidis with bulla formation.

Summary: Toxic shock syndrome
Presentation
Toxic state characterized by an extensive skin rash with multiple organ involvement. Not confined to menstruating women
Diagnosis
Clinical features accompanied by the isolation of a TSST-1 or enterotoxin-producing *S. aureus* from vagina or other site. Less commonly, a β-haemolytic streptococcus, group A, is involved. Bacteraemia is unusual
Management
Intravenous fluids, organ support, removal of infected focus, e.g. tampon, and antibiotics, i.e. flucloxacillin for *S. aureus* or penicillin for streptococci

CASE 41
William and Mary, both aged 30, with blisters on their hands

William and Mary, both aged 30, come separately to your dermatology clinic complaining of the vesicular lesions shown in Figure 41.1. They are otherwise fit and well, with no past medical histories of note, and neither of them is taking any regular medication. William is a sheep farmer; Mary, his wife, is a dental nurse. William's lesions are painless, whereas Mary's is acutely tender and painful. There are no other abnormal physical signs.

Q What are the diagnoses?

A The major clue in these cases, apart from the appearance of the lesions themselves, lies in the occupational histories.

William (Figure 41.1a), is suffering from orf. This is a zoonotic infection acquired from sheep, caused by a pox virus, and is therefore an occupational hazard of farm and

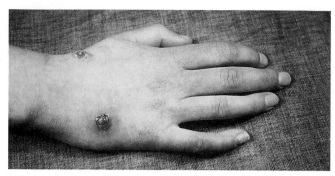

Fig. 41.1A William's hand.   A

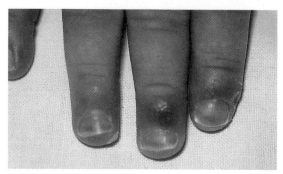

Fig. 41.1B Mary's hand.   B

slaughterhouse workers and veterinarians. Parapox viruses are widespread in sheep, goats and cattle. The lesions they cause in humans are essentially the same, but go under a number of different names. The nomenclature of human disease is based on the identity of the host from which the infection was acquired (see Table 41.1).

Lesions start as erythematous papules and progress to a red centre surrounded by a white halo and an outer inflamed halo, the so-called 'target' stage. This proceeds to a nodular stage, which may have a weeping surface and lasts a week or so before gradually healing. Lesions are surprisingly painless – a useful diagnostic feature – and constitutional upset is slight. Diagnosis is usually based on the history, but can be confirmed by demonstration of pox viral particles by electron microscopy in fluid exuded from the nodule. The host immune response to infection is poor, and recurrent lesions (due to reinfection, not reactivation) may occur.

Mary's middle finger (Figure 41.1b) shows a herpetic whitlow, i.e. infection with herpes simplex virus. Intact skin is an effective barrier to HSV, but if the contiguity of the dermis is broken HSV can gain access. Thus, dental workers are at risk of acquiring dermal infection in their hands because of cuts and abrasions sustained during manipulations in the mouths of patients shedding the virus. Alternative modes of acquisition are by accidental needlestick injury with a contaminated needle (herpetic whitlows are therefore an occupational hazard of many health-care workers) or by autoinoculation of nailfolds in children who bite their nails.

HSV infection of the dermis initiates an inflammatory response. The resultant oedema gives rise to an acutely painful and tender swelling, as the tightness of the skin of the fingers resists expansion. The patient may first notice mild itching and burning at the site of inoculation. Single or multiple vesicles appear, which coalesce into an oozing pustule or abscess filled with

a purulent-looking mixture of serum and debris. The differential diagnosis includes bacterial infection of the skin. Healing occurs gradually over a period of 2 or 3 weeks. If this is the patient's first exposure to HSV (i.e. a primary infection), the whitlow may be accompanied by evidence of systemic upset – fever and lymphadenopathy. As with other forms of HSV infection recurrences may occur at the same site – these are reactivations of the virus, not reinfections (compare with orf, above).

Summary: Blisters on hands

Differential diagnosis

- Orf – painless; reinfections may occur; occupationally associated (farm and animal workers)
- Herpetic whitlow – painful; recurrences may occur; occupationally associated (health-care workers)
- Hand, foot and mouth disease – Coxsackie virus infection; usually in a child (see Case 35)
- Cutaneous anthrax – rare; occupationally associated (e.g. tanning industry)

Diagnosis

Clinical; demonstration of viral particles in vesicle fluid by electron microscopy (orf, HSV)

Table 41.1 Parapox viruses and diseases

Mode of spread	Resulting human disease
Cattle to humans	Pseudocowpox, paravaccinia or milker's nodes
Sheep or goats to humans	Orf, or contagious pustular dermatitis

CASE 42
Skin rash and arthralgia in Eammon, a 25-year-old man

Eammon, a 25-year-old man, presents in mid-September with a 1-week history of arthralgia of the small joins of the hands and a painful elbow. Examination reveals discrete skin lesions on the arms and legs at various stages, which have been present for 3–4 days. Three weeks earlier Eammon and his girlfriend Susan had spent a 2-week holiday camping and fishing in the New Forest, England. Both reported being bitten on numerous occasions by insects and ticks, but she remains well.

Q What do the history and skin rash suggest?

A The combination of tick bites, a migrating skin rash and arthralgia

is consistent with a diagnosis of Lyme disease caused by *Borrelia burgdorferi*, a spirochaete transmitted by the *Ixodes* tick. Although first described in North America, this condition is now recognized in Europe and elsewhere. The initial clinical picture is characterized by erythema chronicum migrans, myalgia, arthralgia and lymphadenopathy. The disease may go undiagnosed and later present with a variety of manifestations, including those of the nervous (meningoencephalitis) and cardiovascular systems (see Figure 42.1).

Q What other infective conditions are tick-borne?

A A number of viral, bacterial and rickettsial conditions are tick-borne and are often travel associated (see Table 42.1).

Q How do you confirm the diagnosis of Lyme disease?

A Isolation of the bacterium from skin lesions is a specialized technique and largely confined to research centres. Serology is the mainstay of diagnosis. A fourfold rise in antibody titres, or a single elevated titre in an enzyme-linked immunoassay (ELISA), confirmed by immunoblotting, clinches the diagnosis.

Q What is the treatment of choice?

A Penicillin, erythromycin, tetracycline and the cephalosporins have all been used to treat Lyme disease. Oral tetracycline to treat early disease is associated with fewer late complications, and should be continued for 10–20 days. Ceftriaxone, a third-generation cephalosporin with a prolonged half-life, has been used successfully to treat CNS disease and has a lower failure rate than benzylpenicillin.

Q Should the patient's partner receive prophylactic antimicrobial chemotherapy?

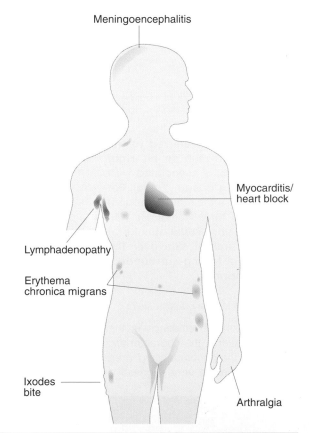

Meningoencephalitis

Myocarditis/heart block

Lymphadenopathy

Erythema chronica migrans

Ixodes bite

Arthralgia

Fig. 42.1 Clinical features of Lyme disease.

Table 42.1 Other tick-borne conditions, with geographical distributions

Condition	Organism	Geographical distribution
Louping ill (encephalitis)	Flavivirus	UK
Omsk haemorrhagic fever	Flavivirus	USSR
Colorado tick fever	Orbivirus	North America
Relapsing fever	*Borrelia recurrentis*	Asia, Europe, Africa
Mediterranean Spotted Fever	*Rickettsia conorii*	Europe, North, Central and South America
Tick-borne encephalitis	Arboviruses, e.g. flavivirus	Worldwide

A No. There is little evidence to suggest that antimicrobial agents administered after possible exposure either prevent or lessen the severity of disease. Those likely to be bitten by ticks in forests or elsewhere should minimize the skin surface area exposed, use insect repellents, and remove ticks likely to be caught in clothing as soon as they come indoors.

Summary: Lyme disease
Presentation
Variable, but skin rash following tick bite is the most common
Diagnosis
Clinical features confirmed by serology; paired sera usually required to demonstrate rise in antibodies
Management
Oral tetracycline but CNS infection more complex

CASE 43
Father Pat, a 45-year-old priest with a skin rash

Father Pat, a 45-year-old Roman Catholic priest, is referred to the dermatology outpatients clinic because of a skin rash on his right forearm. This has been present for some months, is associated with some skin discoloration and is slowly increasing in size. Father Pat has spent most of the past 20 years teaching in a missionary school in Tanzania, but is currently home on holidays for 6 weeks. He has never been seriously ill in the past apart from occasional attacks of malaria. The rash is characterized by a pale area of skin over the forearm (see Figure 43.1). There is some loss of feeling surrounding the lesion but general physical examination is normal.

Q What diagnostic test is indicated?

A A skin biopsy of the central and peripheral areas of the lesion should be taken and should also include some subcutaneous tissue.

Q What is the likely diagnosis?

A The history of residence in the developing world, the characteristic lesion and the accompanying area of anaesthesia are very suggestive

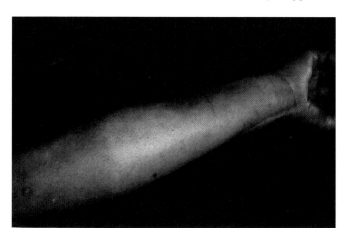

**Fig. 43.1
Skin lesions on forearm.**

of leprosy. Histological examination using haematoxylin and eosin (to show the presence of granuloma) and a modified Ziehl–Neelsen stain (to detect the presence of acid-fast bacilli, see Case 49), is likely to confirm this. The causative agent of leprosy, *Mycobacterium leprae*, has never been grown *in vitro*. Skin and antibody tests are of epidemiological value but are rarely useful in the diagnosis of an individual case because of a lack of specificity.

Q How is leprosy spread?

A It is generally assumed that leprosy is spread by skin-to-skin contact, hence the tradition of ostracizing sufferers over the centuries. The epidermis of the skin is, however, usually intact and free of bacilli. It is more likely that the bacteria are shed from the nose. The number in nasal secretions may approximate to the numbers found in the sputum of patients with 'open' tuberculosis (see Case 49). The disease is almost exclusively confined to humans, but leprosy has been described in armadillos, chimpanzees and monkeys. In endemic areas patients may have both leprosy and tuberculosis, and this has to be considered in diagnosis and management.

Q What are the complications of leprosy?

A The spectrum of disease varies from the lepromatous to the tuberculoid forms, with a number of stages in between (see Box 43.1). Hypersensitivity reactions are a feature of leprosy and these may be cell mediated (type 4 hypersensitivity reaction), giving rise to swollen nerves, or characterized by immune complex formation Recognized complications include:

- erythema nodosum leprosum: more common in forms where bacilli are plentiful and consists of

B43.1 Features of lepromatous and tuberculoid leprosy

	Lepromatous	Tuberculoid
Clinical features		
Nasal destruction	+/-	+
Skin lesions	++	+/-
Nerves	little damage	extensive damage
Response to antimicrobial therapy	poor	good
Pathology		
Baciilli in lesions	++	+/-
Granuloma	-	++
Antibodies to *M. leprae*	++	+/-

erythematous plaques or nodules with endarteritis, phlebitis and leukaemoid reactions due to immune complexes

- physical deformities: nasomaxillary destruction and damage to upper and lower limbs, resulting from loss of sensory function and paralysis
- blindness: occurs in 5% of cases due to corneal ulceration or iridocyclitis.

Orchitis, periosteitis, cutaneous vasculitis (Lucio's phenomenon) and secondary amyloidosis may also occur.

The skin biopsy from Father Pat's lesion reveals mature epithelioid and Langerhans' cells with granulomata, but no bacilli are seen. Infiltration of the nerves and epidermis is seen, however, and it is concluded that Father Pat has a tuberculoid form of leprosy. He is started on antimicrobial chemotherapy and arrangements are made for him to be followed up when he returns to Tanzania.

Q What are the main drugs used to treat leprosy?

A Dapsone, a bacteriostatic agent, is the most useful drug. It is increasingly being used in combination because of the emergence of resistance. A 6–12-month course of dapsone and rifampicin is recommended for patients with tuberculoid forms. Two years' treatment or longer is necessary for lepromatous forms with two or more drugs such as daily dapsone and clofazimine (may cause discoloration of the skin) supplemented with monthly rifampicin. Surgery to correct deformities, such as a collapsed nasal bridge, and referral to an ophthalmologist may be appropriate in more advanced disease.

Summary: Leprosy
Presentation
Raised skin lesions with localized anaesthesia, but extensive destruction of limbs and nasomaxillary area seen in advanced disease
Diagnosis
Clinical features and skin biopsy
Management
Dapsone in combination with other agents for 6–12 months or longer, with surgical treatment of complications

CASE 44
Mary, a 35-year-old engineer with nausea, weakness and rigors

Late on Friday evening Mary, a 35-year-old engineer, is taken to the Accident and Emergency department of her local hospital following consultation with her GP by phone. That afternoon she had become feverish, nauseous and generally weak. Later, she had experienced two episodes of rigors. Four years previously she had a breast lump removed which was benign, and during her two pregnancies had had recurrent urinary tract infections. A week before this presentation she complained of dysuria and frequency, and was prescribed oral ampicillin for presumed cystitis.

Q What is the most likely diagnosis and which physical sign may confirm this?

A Pyelonephritis is the most likely diagnosis, often characterized by renal angle tenderness with fever.

On examination Mary looks flushed, has a temperature of 40°C and a tachycardia of 120/min. General physical examination, including that of the breasts and axillary lymph nodes, is normal apart from acute tenderness in the costovertebral or renal angle. There is protein and blood in a urine sample.

Q What investigations are indicated to confirm the diagnosis?

A A midstream sample of urine (MSU) should be examined microscopically for white and red cells, and cultured. Blood for culture should also be taken (Box 44.1). A white cell count may reveal a polymorph leukocytosis, which would be consistent with a bacterial infection.

Q How many blood culture sets should be taken?

A Two sets of blood cultures (i.e. four bottles, two per set), preferably at different times should be taken. A negative result if one set only is taken may be false due to intermittent bacteraemia. Furthermore, the isolation of a skin bacterium, e.g. *Staphylococcus epidermidis*, may represent a false positive result, if only one set is taken owing to contamination when the blood was taken. In general, the greater the volume of blood cultured the higher the diagnostic yield. It is rarely necessary, however, to take more than two sets, except with a fever of undetermined origin (see Case 50) or infective endocarditis (see Case 46).

Q Is the yield of positive cultures from children, especially small infants, less than that from adults?

A No. It is clearly undesirable to take large volumes of blood from small children but this is compensated for by a higher number of organisms per ml of blood compared with adults. In bacteraemic adults 1 colony-forming unit (cfu) per ml is the norm, but in infants 10–100 times more organisms may be present.

B44.1 Steps in the taking of blood for culture

- Hands should be washed; gloves unnecessary unless inoculation risk (i.e. hepatitis B or HIV patient)
- Inspect skin for suitable peripheral vein and disinfect (e.g. chlorhexidine in alcohol)
- Remove caps from top of blood culture bottles (usually two per set) and disinfect bung with alcohol
- Withdraw 10 ml of blood (for one set), replace needle and inject blood equally into both bottles
- Take blood culture bottles to the laboratory immediately or place in incubator

---

SECTION 6

SYSTEMIC INFECTIONS

On admission, blood cultures and an MSU are taken and Mary is pre-scribed a first-generation cephalosporin, cephradine, which is admin-istered orally. A lactose-positive oxidase-negative coliform is isolated from the MSU, in which there are numerous pus cells seen, and Gram-negative bacilli are seen in blood cultures. Mary's antibiotic therapy is changed as she remains symptomatic.

Q What is the likely identity of the organism in the urine and blood?

A The positive MSU and blood cultures, suggest that Mary has pyelonephritis (upper urinary tract infection with bacteraemia). The commonest cause of urinary tract infection (see Case 26) is *Escherichia coli*, a lactose-positive coliform (see Box 44.2).

Q What is the difference between 'bacteraemia' and 'septicaemia'?

A The terminology is a little con-fusing here! Strictly speaking, 'bacter-aemia' refers to the presence of bacteria in the bloodstream and does not imply anything about the clinical state of the patient. Further-more, transient clinically insignificant bacteraemia is a relatively common everyday occurrence, e.g. following defecation or while brushing teeth. The transient nature of these episodes, the low virulence of the bacteria involved, and the presence of an intact immune system ensures that there are usually no clinical consequences.

In contrast, 'septicaemia' implies that the presence of bacteria in the blood is accompanied by clinical consequences, such as high fever, rigors, low blood pressure. With septicaemia there are greater num-bers of dividing bacteria in the blood, which are more likely to be pathogenic. In recent years the terms 'bacteraemia' and 'septicaemia' have become interchangeable, especially in North America. Which-ever term is used, *E. coli* is the commonest cause (see Table 44.1) and may be community or hospital acquired.

Q What is the most frequent pri-mary source of bacteraemia?

A The urinary tract is implicated as the source in 30% of all cases of clinically significant bacteraemia, and this is especially true when *E. coli*, *Klebsiella* spp., *P. aeruginosa* or other Gram-negative bacteria are involved. Other sources include:

- respiratory tract 15%, *Str. pneu-moniae*, *S. aureus*
- gastrointestinal tract 10%, *E. coli*, *salmonella* etc.
- biliary tract 10%, *E. coli*

- intravascular lines 5%, coagulase-negative staphylococci (e.g. *S. epidermidis*), *S. aureus*

In a proportion of cases, however, no source can be detected clinically, microbiologically or following exten-sive radiological investigations.

Q Is clinically significant bacteraemia or septicaemia always present in septic shock?

A With a greater understanding in recent years of the pathogenesis of septic shock (see Figure 44.1) it is apparent that this is a spectrum of conditions which may or may not be accompanied by the presence of bacteria in the bloodstream. A patient may have overwhelming sepsis with negative blood cultures because of recent antibiotics, intermittent bac-teraemia, or endotoxaemia without bacteraemia. Other terms used to describe patients with serious sepsis, especially if requiring intensive care (see Case 20), include:

- pyaemia: chills, and fever due to an abscess
- sepsis syndrome: clinical evidence of infection, with tachypnoea, tachycardia, hyper- or hypothermia and evidence of inadequate organ perfusion (e.g. hypoxaemia, oliguria)
- septic shock: sepsis syndrome with hypotension (systolic blood

---

B44.2 *Escherichia coli*

- A motile Gram-negative bacillus which grows well on non-selective media
- Virulence may be related to the presence of certain K antigens, especially in urinary tract infection (UTI)
- Predominates amongst the aerobic flora of the intestine, especially the colon
- May also be found in the lower urinary and genital tracts, and occasionally in the upper respiratory tract
- Causes UTI (see Case 26), septicaemia, neonatal meningitis (see Case 1), intra-abdominal infection (see Case 20) and diarrhoea (see Case 19)

Table 44.1 Aetiology of clinically significant bacteraemia

Organism	Hospital (HA) or community (CA) acquired	Incidence (% of total cases)
Escherichia coli	HA = CA	29
Staphylococcus aureus	HA > CA, 2;1	19
Streptococcus pneumoniae	CA > HA, 10;1	13
Klebsiella spp.	HA > CA, 3:1	7
Pseudomonas aeruginosa	HA > CA, 10:1	5
'Viridans' streptococci	CA > HA, 3:1	4
Coagulase-negative staphylococci	HA > CA 20:1	4
Miscellaneous	Varies with the organism	19

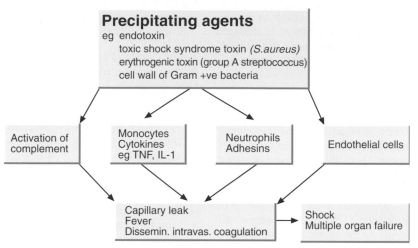

Fig. 44.1 Pathogenesis of septic shock.

bacteraemia. Underlying diseases, e.g. malignancy or accompanying life-threatening conditions, e.g. multiple severe trauma, also contribute to an unfavourable outcome. Factors associated with a high mortality include:

- extremes of age, i.e. very young (premature neonate) or the elderly (>75 years)
- white cell count, i.e. <4 or >30 $\times 10^9$/l
- polymicrobial infection, e.g. *E. coli* and *S. aureus* from pneumonia with bacteraemia
- shock at initial presentation
- significant or severe underlying disease, e.g. diabetic ketoacidosis
- inappropriate or inadequate initial antibiotics.

pressure <90 mmHg) in the absence of other causes.

Q Comment on the choice of antibiotic and route of administration in the treatment of Mary's condition.

A Clinically significant bacteraemia is a potential medical emergency because of complications such as shock and multiple organ failure. Consequently, parenteral antibiotics active against the likely pathogens are indicated, and if the source or organism is not known a broad-spectrum agent should be used. Initial treatment with oral antibiotics is therefore not appropriate, and cephradine is not optimal here because of the possibility that the bacterium may be resistant.

Q What alternatives are there?

A Mary should be changed to an intravenous second- or third-generation cephalosporin, an aminoglycoside (e.g. gentamicin) or a fluoroquinolone (e.g. ciprofloxacin), all of which are appropriate in pyelonephritis as approximately 40–50% of coliforms will be resistant to ampicillin and the earlier cephalosporins. Supportive measures are also important, especially where complications have ensued (see Box 44.3).

Mary is treated with intravenous cefotaxime for 7 days as the *E. coli* isolated from blood and urine is resistant to ampicillin, cephradine and trimethoprim. After 72 hours she is apyrexial and her other symptoms have largely resolved. Before discharge from hospital arrangements are made for investigation of her genitourinary tract (see Case 26), to detect renal tract abnormalities which might explain her recurrent UTIs.

Q What is the mortality from clinically significant bacteraemia?

A Around 30% of patients die directly or indirectly from

Summary: Bacteraemia/ Septicaemia
Presentation
Fever, rigors, shock with or without symptoms related to original focus of infection, e.g. cough, sputum, chest pain with pneumonic bacteraemia
Diagnosis
Usually confirmed by isolating organisms from blood cultures
Management
Reverse shock with i.v. fluids, intravenous high-dose antibiotics (broad spectrum if aetiology unknown or pending). No role for corticosteroids.

B44.3 Management of clinically significant bacteraemia

Supportive therapy	Fluids, e.g. intravenous colloids, saline etc. Inotropes, e.g. dobutamine with monitoring Organ support, e.g. ventilation, haemofiltration
Removal of infected focus	Surgery to drain abscess Removal of infected intravascular catheter Wound debridement
Antibiotics	Must be intravenous at least initially and in high dose *Broad spectrum*: if aetiology unknown and focus cannot be removed, e.g. cefotaxime + metronidazole for intra-abdominal sepsis *Narrow spectrum*: when organism known, e.g. flucloxacillin for *S. aureus*
Immunotherapy	? corticosteroids: no current evidence of benefit ? monoclonal antibodies, e.g. antiendotoxin (HA-1A) not effective, others being evaluated

CASE 45
Tony, a 65-year-old man with vomiting, abdominal pain and fever

Tony, a 65-year-old man, presented to hospital with vomiting, right-sided abdominal pain and fever. At laparotomy a mass was detected in the ascending colon, with perforation of the bowel and generalized peritonitis. The tumour was resected and a right hemicolectomy performed. Histological examination revealed a poorly differentiated adenocarcinoma. His postoperative course was characterized by fever, a leukocytosis (white cell count $24 \times 10^9/l$) and a wound infection caused by *Staphylococcus aureus* and *Bacteroides fragilis*. Despite a 10-day course of intravenous cefotaxime, flucloxacillin and metronidazole, he remains pyrexial with a temperature of 39–40°C and is generally unwell 2 weeks after surgery. He is unable to tolerate oral feeds, is being fed parenterally via a central line, and he also has a urinary catheter.

Q What are the possible causes of the persistent fever and leukocytosis?

A Infection is the most likely cause. Possible sites of infection include the wound, abdomen (persistent peritonitis or an intraabdominal abscess requiring drainage), intravascular line, bloodstream, urinary tract (especially as he is catheterized) and chest. Other possible causes include the effects of the tumour, deep venous thrombosis or pulmonary embolism and a drug-related fever.

Q What steps should be taken to identify the source and aetiology of the probable infection?

A Despite the antibiotics, a full septic screen should be taken, which includes two to three sets of blood cultures, a wound swab or pus (preferable if present), urine, sputum if productive cough, and removal of intravascular lines for culture if line infection is possible. These specimens should preferably be taken just before antibiotics are given, when serum and tissue antibiotic levels are at their lowest, to maximize the chances of isolating a pathogen. A chest X-ray may help to exclude lower respiratory tract infection, and an ultrasound examination or an isotope or CT scan may help diagnose an intra-abdominal collection.

The initial results of Tony's investigations are as follows: blood cultures are sterile after 48 hours; a scanty growth of an enterococcus is isolated from the wound swab; a catheter urine specimen is sterile; *Candida albicans* is isolated from a pharyngeal swab; and respiratory commensals only are grown from a mucoid specimen of sputum. The chest X-ray reveals right basal atelectasis but no gross evidence of infection, and both an ultrasound and CT examination of the abdomen are negative for an intra-abdominal collection. Topical nystatin is prescribed for the oral candidiasis but the antibacterial agents are discontinued.

Q Was it a good decision to stop the antibiotics?

A Unless there is overwhelming infection it is reasonable to discontinue antibiotics now after 10 days, reassess the clinical situation and reculture. Prolonged courses of antibiotics result in the selection of resistant bacteria and superinfections. Enterococci, as isolated here, rarely cause wound infection but are selected for by the use of cephalosporins to which they are resistant.

Q Is the oral candidiasis likely to be the cause of his persistent pyrexia?

A Oral or vaginal candidiasis is quite common in patients who have been on antibiotics owing to selective pressures on the normal flora, but rarely result in systemic signs or symptoms. Colonization or superficial infection (see Case 20) is not a reliable predictor of systemic candida infection, except perhaps with *C. tropicalis* in immunocompromised patients during an outbreak.

Three days later it is noticed that the site of the central line is inflamed and pus is present. A sample of this is sent to the microbiology laboratory for culture and repeat blood cultures are taken. The following day the laboratory calls to say that yeasts are present in one of the blood culture bottles.

Q Is the presence of yeasts in only one set of blood cultures likely to represent contamination?

A The isolation of *Candida* from blood cultures should always be regarded as significant until proven otherwise. Although yeasts may colonize the skin, especially in a patient who has been on broad-spectrum antibacterial agents, they should not be considered as contaminants in the blood, unlike coagulase-negative staphylococci (e.g. *Staphylococcus epidermidis*), micrococci and diphtheroids. Furthermore, Tony has a number of risk factors for systemic Candida infection or candidaemia (see Box 45.1).

Q What should be done next to confirm this diagnosis?

A Further blood cultures should be taken and, where possible (i.e. if an intra-arterial or triple-lumen intravenous catheter is present), these sets should be taken through the catheter if this is suspected as the source. Isolation of *Candida* from pus taken around the catheter site

B45.1 Risk factors for systemic candida infection

- Immunocompromised state, e.g. neutropenia, malignancy, corticosteroids
- Presence of a foreign body, e.g. intravascular catheter (see Figure 45.1), urinary catheter
- Major surgery, e.g. bowel resection, ruptured aortic aneurysm
- Broad-spectrum antibacterial agents, e.g. cephalosporins such as cefotaxime, quinolones such as ciprofloxacin
- Extensive burns
- Parenteral nutrition

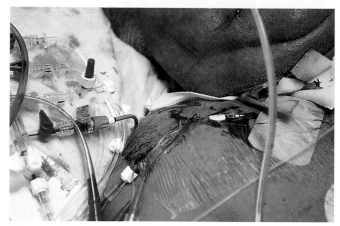

Fig. 45.1 Central line, a possible source of candidaemia.

and from the tip of the central line, if removed, will also confirm this as the likely source. Removal of the infected line tip in addition is usually necessary for effective eradication.

Q How is systemic candida infection usually diagnosed?

A Clinical suspicion in patients with one or more risk factors is the first requirement for early diagnosis. Laboratory confirmation may be achieved by:

- Blood cultures: only about 50% of blood cultures are positive in candidaemia. Specialized techniques such as lysis centrifugation (releases yeasts from inside white cells) are recommended by some as this increases the yield, but these are not always available
- Tissue biopsy: skin lesions may accompany candidaemia and yeasts may be isolated from these or visualized on histology. Similarly, internal organs such as the liver, kidneys may be biopsied if these are involved
- Antibody detection: some patients may develop serum precipitins to *C. albicans*, but this is dependent on a normal immune response, which may be absent in immunocompromised patients. The presence of antibodies is suggestive but not diagnostic

- Antigen detection: during candidaemia a variety of metabolites (e.g. D-arabinitol) or antigens (e.g. enolase, mannan) may be detected in the serum of systemically infected patients, but the presence of these is usually transient and may be missed when the sample is taken. In addition, these tests are not readily available
- Polymerase chain reaction: an ultrasensitive technique for the detection of genomic material which is increasingly being used in the diagnosis of many other infectious conditions and offers considerable promise for the future. However, there is no routine service available at present.

Q What options are there for the treatment of systemic candida infection?

A Intravenous amphotericin B with or without flucytosine is still considered the treatment of choice for systemic candida infection. Renal failure due to amphotericin B, acquired candida resistance to flucytosine, liver toxicity or bone marrow failure with flucytosine, and the many side effects of amphotericin B, such as rigors, thrombocytopenia, hypokalaemia, hypomagnesaemia and rising creatinine, are significant problems.

Liposomal or colloidal amphotericin B, which are new preparations, are said to be more effective because higher doses can be administered with a lower incidence of side-effects. However, these compounds are still being evaluated and are very expensive. The newer triazole drugs fluconazole and itraconazole are interesting additions to the repertoire of antifungal chemotherapy. They have a role to play in the treatment of oesophagitis and some systemic candida infections, but should not be regarded as agents of choice, especially in the severely immunocompromised host. Furthermore, some *Candida* species, e.g. *C. kruzei*, are resistant to fluconazole. These agents are, however, increasingly used in the treatment of less severe fungal infections such as superficial (i.e. oral, vaginal and skin) candidiasis.

Q What other systemic candida infections do you know of?

A *Candida spp.* can infect almost any organ in the body but endocarditis, meningitis and infection of the liver and spleen are especially difficult to treat. Some features of these and other infections are outlined in Table 45.1.

Table 45.1 Other deep-seated candida infections (may be accompanied by candidaemia)

Infection	Clinical features	Comments
Peritonitis	Cloudy dialysate with CAPD (see Case 27)	Removal of catheter required
	Usually following bowel surgery	Antifungal agents not essential if adequate drainage
Urinary infection	Often asymptomatic if lower renal tract involved in catheterized patient	Removal of catheter usually followed by clearance
	Renal abscess may be a feature of disseminated candidiasis	Poor prognosis if immunocompromised
Hepatosplenic candidiasis	Fever of undetermined origin in leukaemic/ neutropenic patient with elevated liver function tests	Diagnosis made by liver scan or biopsy Prolonged antifungal chemotherapy required
Endocarditis	Occasional cause of endocarditis. Acute presentation with fever and emboli in at-risk patient, e.g. intravenous drug abuser	Multiple blood cultures may be sterile and echocardiogram often negative (see Case 46)
Arthritis, osteomyelitis, meningitis, ophthalmitis	Localized signs and symptoms	Often associated with trauma and diagnosed on tissue culture. Prognosis variable

The central line is removed and *C. albicans* is isolated from the tip and pus at the site. Repeat blood cultures are also positive. Tony is started on intravenous fluconazole but remains pyrexial. Later that week he starts to vomit, his abdomen becomes distended, his urine output declines and his serum urea and creatinine increase. He undergoes a laparotomy, which reveals that the bowel anastomosis has broken down, with resultant peritonitis. In the intensive therapy unit, he rapidly goes downhill with respiratory failure due to the adult respiratory distress syndrome, renal failure and jaundice. He dies shortly afterwards, 3 weeks after admission. At postmortem, micrometastases from his bowel tumour are detected in his liver and a vegetation, from which *C. albicans* is isolated, is seen on his tricuspid valve.

Table 45.2 Other systemic fungal infections

Disease	Pathogen	Location	Features
Aspergillosis	*A. fumigatus, A. flavus* (moulds)	Worldwide	Pneumonia, disseminated disease, aspergilloma, allergic lung disease
Cryptococcosis	*C. neoformans* (true yeast)	Worldwide	Meningitis, occasionally respiratory or disseminated
Histoplasmosis	*H. capsulatum* (dimorphic fungus)	River valleys of eastern USA	Pneumonia disseminated in AIDS
Coccidioidomycosis	*C. immitis* (dimorphic fungus)	USA and Mexico	Respiratory, skin or subcutaneous involvement

Q Is it surprising that Tony died despite the fluconazole?

A The prognosis from candidaemia is disappointing when the underlying state of the patient is poor. The development of multiple organ failure heralds an especially poor prognosis and makes treatment more difficult. It is unlikely that conventional or liposomal amphotericin B, although perhaps preferable would have altered the outcome here.

Q Which patients should be considered for prophylactic antifungal chemotherapy?

A This is a difficult question. The increasing number of patients at risk of systemic candida and systemic fungal infections (see Table 45.2) has stimulated interest in targeting certain patients for chemoprophylaxis e.g. those with neutropenia. Oral fluconazole is often prescribed as part of a selective gut decontamination regimen for the duration of the risk period, i.e. just before the onset of neutropenia and until the white cell count begins to increase. Itraconazole has been used prophylactically for neutropenic patients at risk of invasive aspergillosis, e.g. during building construction work, when there will be dissemination of fungal spores.

Summary: Systemic candida infection
Presentation
Fever with or without localizing signs in an at-risk patient, e.g. neutropenia, broad-spectrum antibiotics, leukaemia etc.
Diagnosis
Blood cultures (positive in only 50%), isolation from deep site, e.g. liver biopsy, serum positive for antibodies, antigens or metabolites (where available)
Management
Correction of underlying risk factors (if possible), intravenous amphotericin B or fluconazole

CASE 46

Eric, a pyrexial 76-year-old war veteran with a heart murmur

Eric, a 76-year-old retired war veteran, is seen in the medical out-patients clinic for evaluation of persistent fever, malaise, anorexia and weight loss. He has been fit and healthy throughout his life, apart from a 'touch of malaria' during the war! During the past 3–4 months, however, he and his wife Doris have noticed that he has 'slowed up', and that he has been hot and sweaty on occasions. He has no respiratory symptoms and there has been no change in bowel habit. On examination he has a tachycardia of 100/min and a temperature of 37.5°C, but his blood pressure and respiratory rate are normal. He has extensive gum disease and dental hygiene is poor. There is a soft diastolic murmur at the sternal border but examination of the lungs, abdomen and rectum is normal. There is no lymphadenopathy.

Q Is this man sufficiently ill to warrant admission to hospital?

A Yes. Although Eric is not critically ill he requires observation and investigation, which is best done in hospital.

Q What diagnosis should be considered first?

A Infective endocarditis. The combination of fever, systemic symptoms such as weight loss, and a changing or recently diagnosed murmur should immediately alert one to this diagnosis. A minority of patients have a history of a recent precipitating procedure, such as dental extraction, and there may be no record of damaged heart valves such as that following rheumatic valve disease (see Figure 46.1).

Q How may a diagnosis of infective endocarditis be confirmed?

A Three sets of blood cultures should be taken, at least 30 minutes apart and preferably from different sites. It is usual in endocarditis for all three to be positive, as a continuous bacteraemia is typical of this condition (see also Case 44). Sometimes it may be necessary to take more than three sets, e.g. if the patient has recently been on antibiotics, or if a fastidious organism is suspected as the cause. It is important to delay antimicrobial therapy if possible until a microbiological diagnosis has been made, to ensure that the most appropriate treatment is started. Vegetations seen on an echocardiogram are very suggestive of infective endocarditis, but a negative result does not exclude the diagnosis because in early disease they may not be visible or they may be difficult to see in right-sided disease. Other helpful investigations include a full blood count (raised white cell count due to bacterial infection, anaemia due to chronic disease), ESR, urinalysis (haematuria indicative of glomerulonephritis, see Figure 46.1) and an immunology profile, which might include C_3 and C_4 levels (both low), C_3 degradation products (elevated) and assays for the presence of immune complexes.

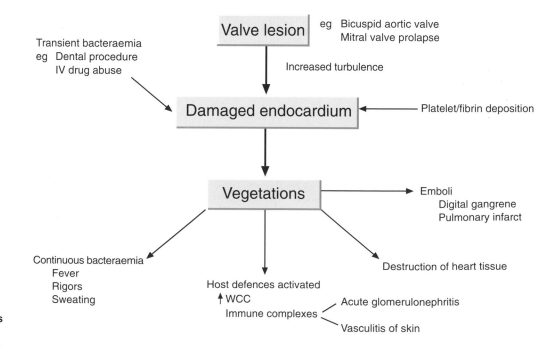

Fig. 46.1 Pathogenesis of infective endocarditis.

Q What is subacute bacterial endocarditis (SBE) and is it different from infective endocarditis?

A In the pre-antibiotic era SBE was characterized by a prolonged illness of 3–6 months with many of the classic clinical manifestations, such as Osler's nodes, Roth spots. This illness was due to low-grade pathogens such as 'viridans' streptococci. This was in contrast to acute bacterial endocarditis caused by more virulent bacteria such as *Staphylococcus aureus* or *Streptococcus pyogenes* (β-haemolytic streptococci group A), where the course of the illness was uniformly fatal within a matter of days to weeks. This clinical distinction is less relevant now, and the term 'infective endocarditis' is used to encompass both of the previously used terms and also to acknowledge that there are non-bacterial causes.

Q What groups of organisms are most commonly implicated in the aetiology of infective endocarditis?

A Streptococci, especially 'viridans' streptococci (see Case 36) and *Staphylococcus aureus* are the most common causes (see Table 46.1).

Eric is admitted to a bed in the cardiology division for observation and evaluation. He is persistently pyrexial over the next 48 hours, and although his white cell count is normal he is mildly anaemic (Hb 9.7 g/dl). *Streptococcus mitis* **is isolated from three sets of blood cultures (six bottles). The echocardiogram reveals an aortic valve with regurgitation, and a vegetation (see Figure 46.2). Urinalysis and a complement profile are normal.**

Q What is *S. mitis* and where may it have come from?

A *S. mitis*, usually an α-haemolytic 'viridans' streptococcus, is a normal inhabitant of the oral cavity and the upper respiratory tract. It accounts

Table 46.1 Organisms implicated in the aetiology of infective endocarditis

Organisms	Incidence (%)
Streptococci	**65**
'Viridans'	50
Enterococci	10
Others	5
Staphylococci	**20**
S. aureus	14
Coagulase negative	6
Others	**5**
e.g. Gram-negative bacilli, fungi	
No organism identified	**10**

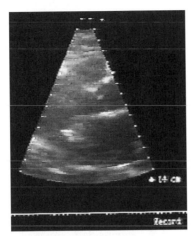

Fig. 46.2 2D echocardiogram of aortic valve vegetation.

for 15–20% of infective endocarditis and may gain access to the bloodstream during dental procedures, such as tooth extraction or even during scaling. Eric's extensive gum disease is likely to be significant as a possible source. In the majority of patients, however, no predisposing event is identifiable.

Q What is the role of the microbiology department in the management of endocarditis?

A The medical microbiologist, using all the resources of the laboratory, has an important role to play in the diagnosis and treatment of infective endocarditis. This includes:

- isolation and identification of the organism to indicate the possible source (e.g. 'viridans' streptococci from the oral cavity, *S. bovis* from a bowel tumour) and what

measures may be necessary to prevent recurrence (e.g. dental hygiene)
- sensitivity testing, minimum inhibitory and minimum bactericidal concentrations (MIC and MBC) as well as routine tests to assess how sensitive the bacterium is, especially to penicillin. Dosages of antibiotics will be influenced by what serum concentrations are required to kill and not just inhibit the bacteria
- serum bactericidal test. The patient's serum, taken while he or she is on antibiotics, is assessed to determine how effective the antibiotics and the host defences are in inhibiting the growth of and killing the bacteria. An eight fold dilution of serum that is capable of killing the organism is said to be predictive of clinical success
- antibiotic assays. Because of the low therapeutic index of aminoglycosides and vancomycin, key agents used in treatment (see Case 20), it is essential to monitor serum levels regularly to ensure adequate but non-toxic levels
- C-reactive protein (often assayed in immunology or biochemistry departments) may be used to monitor response to treatment.

The isolate of *S. mitis* has an MIC and MBC to penicillin of 0.03 mg/l, i.e. very sensitive. Eric is started on high-dose intravenous penicillin and gentamicin. A serum bactericidal test performed 4 days into therapy shows a

predose titre (sample of blood taken just before administration of antibiotics) of 1 in 16 and a post-dose titre of 1 in 32. Eric's temperature gradually falls over the next 3 days, he is seen by a dentist and his general condition improves.

Q Why is gentamicin used when the isolate is very sensitive to penicillin?

A The aminoglycosides, including gentamicin, have poor activity against streptococci but act synergistically when combined with a β-lactam antibiotic such as penicillin. This probably relates to different modes of action: penicillin disrupts the cell wall, facilitating the entry of gentamicin into the cell and its action on protein synthesis. Synergistic antibiotic activity is important in eradicating bacteria from the vegetations.

Q What is the normal duration of therapy for infective endocarditis?

A Where a 'viridans' streptococcus is very sensitive to penicillin, 2 weeks of i.v. followed by 2 weeks of oral antibiotics is usually adequate. With a less sensitive isolate, e.g. an enterococcus, 4 or even 6 weeks of i.v treatment is recommended. Four weeks of parenteral treatment with flucloxacillin and an aminoglycoside or fusidic acid is preferred for staphylococcal endocarditis. Vanco-mycin or teicoplanin are indicated if there is allergy to penicillin or if resistant bacteria (e.g. methicillin-resistant *S. aureus*) are respon-sible. These are, however, only general guidelines and therapy should be individualized to the patient's circumstances, response to treatment and underlying cardiac abnormality.

Q What is the mortality from infective endocarditis?

A Since the start of the antibiotic era mortality has declined significantly to around 30%, largely due to earlier diagnosis, more aggressive treatment and surgery. The outlook is better

B46.1 Prosthetic valve endocarditis (incidence 2%)	
Early	Within the first 3 months of surgery Organisms acquired during surgery and hence preventable Staphylococci predominate 70% mortality
Late	Occurs 3 months or later after surgery Aetiology similar to native valve endocarditis 10% mortality

for native valve as opposed to prosthetic valve endocarditis (see Box 46.1) and the prognosis is also influenced by the aetiology (staphylococcal and Gram-negative endocarditis have a higher morality), the age of the patient, presentation (significant cardiac decompensation and embolic phenomena herald a poorer outcome), and response to treatment. Other recent changes in the epidemiology of infective endocarditis include:

- endocarditis in intravenous drug abusers (right-sided relatively more common) due to *S. aureus*, yeasts or *Pseudomonas aeruginosa* is increasingly common.
- Clinical presentation characterized by fewer of the classic stigmata, such as splinter haemorrhages, Osler's nodes, due to earlier diagnosis and treatment.
- Now more a disease of the elderly rather than the young or middle-aged, due to increasing life ex-pectancy and the declining incidence of rheumatic fever.
- 'Viridans' streptococci account for proportionally fewer cases and enterococcal and staphylococcal infection increasing in incidence.

A week after the start of anti-biotics, however, Eric's temp-erature spikes to 38.5°C but his general condition, including cardiac status, remains unchanged.

Q What are the possible reasons for the recurrence of Eric's pyrexia?

A Possible explanations:

- extensive infection of the valve ring and adjacent structures, re-quiring surgery and immediate valve replacement
- metastatic infection involving bones, kidneys; more likely with *S. aureus* endocarditis than with streptococcal infection
- systemic or pulmonary emboli, the latter more common in right-sided infection, as with i.v. drug abusers
- drug hypersensitivity or allergy
- a second infection, e.g. intra-vascular line
- antibiotic resistance: relatively rare when patients are on combined treatment.

Most patients respond fairly quickly to i.v. antibiotics if the organism isolated is sensitive to conventional antibiotics. In culture-negative endo-carditis it is always possible that treatment is not appropriate or that a rare cause is responsible (see Box 46.2). Failure to respond to treatment or recurring pyrexia re-quires a careful and multidisciplinary approach involving cardiologist, microbiologist, infectious diseases physician and cardiac surgeon (urgent valve replacement may be required).

B46.2 'Culture negative endocarditis'
Refers to cases of infective endocarditis where no organism is isolated or an atypical cause is identified
Causes
• Recent antibiotics, especially if taken for >3 days • Fastidious organisms, e.g. haemophilus–actinobacillus–cardiobacterium–eikenella–kingella (HACEK) group, brucella (see Case 50), legionella (see Case 13) • Fungi, e.g. *Candida* spp. in drug abusers, *Aspergillus* following valve surgery • *Coxiella burnetii* (Q fever) and *Chlamydia psittaci*, both diagnosed serologically

CASE 46

Eric is assessed for local or systemic spread of infection, clinically and by echocardiogram. Repeat blood cultures are negative. The site of the peripheral line through which he is receiving the i.v. antibiotics is a little inflamed. Consequently, the line is removed and a central one inserted for the duration of i.v. antibiotic therapy. *S. epidermidis*, resistant to penicillin, gentamicin and flucloxacillin but sensitive to vancomycin, is isolated from the removed peripheral vascular catheter tip and the fever resolves without a change in his antibiotics. After 2 weeks of parenteral penicillin and gentamicin his treatment is changed to oral amoxycillin, and 3 days later Eric is discharged from hospital to be followed up in the clinic.

Q What advice should Eric be given regarding future visits to the dentist?

A He should receive prophylactic antibiotics when undergoing dental extractions, scaling or periodontal surgery. Patients with prosthetic valves, patients with a previous attack of endocarditis, and patients due to have a general anaesthetic who have damaged heart valves, are all at increased risk. These patients should receive parenteral amoxycillin at induction and orally 6 hours later, plus gentamicin 120 mg at induction. Other at-risk patients, i.e. those with rheumatic or congenital heart disease and mitral valve prolapse, should receive high-dose oral amoxycillin, i.e. 3 g 1 hour before the procedure. Clindamycin is preferred for patients allergic to penicillin.

Summary: Infective endocarditis
Presentation
Fever in a patient with a new or changing murmur, pyrexia of unknown aetiology, embolic phenomena
Diagnosis
Clinical features and repeated positive blood cultures with or without a positive echocardiogram
Management
Intravenous followed by oral antibiotics for 4 or more weeks, with close liaison between all involved in management

CASE 47
Margaret returns from Africa with a fever and headache

Margaret arrives in A and E at 3 o'clock in the morning, with a high fever, headache and backache. She first felt ill on the previous day, with nausea, vomiting and anorexia, and what she describes as bouts of shivering and feeling cold. She is 25 years old, a qualified nurse, and has been working at a mission hospital in Zimbabwe for the previous 6 months, returning to England 2 weeks ago. Prior to her departure from England she received vaccinations against hepatitis A and typhoid, and she had been taking chloroquine prophylaxis against malaria, although she admits to having missed occasional doses. She was previously fit and well, and on no regular medication. On examination her temperature is 39.6°C, she has a tachycardia of 120, but there are no other physical signs.

CASE 47

Q What is the differential diagnosis and initial management?

A Malaria must be the first consideration in a patient developing fever within a year of visiting an endemic area, despite the history of prophylaxis. Other possibilities include bacterial meningitis, influenza and typhoid.

A diagnosis of malaria constitutes a medical emergency, as there are a number of life-threatening complications, the risks of which increase with delay in instituting appropriate therapy. Therefore Margaret must be admitted to hospital, and a range of diagnostic tests performed.

Q What is the cause of malaria?

A Infection with one or more of the four plasmodia that infect humans:

- *P. falciparum* (malignant tertian malaria, throughout the tropics, especially Africa, southeast Asia, south America)
- *P. vivax* (common cause of benign tertian malaria, Indian subcontinent, Africa, southeast Asia)
- *P. ovale* (uncommon cause of benign tertian malaria, Africa)
- *P. malariae* (quartan malaria, throughout the tropical world).

Q How is the diagnosis of malaria made in the laboratory?

A By examination of unfixed thick films stained by Field's stain, and thin blood films stained at pH 7.2 by Giemsa or Leishman stains. The thick films are for the rapid detection of parasites, especially if these are few in number, whereas the thin films allow identification of the species of plasmodium. The films must be examined by an experienced observer using oil immersion magnification. If initial films are negative but malaria remains a possible diagnosis, then repeat films should be taken.

Parasites are seen on a thick film from Margaret. The appearance of a thin film is shown in Figure 47.1.

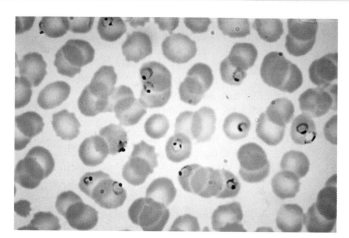

**Fig. 47.1
Thin film of
Margaret's
blood.**

Q What does this show?

A Multiple red cells infected with ring forms (see below) of a plasmodium parasite. The frequency of red-cell parasitaemia and the absence of mature forms of the parasite make this most likely to be *P. falciparum*.

Q What is the treatment for malaria?

A (i) Specific antimalarial chemotherapy must be given as soon as a diagnosis of malaria is suspected. Severe or complicated disease due to *P. falciparum* should be assumed to be chloroquine-resistant and treated with intravenous quinine or quinidine, with subsequent oral maintenance therapy. Chloroquine is the drug of choice for *P. vivax*, *P. ovale* and *P. malariae* infections. Intravenous administration is indicated for severe cases, especially with heavy parasitaemias, but care is necessary because of potential cardiotoxicity. *P. vivax* and *P. ovale* infections must also be treated with primaquine, to eliminate the reservoir of organisms in the liver (see below) and thereby prevent later relapses.

Drugs for uncomplicated infection, given orally, include quinine, mefloquine and halofantrine (contraindicated in pregnancy). All these drugs, especially halofantrine, may result in cardiotoxicity; mefloquine may cause neuropsychiatric side-effects. Tetracycline, clindamycin and pyrimethamine–sulfadoxine have some activity, but are unreliable when used alone. Patients should not be treated with the same drugs they were taking as prophylaxis, as the organisms may be resistant to those agents. Derivatives of artemisinin are being developed.

(ii) Supportive therapy for the various life-threatening complications (see below).

Therapy with intravenous quinidine is initiated. Later that night the following results are received:

**Hb 7.3 g/dl (MCV 105 fl, normal range 76–96), 10% reticulocytes
White cell count 4.5 × 10⁹/ml
Platelets 57 × 10⁹/ml**

**Urea 25.2 mmol/l (normal range 2.5–7.0)
Electrolytes normal
Glucose 2.6 mmol/l (normal range 3.3–5.4).**

Margaret is now sweating profusely and her fever is declining. She manages to pass a small urine sample, which is very dark in colour. However, she has become drowsy and difficult to communicate with.

Q What complications of malaria may now be developing?

A These include:

• Anaemia – due mainly to acute haemolysis, and cytokine-induced suppression of bone marrow function
• Acute renal failure – usually oliguric; dark urine arises from free haemoglobin and malarial pigment filtered from blood into urine
• Cerebral malaria – seizures, impairment of consciousness, coma
• Hypoglycaemia – due to depletion of liver glycogen from decreased oral intake prior to seeking medical attention; glucose consumption by the large number of malarial parasites; hypoglycaemic effects of inflammatory cytokines.

Rare complications include pulmonary oedema, disseminated intravascular coagulation, severe impairment of liver function and splenic enlargement (chronic *P. falciparum*, *P. vivax*).

Q What is the pathogenesis of the multiorgan failure seen in severe *P. falciparum* malaria?

A The pathogenesis of many of the complications of malaria is not fully understood. The most important factors are:

• cytoadherence of parasitized red cells to endothelial cells in the small vessels of the brain, kidneys and other affected organs, leading to occlusion and impairment of organ function. The ability to sequester infected red cells in the microcirculation is unique to *P. falciparum*, which explains why this species causes malignant disease, and the absence of mature forms of *P. falciparum* in peripheral blood smears
• induction of cytokine release from macrophages. Tumour necrosis factor (TNF) -α levels are increased in severe *P. falciparum* malaria. Cytokines have a wide range of inflammatory effects

- at the tissue level, the roles of nitric oxide and free radicals in causing oxidative damage are the subjects of current research.

Q What is the route of infection of malaria?

A Malaria is spread by bites from female anopheline mosquitoes. Plasmodia have a complicated life-cycle, involving replication within both the mosquito vector and the human host (see Figure 47.2):

- *Sporozoites* acquired from the mosquito infect hepatocytes, where they mature to form *tissue schizonts* or become dormant *hypnozoites* (*P. vivax, P. ovale*)
- *Tissue schizonts* produce several thousand *merozoites*, which are released into the bloodstream and infect red cells
- each *merozoite* matures through an asexual cycle of 48–72 hours, involving a *ring form*, a *trophozoite* and a *schizont*, ultimately producing 8–24 new merozoites which are released as the red cells lyse, thus initiating another cycle of red-cell infection
- some parasites within red cells differentiate into male and female *gametocytes* (sexual forms)
- these sexual forms are taken up during a blood meal by the mosquito, where the sexual cycle involves the formation of *gametes*, *zygotes*, *ookinetes*, *oocysts* and ultimately *sporozoites*, which migrate to the salivary gland ready to be injected into the next human host

The hypnozoites may remain dormant for several months before eventually maturing to tissue schizonts and initiating a clinical relapse. This exoerythrocytic liver cycle is not part of the lifecycle of *P. falciparum*. Thus, late relapses do not occur with this plasmodium and there is no need for a course of primaquine to eliminate liver organisms. The same is possibly true of *P. malariae*.

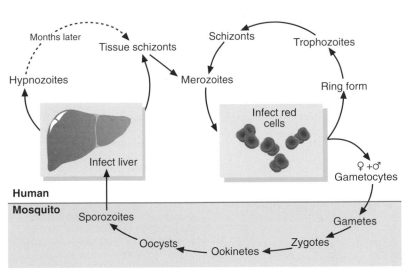

Fig. 47.2 Life cycle of malarial parasite.

Q What do the terms 'tertian' and 'quartan' mean?

A The periodicity (tertian, quartan) of malarial fevers in days, which is related to the red cell cycle. The malarial paroxysm of fever typically includes a 'cold or chilling stage', then a 'hot stage' coincident with red cell lysis and the release of merozoites and lasting several hours, and finally a 'sweating' phase with resolution of fever and marked fatigue. Since erythrocytic parasites of *P. falciparum* do not become synchronized, typical tertian fevers are unusual in falciparum malaria and their absence does not exclude the diagnosis.

Q How may malaria be prevented?

A Elimination of the mosquito vector would prevent transmission of disease. Swamp drainage and the use of insecticides has resulted in a degree of success in some areas.

For travellers to endemic areas, the three principles of prevention are:

- Be aware of the risk of malaria
- Avoid being bitten by mosquitoes, e.g. by using bed-netting (impregnated with insecticide if possible) and insect repellents

- Take appropriate antimalarial prophylaxis
- Even if all these precautions are taken, urgent medical advice must be sought in the event of a fever or flu-like illness within a year of travel, remembering to relate the travel history.

Q When should chemoprophylaxis begin?

A Shortly *before* travel (in case of unacceptable side-effects, and to ensure adequate levels on arrival in an endemic area). It should be continued religiously throughout the period of travel, and for at least 4 weeks after return. The exact choice of drugs is a complex issue, with the emergence of drug-resistant plasmodia and the toxicity of some of the recommended agents. Expert advice should be sought. Guidelines are issued and updated at intervals by national or other bodies. Typical regimens include:

- chloroquine once weekly plus proguanil daily
- pyrimethamine and dapsone (Maloprim) plus chloroquine
- mefloquine once weekly.

Chloroquine should not be taken long term (>5 years) because of the risk of retinopathy. Mefloquine should not be taken for more than 1 year.

Note that, as in Margaret's case, prophylaxis may not be 100% effective due to poor compliance and the emergence of resistant strains; hence the need for other precautions to try and avoid infection.

Summary: Malaria
Presentation
Cyclical fever, headache, nausea, diarrhoea and vomiting, in a patient with an appropriate travel history
Complications
Cerebral malaria; renal failure; anaemia; metabolic upset (hypoglycaemia, lactic acidosis)
Management
A medical emergency; seek urgent diagnosis by examination of thick and thin blood films; initiate therapy, dependent upon the likelihood of encountering resistant organisms

CASE 48
Thomas, a 35-year-old school teacher who is anti-HIV positive

Thomas, a 35-year-old schoolteacher, is homosexual and first tested positive for anti-HIV 5 years ago. He is seen at roughly 6-monthly intervals, and thus far there have been no additional medical problems. His CD4 count 6 months ago was $700 \times 10^9/l$. He now complains of a painful vesicular rash on the right side of his abdomen. On examination, there is the typical appearance of herpes zoster affecting the T10 dorsal root.

Q Does the presence of herpes zoster now mean that Thomas has AIDS?

A No. The different stages of HIV infection, as defined by the Centers for Disease Control (CDC) in the USA, were referred to earlier in Case 30 (see Table 30.1 p. 71). CDC have also produced an extensive case definition for the acquired immunodeficiency syndrome (AIDS), which has been adopted worldwide to assist in the diagnosis of AIDS in individual patients (see Appendix 4). Herpes zoster, recurrent mucocutaneous herpes simplex, oral candidiasis and oral hairy leukoplakia (see Box 48.1) are all considerably more common in HIV-infected individuals than in age- and sex-matched controls. These manifestations reflect

an underlying immunodeficiency and may herald the imminent onset of AIDS, but they do not of themselves constitute AIDS-defining illnesses. Persistent generalized lymphadenopathy (PGL), another

B48.1 Oral hairy leukoplakia
• Whitish lesions on oropharyngeal mucosal surfaces, usually on the side of the tongue
• May resemble oral candidiasis
• Caused by extensive replication of Epstein–Barr virus in epithelial cells
• May occur in any immunosuppressed patient, although rare in absence of HIV infection
• Lesions resolve with acyclovir therapy, but may recur once therapy is stopped

common clinical feature in HIV-infected patients, is not associated with an increased risk of developing AIDS, than is asymptomatic infection without lymphadenopathy.

Thomas' herpes zoster rash is treated with high-dose oral acyclovir (see Case 38) and after 2 weeks the rash resolves. His CD4 count is down to $250 \times 10^6/l$. The possible use of azidothymidine (AZT) at this stage is discussed, but Thomas is unwilling to take this step. At his next visit, 4 months later, Thomas is looking ill. He has lost weight (8 kg) and complains of an incessant dry cough. On examination he has a low-grade fever (37.8°C), but examination of the chest is unremarkable, with only a few crackles at both lung bases. There are no other abnormal physical signs. An urgent chest X-ray, and blood gases are ordered. The blood gases reveal a PaO_2 of 7.0 kPa (normal range 10.6–13.3) and a $PaCo_2$ of 3.1 kPa (normal range 4.6–6.0).

Q What is the likely diagnosis?

A Although it is possible that Thomas has a lower respiratory tract infection due to conventional

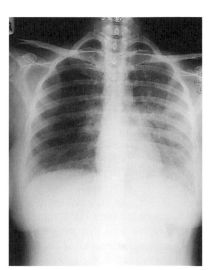

Fig. 48.1 Chest X-ray of Pneumocystis pneumonia.

organisms such as *S. pneumoniae* or *H. influenzae*, the most likely diagnosis is *Pneumocystis carinii* pneumonia (PCP). This frequently presents as an insidiously progressive but non-productive cough in association with systemic manifestations such as fever and weight loss. The chest X-ray features (see Fig. 48.1), of PCP are diffuse interstitial shadowing. X-ray abnormalities are often considerably more dramatic than those detected by physical examination.

Q When do you think Thomas might have acquired his pneumocystis infection?

A *Pneumocystis carinii* infection commonly occurs in early life, without resulting in clinical disease. The organism (now believed to be a fungus) remains in the lung for life. Disease only arises when the host is immunosuppressed, from whatever cause, with reactivation resulting in a life-threatening intra-alveolar pneumonitis.

Q How would you confirm the diagnosis?

A Diagnosis is by demonstration of *P. carinii* cysts in clinical material. The cysts can be identified by silver staining, or by immunofluorescence using monoclonal antibodies. However, spontaneously produced sputum is not optimal for diagnosis – the cysts may not be coughed up from their location deep in the lower respiratory tract. An induced sputum sample (obtained following inhalation of nebulized saline) or bronchoalveolar lavage (BAL) fluid obtained at bronchoscopy, are necessary for accurate diagnosis. Although bronchoscopic diagnosis is desirable, the availability of suitable expertise and dedicated equipment may vary. In a case such as Thomas', in which the HIV status of the patient is known and the clinical presentation so typical, it would be reasonable to make a presumptive diagnosis of PCP and treat accordingly, if bronchoscopy was not possible.

Q How would you manage a patient with PCP?

A First-line therapy is high-dose co-trimoxazole, but there is an increased incidence of allergic reactions (e.g. rash) to this drug in HIV-positive individuals. Alternatives include intravenous pentamidine, clindamycin plus primaquine, dapsone plus trimethoprim.

Thomas is treated with high-dose co-trimoxazole, which results in considerable clinical improve- ment. After 2 weeks in hospital Thomas is ready to be discharged.

Q How should Thomas be managed now?

A The immunodeficiency in AIDS is not reversible, and the emphasis in managing HIV-infected patients is therefore directed towards the prevention of opportunist infections (see Table 48.1) by appropriate prophylactic therapy. This may result in HIV-positive patients being

---

Table 48.1 Features of six common opportunist infections in AIDS

Cytomegalovirus

Multisystem disease including one or more of the following: retinitis, leukopenia, hepatitis, pneumonitis, oesophagitis, colitis, painful peripheral neuropathy, encephalitis
Disease may respond to ganciclovir (toxic to bone marrow) or foscarnet (nephrotoxic). Long-term therapy is necessary to prevent reactivation

Cerebral toxoplasmosis

Commonest cause of intracranial mass lesions
CT scan features include multiple ring-enhancing lesions. MRI scan is more sensitive
Initiation of therapy (pyrimethamine with folinic acid, plus sulfadiazine) usually empirical
Serology is of little diagnostic value

Cryptococcal meningitis

Caused by *Cryptococcus neoformans*, a fungus
Seen in CSF by India ink staining
More reliable diagnosis by isolation of the organism or cryptococcal antigen detection
Measurement of antigen titre useful in monitoring response to treatment, and the emergence of relapsing disease

Mycobacterium avium complex disease

Causes fevers, night sweats, abdominal pain and diarrhoea, fatigue and weight loss
Hepatosplenomegaly and diffuse lymphadenopathy
Continuous bacteraemia, therefore diagnosis by isolation from blood culture

Progressive multifocal leukoencephalopathy (PML)

Due to reactivation of polyomavirus infection (JC virus)
Primary infection acquired in childhood
CNS infection causes multiple white matter lesions
May respond to cytosine arabinoside therapy

Cryptosporidiosis

Protozoan
Cause of chronic (>1 month) diarrhoea
Diagnosis by microscopy of faeces
No proven form of therapy available

on multiple antimicrobial agents, e.g. co-trimoxazole (for the prevention of pneumocystis infection), acyclovir (for the prevention of HSV and VZV reactivations), and fluconazole (for the prevention of cryptococcal disease), in addition to specific anti-HIV drugs. Thomas certainly requires PCP prophylaxis. In fact, he should have been offered this at his previous outpatient visit. His declining CD4 count and his earlier attack of herpes zoster were indicative that

he was progressing towards the development of an AIDS-defining illness, of which PCP is the commonest. Ideally, PCP prophylaxis should begin *before* the occurrence of disease. This may be difficult to predict, but patients should be offered prophylactic therapy as their CD4 count declines towards 200.

Q What specific anti-HIV agents are currently available?

A There are a large number of

experimental drugs undergoing clinical trials in HIV infection. Thus far, only the reverse transcriptase inhibitors have been shown to be of therapeutic value. However, there are several unresolved issues surrounding the use of these agents. Long-term use is associated with the emergence of resistant mutants of HIV, and any benefit is thus likely to be short-term only. The ones in current usage, and their principal side-effects, are listed in Appendix 3. Future advances in anti-HIV therapy are likely to arise through the use of combination regimens, incorporating drugs with different sites of action in the HIV replication cycle e.g. protease inhibitors.

Q List some other clinical manifestations of AIDS.

A The clinical manifestations of AIDS are protean. For epidemiological and comparative purposes they are broadly categorized into infectious, malignant and neurologic complications. A list of common manifestations is given in Table 48.2. The relative frequency of these will vary in different patient groups. The spectrum of opportunistic infections in particular will reflect the pattern of infectious organisms extant in a given geographical location.

Table 48.2 Common clinical manifestations of AIDS

Opportunistic infections

Pulmonary	*Central nervous system*
Pneumonia	Multiple brain abscesses
Pneumocystis carinii	*Toxoplasma gondii*
Cytomegalovirus	Meningitis
Cryptococcus neoformans	*Cryptococcus neoformans*
Tuberculosis	Retinitis, encephalitis
Mycobacterium tuberculosis	Cytomegalovirus
	PML
Gastrointestinal	JC polyomavirus
Oral and oesophageal thrush	
Candida albicans	*Skin and mucous membranes*
Oral hairy leukoplakia	Prolonged recurrent ulceration
Epstein–Barr virus	Herpes simplex virus
Oral ulcers, oesophagitis	Herpes zoster
Herpes simplex virus, CMV	Varicella-zoster virus
Diarrhoea	Multiple skin lesions
Salmonella spp.	*Cryptococcus neoformans*
Shigella	
Giardia lamblia	*Reticuloendothelial system*
Cryptosporidium	Lymphadenopathy
M. avium complex	*Toxoplasma gondii*
Colitis	*M. avium* complex
Cytomegalovirus	Epstein–Barr virus

Malignant disease

Kaposi's sarcoma	Hodgkin's lymphoma
Non-Hodgkin's lymphoma, cerebral	Squamous carcinoma
or peripheral	Testicular cancers
EBV-associated lymphomas	Basal-cell cancer
polyclonal lymphoproliferation,	Melanoma
Burkitt's lymphoma	Carcinoma of the uterine cervix

Neurologic disease

Aseptic meningitis	Intracranial mass lesions
May be HIV-related	Cerebral toxoplasmosis
HIV encephalopathy	Primary CNS lymphoma
HIV	Metastatic lymphoma
	Kaposi's sarcoma
	PML
	CMV or HSV encephalitis
	Cerebral tuberculosis

Summary: PCP in AIDS

Presentation

Fever, cough, breathlessness in a patient known to be anti-HIV positive or in a risk group

Diagnosis

Clinical; chest X-ray; demonstration of cysts in clinical material – bronchoalveolar lavage may be necessary

Management

Co-trimoxazole in high dose and subsequently in lower dose as prophylaxis; pentamidine; consider AZT, especially if low CD4 count

CASE 49

Karim, a 65-year-old cachectic man with fever

Karim, a 65-year-old man, is admitted to hospital because of a 2–3-month history of increasing lassitude, weight loss, anorexia and intermittent pyrexia. Eight years ago Karim made an uncomplicated recovery from an inferior myocardial infarction, and non-insulin dependent diabetes mellitus was diagnosed 3 years before this presentation. His father died of tuberculosis at the age of 45 and one of his two brothers also has diabetes mellitus. On examination he is a pleasant, if slightly confused, cachectic man. His temperature is 38.5°C but his blood pressure, respiratory rate and heart rate are all normal. The rest of his physical examination is unremarkable. There is no neck stiffness.

Q What initial investigations should be carried out?

A Full blood count, erythrocyte sedimentation rate (ESR), urea and electrolytes, electrocardiogram (ECG), blood sugar and chest X-ray are initially indicated. Culture of urine, blood and sputum (if available) should also be carried out. A lumbar puncture and/or CT scan may be considered because of Karim's confusion, to rule out intracranial pathology such as a cerebral abscess (see Case 3) or encephalitis (see Case 2).

The urea and electrolytes are normal and the FBC reveals a mild normochromic normocytic anaemia. Evidence of the previous myocardial infarct is present on the ECG and the random blood sugar is elevated, at 10 mmol/l.

The chest X-ray (see Figure 49.1) is abnormal.

Q What comments can be made about the chest X-ray?

A A patten of fine opacities is present throughout both lung fields, for which there are a number of possible explanations. These include lymphangitis carcinomatosis, occupational lung disease, idiopathic pulmonary fibrosis, sarcoidosis and miliary tuberculosis. The appearance of the X-ray, the recent history of deteriorating health and a positive family history of tuberculosis indicates

B49.1 Miliary tuberculosis
Extensive haematogenous spread involving multiple organs which is most commonly seen in the very young or the elderly
Risk groups
Immigrants from the developing world, the socially deprived, alcoholics, intravenous drug addicts, patients with liver disease or cirrhosis, neoplasia, HIV disease, diabetes mellitus and pregnancy
Features
Fever, malaise and weight loss occurring over 10–15 weeks Previous history of tuberculosis present in only 5% Meninges involved in 20% of cases Hyponatraemia if adrenals infected, raised alkaline phosphatase if liver involved

that miliary disease (see Box 49.1 and Figure 49.2) must be excluded.

Q How may the diagnosis be confirmed?

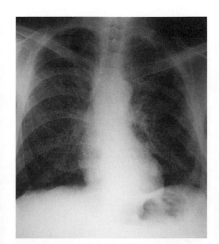

Fig. 49.1 Karim's chest X-ray at presentation.

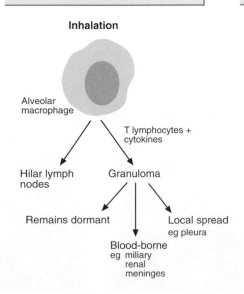

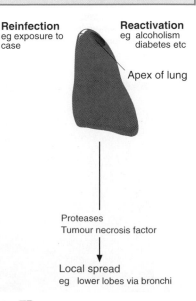

Fig. 49.2 Pathogenesis of primary and post-primary TB.

A Investigations to confirm the diagnosis should include:

- tuberculin skin test (see Box 49.2)
- microscopy (Ziehl–Neelsen or auramine stains) and culture of sputum or pulmonary lavage obtained at bronchoscopy, urine (24-hour collection), bone marrow and liver biopsy material

B49.2 Tuberculin skin tests (Heaf, Tine or Mantoux)

- Purified protein derivative (starting at 1 and then moving to 10 and 100 IU if necessary) administered intracutaneously by a needle or 'gun' and read at 48–72 hours
- Positive result, which is graded, indicated by significant erythema, swelling and induration around the puncture site (type IV hypersensitivity reaction)

Result and interpretation

- *Positive*: infection (current or previous)
  previous vaccination (see below)
  asymptomatic exposure to *Mycobacterium tuberculosis* or other mycobacteria in the past
- *Negative*: not infected, no previous exposure
  very early infection,
  infection but negative response due to immunosuppression (e.g. HIV disease, steroids)
  overwhelming infection suppressing the type IV response

- histological examination for caseating granulomata (see Figure 49.3) of lung, lymph nodes, liver etc.

A Heaf test carried out on Karim is strongly positive. Acid-fast bacilli are not seen on mciroscopy of either lung aspirates or biopsies obtained during bronchoscopy, but granulomata are seen in histological sections of lung and liver biopsies. *M. tuberculosis* (see Box 49.3) is isolated from lung and liver biopsies after 2–3 weeks' incubation on Löwenstein–Jensen medium.

Q What are the main principles of the treatment of tuberculosis?

A Unlike most other bacterial infections, this involves the use of more than one agent for a period of months. Uncomplicated pulmonary tuberculosis is treated with four agents (e.g. rifampicin, isoniazid, pyrazinamide and ethambutol) for an initial 2-month period to be followed by 4 months of dual therapy (e.g. rifampicin and isoniazid). Treatment is continued for longer if the disease is extrapulmonary, the isolate is resistant to one or more of the agents used, or there is non-compliance. Because of the widespread nature of infection in this patient, treatment should probably be continued for 9–12 months.

B49.3 Mycobacteria

- Non-motile, slowly growing curved rods (take 2–8 weeks to isolate on artificial media), obligate aerobes
- Possess a thick complex lipid-rich cell wall; will only take up carbol fuchsin following heating and difficult subsequently to decolorize with mineral acids or alcohol (acid-fast). *Not* therefore visualized with Gram stain
- Mycobacteria are pathogens of humans (e.g. *M tuberculosis*) and animals (e.g. *M. bovis*) but are also found in the environment, e.g. water

Q What is the risk of Karim having transmitted tuberculosis to contacts?

A Karim's tuberculosis is not 'open', that is, he does not have a productive cough which is Ziehl–Neelsen-positive or an open lesion in which acid-fast bacilli are seen. Consequently he does not represent a significant infectious risk and an isolation cubicle is not essential.

Q Who are most at risk from 'open' tuberculosis?

A Family members, other household members with whom the patient lives, and friends and work colleagues who are in regular and frequent contact. Young contacts, i.e. those less than 35 years of age, can be screened with a Heaf test

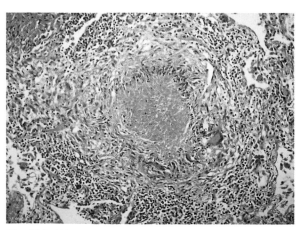
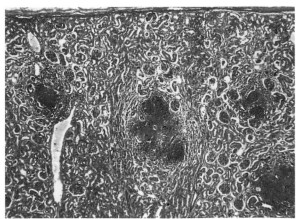

A   B

Fig. 49.3 **(A) caseating granuloma in lung with giant and epithelioid cells; (B) multiple granulomata in kidney.**

only, but if positive should have a chest X-ray. Those older than 35 are screened with a chest X-ray at initial contact and possibly subsequently. Such contact tracing, which is usually carried out by public health authorities, emphasizes the importance of notifying diagnosed or suspected tuberculosis.

Q Is nosocomial spread common?

A Not usually. Although nosocomial spread may occur if the diagnosis of 'open' tuberculosis is unsuspected and therefore delayed, most contacts are at relatively low risk, but their doctors should be informed. Patients with suspected tuberculosis should be isolated in a side room or infectious disease unit until the result of microscopy is negative. Staff in hospitals in many parts of the world receive BCG vaccination (see Box 49.4) and are therefore relatively protected. Where this is not routine, occupational acquisition is a recognized hazard and the use of masks or respirators is recommended, especially if aerosol dispersion is likely (e.g. suctioning of airways) or multidrug-resistant strains are prevalent.

Q Is chemoprophylaxis indicated for any of Karim's contacts?

A No. This is reserved for contacts of 'open' cases, including the patient's children and at-risk individuals, e.g. HIV-positive individuals, neonates and other contacts who have not been vaccinated with BCG but who, following exposure, have become tuberculin skin test-positive and may therefore be incubating the infection.

Q Which other organs or systems may *M. tuberculosis* infect?

A Tuberculosis can affect almost any system in the body, as may be deduced from its pathogenesis (see Figure 49.2). Extrapulmonary tuberculosis, including miliary disease, is more common in immigrants than the indigenous population of most western countries, and is a recog-

---

B49.4 BCG (Bacille Calmette-Guérin) vaccine

- Live attenuated vaccine derived from *M. bovis*
- 75% protective in the UK but less elsewhere, e.g. India, because of exposure to other mycobacteria or malnutrition
- Excellent protection against disseminated (miliary) or meningeal tuberculosis
- Affords some protection against leprosy (see Case 43)

---

nized cause of fever of unknown origin (FUO, see Case 50). The more common organs infected include:

- lymph nodes: not an uncommon initial presentation of tuberculosis. Cervical glands most commonly involved, and are usually painless
- genitourinary: recognized cause of 'sterile pyuria' and infertility or other gynaecological problems in females
- bones and joints: may present with septic arthritis or spinal abscess and tuberculosis should be excluded by Ziehl–Neelsen stain and culture of all bone and joint specimens
- brain: TB meningitis should be suspected in any case of meningitis characterized by a high CSF lymphocyte count and a low CSF glucose (see Case 1). Delayed diagnosis contributes to the poor outcome.

Q What is meant by the term 'atypical mycobacteria', and what diseases do these organisms cause?

A In the past these were also referred to as 'environmental mycobacteria', as they are found in water, soil etc., and it was assumed that they were harmless or of low pathogenicity. In recent years, however, they have been increasingly described as pathogens in the compromised host and cause a range of illnesses in a variety of patient groups. Consequently, they have

also been referred to as 'opportunist mycobacteria'.

These bacteria may cause:

- Lymphadenitis: most commonly seen during childhood and may be caused by *M. avium complex* or *M. scrofulaceum*, not unlike that due to *M. tuberculosis*
- Skin lesions and ulcers: abscesses (*M. chelonei*) or 'fishtank granuloma' (*M. marinum*).
- Pulmonary infection: similar presentation to tuberculosis but usually seen in previously damaged lungs, such as chronic obstructive or industrial lung disease (*M. kansasii*)
- Disseminated infection: seen in severely immunocompromised states, such as the terminal stages of AIDS (*M. avium complex*).

Unlike *M. tuberculosis*, patient-to-patient transmission is extremely uncommon with these mycobacteria and attempts should be made to isolate the organism from repeat specimens because of the chance of specimen contamination, causing a false positive result. Management often involves surgery. Antimicrobial chemotherapy is less predictable because many strains are resistant to a number of antimycobacterial agents *in vitro*, but these may be effective *in vivo*.

Summary: Tuberculosis
Presentation
Cough, respiratory tract infection (pulmonary), systemic signs and symptoms, e.g. fever, weight loss if miliary or extrapulmonary
Diagnosis
Microscopy and culture of specimens, histology, radiology and skin testing (Heaf, Mantoux etc.)
Management
Combination chemotherapy for 6 months or longer, chemoprophylaxis for at-risk groups

CASE 50
Gordon, a 35-year-old Scottish vet with fever

Gordon is a 35-year-old Scottish vet who has been in hospital for 7 days for investigation of fever, malaise and weight loss. Apart from fracturing his arm during a game of rugby 4 years earlier, he has never been ill or required admission to hospital. He is on no medications, has no relevant family history and does not smoke. On initial examination he appears somewhat pale and his vital signs are normal. There are no skin rashes, enlarged lymph nodes, heart murmurs or hepatosplenomegaly.

Q Does Gordon have a FUO (fever of unknown origin)?

A No. Strictly speaking FUO (previously known as a PUO, referring to pyrexia) as originally described is an illness characterized by a fever of 38.5°C or higher on several occasions of more than 3 weeks' duration, despite appropriate investigations in hospital or as an outpatient. Gordon has only been an inpatient for 7 days and we are not told how high the fever is or long he has had it. The term is often loosely used to describe patients under investigation for shorter periods with a fever for which there is no obvious cause.

Q What other information might it be useful to know about Gordon?

A Specific questions Gordon should be asked are:

- What vaccinations has he received, e.g. BCG for TB?
- What does his work as a vet involve: is he in direct contact with sick animals rendering him vulnerable to acquiring a zoonosis (see Box 50.1)?
- Has he been abroad recently, i.e. in the last year? If so, when, where and for how long. Did he take malaria prophylaxis (see Case 47) if appropriate, or receive additional immunizations, e.g. typhoid?
- Has anybody with whom he lives or has close contact, i.e. work colleagues, had a similar illness recently?
- What are his pastimes or hobbies, e.g. does he keep budgies or

parrots (see Case 13) or walk through 'tick-infested forests' (see Case 42)?
- What is his lifestyle? Does he have risk factors such as intravenous drug abuse which predispose him to acquiring HIV (see Case 48)?

Gordon has daily contact with farm animals, including cattle and sheep, but none of his veterinary colleagues have been ill recently. He has had a booster tetanus dose in the last year. He has not been abroad since a trip to Majorca 3 years earlier, and apart from rugby his only other hobby is collecting antique teapots! He has never injected intravenous drugs and has been living with his current girlfriend for the last 2 years. He denies any homosexual encounters or other heterosexual relationships, apart from on one occasion 8 years previously when he was very drunk during a rugby tour! His girlfriend has not had sexual intercourse with anybody else for the last 2 years and has no risk factors for HIV disease.

Q What aspects of the physical examination are especially important here?

A In addition to his vital signs, i.e. pulse, blood pressure, respiratory rate and temperature (should be monitored initially every 4–6 hours), a comprehensive phyical examination should be carried out looking for evidence of anaemia, jaundice, weight loss, lymphadenopathy and

B50.1 Some features of zoonoses

Definition

Infections acquired by man through contact with animals (usually vertebrate) or animal products

How acquired

Directly, e.g. farmer, vet in contact with cows or sheep
Inhalation, e.g. infected droppings or excreta
Saliva, e.g. bite or lick from a dog
Faeces, e.g. chicken faeces contaminating eggs
Urine e.g. urine from animal contaminating recreational waters
Blood/tissues, e.g. animal house attendants involved in research

Common examples

Tuberculosis (see Case 49), salmonellosis (see Case17), brucellosis, leptospirosis, listeriosis (see Case 54) Q fever (see Case 13), rabies (see Case 5), Lassa fever (see Case 63), toxoplamosis (see Case 59), Leishmaniasis (see Case 52)

hepatosplenomegaly. Localizing signs in the respiratory tract and abdomen should also be sought. Particular attention should be paid to the presence of skin rashes and a new or changing heart murmur, indicative of endocarditis (see Case 46).

On repeat examination Gordon appears pale, but his vital signs are normal apart from an elevated temperature of 39°C. Fundoscopy is normal and there is no evidence of peripheral vein injection sites, indicative of intravenous drug abuse. There are no skin rashes, enlarged lymph nodes, heart murmurs or hepatosplenomegaly. Rectal examination and examination of the external genitalia is normal. Repeat physical examinations over the next few days are unremarkable. He continues to remain pyrexial 3 weeks after admission for investigation, and by now has lost 3 kg.

Q What is the relevance of fundoscopy here?

A Fundoscopy is part of the normal physical examination and may reveal abnormalities such as exudates consistent with candidaemia (as may occur in i.v. drug abusers (see Case 45)), infective endocarditis and cyto-megalovirus infection (HIV disease).

Q What initial investigations should be undertaken in a patient with FUO?

A These may be classified as general and microbiological. General investigations include a full blood count (including blood film for atypical mononuclear cells or patho-gens such as malaria, trypanosomes), ESR, C-reactive protein (C-RP), urea and electrolytes, liver function tests, chest X-ray, ECG and echo-cardiogram. These tests will both reflect the general state of Gordon's health and may point to specific areas requiring further investigation, e.g. abnormal liver function tests indicating the need for liver biopsy. Initial microbiological tests will include the following:

- Blood cultures: At least two sets from different sites and taken at least half an hour apart. If endo-carditis (see Case 46) is suspected three sets should be taken, or more if the patient has recently been on antibiotics. If the patient remains pyrexial, repeat cultures should be taken.
- Urine microscopy and culture: Red blood cells and casts may be indicative of endocarditis, pyuria reflect a renal abscess, and a 24-hour collection should be made for Ziehl–Neelsen staining and TB culture.
- Serology: There is a multitude of tests that one might carry out to investigate a FUO. 10–20 ml serum should be taken and 5–7 ml stored for later to serve as a baseline serum if initial screening tests are negative. Initial tests should include monospot for infectious mononucleosis, com-plement fixation tests for *Myco-*

plasma pneumoniae, *Chlamydia* spp., influenza and adenoviruses, and serology for *Legionella pneu-mophila*. Serology for Lyme disease, brucellosis, leptospirosis, toxoplasmosis and syphilis should also be undertaken early on.

- Skin Tests: A Heaf or Mantoux test for tuberculosis is important. Skin tests to detect anergy (present in sarcoidosis and HIV disease) may also be relevant, as may skin tests to diagnose hydatid disease (see Case 23) and histo-plasmosis (see Case 45), if recently abroad in certain parts of North America or elsewhere.

Q What proportion of FUOs are due to infection?

A Approximately 30%, but this will vary according to the population or ethnic group, geographical location, i.e. temperate or tropical climate, and the age of the patient (see Table 50.1). In children less than 6 years of age viral respiratory infection is the commonest cause, but after this connective tissue diseases such as juvenile rheumatoid arthritis are more common. After 14 years of age the aetiology reflects that of adults. In 30% of adults no aetiology is identified, and the remainder may be categorized into infective, neoplastic and con-nective tissue or 'autoimmune'.

In the HIV-infected or neutropenic patient opportunist pathogens such as *Pneumocystis carinii* (see Case 48), systemic or fungal infection (see Case 45) are more likely. If the patient has been hospitalized for some time, nosocomial infections

such as wound, catheter-associated urine and intravascular line (see Case 27) infections are relatively more important. After extensive investigation, and especially in some patients with a psychiatric disorder, a factitious temperature must be considered, e.g. self-injection with pyrogens, and the patient closely observed.

The results of Gordon's initial investigations are not very helpful. His ESR is elevated at 50 mm/h and his C-RP is also high, at 25 mg/l (normal <10 mg/l) but full blood count, examination of repeat blood films, urea and electroytes, liver function tests, ECG, echo-cardiography, ultrasound and CT scan of the abdomen are normal. Urinalysis and culture of three samples of urine is negative, as are blood cultures. He also undergoes a bone marrow biopsy, which reveals normal architecture and cells is sterile, and Ziehl–Neelsen staining is negative. His chest X-ray shows some 'tenting' of the right diaphragmatic pleura, but without a previous chest X-ray, it is not clear whether this is long-standing or not. CT scans of his thorax are no more helpful and bronchoscopy is unremarkable. Bronchial aspirates are sterile and Ziehl–Neelsen stains are negative (TB culture negative so far). His Heaf test is moderately reactive, with 10IU (see Case 49) but he has a scar indicating previous BCG vaccination on his left upper arm.

	Infective	Neoplasia	'Autoimmune'
Incidence	30%	25%	15%
Examples	Occult abscess, e.g. liver	Hodgkin's disease	Systemic lupus
	Endocarditis	Abdominal lymphoma	Polyarteritis nodosa
	Tuberculosis	Renal-cell carcinoma	Polymyalgia rheumatica
			Sarcoidosis
	Epstein–Barr virus Toxoplasmosis	Atrial myxoma	

Table 50.1 Some of the more common causes of FUO in temperate climates

Q What options should now be considered?

A There is often no obvious diagnosis following intitial and repeated investigations of FUO. The negative ultrasound and CT scans, with a normal white cell count, probably exclude an occult abscess, but a white cell-labelled scan is more sensitive and might be considered. The normal biochemistry, e.g. liver function tests, is consistent with the absence of a malignancy but non-Hodgkin's lymphoma may present like this if abdominal lymph nodes are involved without marked lymphadenopathy. The minor abnormalities on the chest X-ray and the positive Heaf test indicate that tuberculosis must be considered possible. The negative Ziehl–Neelsen stains and the negative culture results to date do not rule this out. Finally, we are not told the results of any investigations to exclude a connective tissue disorder or serology results.

Rheumatoid factor and antibodies to DNA, histones, non-histone antigens and nuclear antigens are negative, all of which probably excludes a connective tissue or 'auto-immune' disorder. A monospot is negative, as are antibodies to Epstein–Barr virus. Antibodies to the following from paired samples of sera are also negative: *Mycoplasma pneumoniae*, *Chlamydia* spp, *Legionella pneumophila*, *Coxiella burnetii* (Q fever), *Borrelia burgdorferi* (Lyme disease), adenovirus, influenza virus, *Toxoplasma gondii*, *Toxocara canis*, syphilis and leptospira. Following discussion with the patient he agrees to have an HIV antibody test, which is also negative. Three days later his case is discussed at the hospital's medical conference, where the physican looking after Gordon seeks advice from her colleagues about how to proceed from here. The negative rheumatoid factor and other immune parameters, it is agreed, points against a connective tissue disease. There is also a consensus that because he is not acutely ill, has not lost a great deal more weight and the various scans are negative, a malignancy is down the list of likely diagnoses.

There is much discussion about the abnormal chest X-ray and the positive Heaf test. These findings, combined with the elevated ESR and C-RP, suggest to many present that an infective process, most likely bacterial, is present and the idea of a therapeutic trial with antituberculosis chemotherapy is favoured by some. Finally, just before the conference concludes, a recently retired general physician who is a regular attender at these conferences, requests the results of one test outstanding, especially relevant here.

Q What test is he referring to?

A Serology for brucellosis (see Box 50.2). In a farmer, vet or abattoir worker one must consider this together with tuberculosis (see Case 49), Q. fever (see Box 50.3) and leptospirosis (see Box 50.4).

The results of Gordon's brucella serology indicate a rise in antibodies to *Brucella abortus*: serum on admission had antibodies at a dilution of 1 in 16 (barely raised), but 2 weeks later this had risen to 1 in 256, indicative of acute brucellosis. He is started on oral tetracycline and a week later his temperature is almost normal. He is discharged home and arrangements are made for him to be seen in the outpatients in 3 weeks' time.

B50.2 Brucellosis

- Caused by small fastidious Gram-negative bacilli, i.e. *Brucella abortus* (from cattle), *B. mellitensis* (from goats and sheep) and *B. suis* (from pigs). Acquired by contact with animal tissues, blood, e.g. abortions, or consumption of unpasteurized milk
- Acute illness, incubation period of 2–3 weeks with fever, headaches, sweating attacks and arthralgia. May be recurrent or chronic, presenting with depression
- Diagnosis by serology (more than one technique required, e.g. complement fixation, agglutination) or culture (blood, liver biopsy), which is difficult and hazardous to laboratory staff
- Treatment is with tetracyclines for 3 months

B50.3 Q fever (Query fever)

- Rickettsial disease caused by *Coxiella burnetii* which is acquired by inhalation of aerosols or contact with animals
- Presents with FUO (often with splenomegaly), atypical pneumonia (see Case 13) or infective endocarditis (see Case 46)
- Diagnosis by demonstrating a rise in complement fixing antibodies to phase 1 (chronic disease or endocarditis) or phase 2 (Q fever or pneumonia) antigens
- A tetracycline is the treatment of choice

B50.4 Leptospirosis

- Caused by spirochaetes (*Leptospira icterhaemorrhagiae*, *L. canicola*, *L. hardjo*) from contact with rodent urine, livestock or contaminated water (such as during farming or water sports, e.g. canoeing)
- Presents with fever and sometimes jaundice, proteinuria and renal failure (Weil's disease)
- Diagnosis usually by demonstration of a rise in antibodies, but bacteria may be cultured with some difficulty from urine and blood
- Benzylpenicillin is the treatment of choice

Q How long should Gordon receive antibiotics for, and what is the likely prognosis?

A Three months' treatment is usually adequate. In the past, combined treatment with a tetracycline and streptomycin has been advocated but it is doubtful whether this is more efficacious than tetracycline alone. Co-trimoxazole is an alternative for those patients who should not receive tetracycline antibiotics, e.g. growing children. The majority of patients with acute brucellosis respond but a minority develop recurrences or develop chronic brucellosis. Chronic brucellosis is difficult to diagnose clinically and serologically (elevated antibodies from acute infection may be lifelong), and the differential diagnosis includes many of the other causes of the chronic fatigue syndrome.

Summary: Fever of unknown origin
Presentation
Persistent temperature of 38.5°C for 3 weeks or more with no obvious cause after initial investigations. Physical examination is often completely normal
Diagnosis
Comprehensive history including that of occupation, family, travel and pastimes with repeated physical examinations. The number and type of investigations are almost infinite but should be directed to the most likely cause, i.e. whether infective, neoplastic or connective tissue disease
Treatment
Will depend upon the cause: antimicrobial chemotherapy if infective (a therapeutic trial, e.g. TB or endocarditis may be necessary), chemotherapy for neoplastic disease or immunosuppressive therapy, e.g. corticosteroids for connective tissue or 'autoimmune' diseases

CASE 51
Complications of a road traffic accident in Brian, a retired 63-year-old barrister

Brian is a 63-year-old retired barrister who was involved in a serious road traffic accident 3 months ago. He was in a head-on collision and sustained injuries to his chest (four fractured ribs), head (subdural haematoma with cerebrospinal fluid leak), abdomen (lacerated liver, and lacerated spleen requiring removal) and lower limbs (compound fracture of his right femur). He spent 5 weeks in the intensive care unit and was ventilated because of adult respiratory distress syndrome (ARDS) and bronchopneumonia. This was followed by 3 weeks in the orthopaedic ward for management of his fractured femur and a wound infection due to *Escherichia coli*, treated with oral co-amoxyclav. Tragically, Brian's wife died in the accident and he himself has had difficulty coping since.

At the orthopaedic clinic Brian is apyrexial but there is some discharge at the leg wound site, where an intramedullary nail was inserted, and he complains of a dull ache there in the last couple of days. A wound swab is sent to the microbiology laboratory and a provisional report indicates that *Staphylococcus aureus* has been isolated, with sensitivities to follow. Brian has not been on antimicrobial agents for almost 4 weeks.

Q Is it surprising that Brian is on no antibiotics whatsoever?

A Brain had his spleen removed, and therefore he is at increased risk of fulminating infection with *Streptococcus pneumoniae* and other capsulated bacteria for the remainder of his life. Consequently, he should receive pneumococcal, and *Haemophilus influenzae* type B vaccines (see Case 7). Should he travel to a meningococcal-endemic area, e.g. the Middle East, a meningococcal vaccine, which will protect him against non-group B strains prevalent there, is especially important. Malaria prophylaxis is also essential when travelling to endemic areas. It is also widely recommended that he receive lifelong oral penicillin to protect against pneumococcal bacteraemia. His GP should be informed of his increased susceptibility to infection, and finally, he should always carry a card in case of emergency, indicating that his spleen has been removed.

Q What is the significance of the *S. aureus*?

A Staphylococci, especially coagulase-negative staphylococci such as *S. epidermidis*, are part of the normal flora of the skin. *S. aureus* readily colonizes or infects damaged skin or wounds (see Case 36), and isolation may represent a wound infection, but the significance of this bacterium here, especially from a swab, is difficult to interpret. A sample of the discharge fluid or wound debridement tissue is likely to be more representative of what is happening in the deeper tissues.

Brian is admitted to hospital. An X-ray of his right femur indicates increased sclerosis of the bone and periosteum beneath the site of the wound (Figure 51.1 shows similar changes in a child) with accompanying soft tissue swelling. The *S. aureus* isolated from the swab is resistant to penicillin, flucloxacillin,

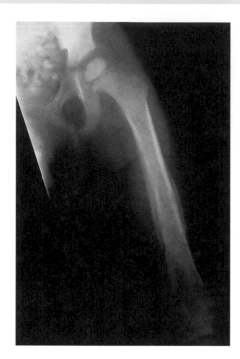

Fig. 51.1 X-ray of femoral osteomyelitis showing extensive sclerosis.

erythromycin and gentamicin. Brian is taken to the operating theatre, where the wound and underlying tissue is explored. A specimen of bone taken during debridement is sent to the microbiology laboratory and *S. aureus* with similar sensitivities is isolated.

Q What is the likely diagnosis?

A Brian almost certainly has osteomyelitis, as indicated by the radiological features and the isolation of a pathogen from tissue taken at operation. Other investigations which may contribute to this diagnosis include a peripheral white cell count, ESR or C-reactive protein, and MRI or CT scans.

Q How may osteomyelitis be classified?

A Bone and joints are remarkably vascular, especially during childhood and early adolescence, when infection is often blood-borne. Osteomyelitis and septic arthritis may be considered as acute or chronic, but a more useful classification is based upon pathogenesis (see Box 51.1). Patients with sickle cell

disease are at greater risk of Gram-negative osteomyelitis due to infarction and deficient phagocytosis. Tuberculosis (see Case 49) usually arises from dissemination via the bloodstream, even if infection does not manifest for some years after the initial exposure. Bones commonly infected in tuberculosis are the spine, hips and knees, reflecting the volume of blood flow there.

Q Are antibiotics required in non-acute, non-haematogenous osteomyelitis where infected tissue is removed during surgery?

A Yes. Although it is essential that as much infected tissue as possible be removed during surgical debridement (this also provides specimens

for microbiological diagnosis), antibiotics are also necessary to eradicate any bacteria remaining. Few if any well-conducted clinical trials on the choice of antibiotics, routes of administration or total duration of treatment have been carried out in osteomyelitis/septic arthritis, but the following recommendations can be made:

- Acute osteomyelitis: 3–4 weeks antibiotics in total, with the first 2 weeks by the intravenous route

- chronic osteomyelitis: longer course required, 3–4 weeks intravenous followed by 1–2 months oral antibiotics.

Q Is there anything unusual about the *S. aureus* recovered from Brian?

A The isolate is resistant to many of the commonly used antibiotics used to treat staphylococcal infection, including flucloxacillin, erythromycin and gentamicin. In fact, it is an MRSA (methicillin-resistant *S. aureus*). Methicillin rather than flucloxacillin is used in the laboratory to assess susceptibility to the antistaphylococcal penicillins and resistance implies the unsuitability of all β-lactam agents in treatment. As some of these strains are resistant to almost all antistaphylococcal antibiotics and are epidemic in distribution, other synonyms have been used, e.g. multiresistant *S. aureus* or epidemic MRSA (EMRSA); see Box 51.2. For many patients, isolation of MRSA from the skin or a superficial site represents asymptomatic colonization rather

B51.1 Pathogenesis of osteomyelitis and septic arthritis		
Primary	*Haematogenous*, usually acute disease, largely of childhood, with abrupt onset and systemic illness	*S. aureus* (long bones), *H. influenzae* type B (<5 years), β-haemolytic streptococci
Secondary	*Contiguous focus*, e.g. pressure sore, trauma, local signs	Often polymorphic, with *S. aureus*, coliforms, *P. aeruginosa*, anaerobes, etc.
	Vascular problems, elderly patients involving feet, local signs, cellulitis	

B51.2 Features of methicillin resistant *S. aureus*

MRSA

Implies resistance to methicillin, flucloxacillin and other β-lactam agents. Some strains also resistant to aminoglycosides (e.g. gentamicin), macrolides (e.g. erythromycin) and quinolones (e.g. ciprofloxacin).

Resistance

Gene responsible is chromosomal and results in the production of a penicillin-binding protein with low affinity for β-lactams. MRSA strains believed to be clonal in origin

Epidemiology

- Hospital-acquired, especially prevalent in ITUs and trauma units
- Common carriage sites include nose, axilla, perineum and broken skin
- Spread is by contact, e.g. hands, and both patients and staff may be asymptomatic carriers
- Different EMRSA strains denoted by number, e.g. EMRSA 16, and characterized by similar genotype and often geographical distribution

than infection requiring systemic antibiotic treatment.

Q Is it likely that Brian acquired the MRSA while at home?

A No. Methicillin-resistant *S. aureus* is predominantly a hospital pathogen. Brian probably acquired MRSA during his previous admission to the orthopaedic ward, but it was not detected until now. MRSA is especially prevalent in the larger teaching or tertiary referral hospitals, where vulnerable patients congregate from a wide variety of hospitals or geographical areas. MRSA is not uncommon in London and the southeast of England, Ireland, many parts of Southern Europe, Australia and the Middle East.

Q What options are available for the treatment of Brian's osteomyelitis?

A Strains of MRSA are usually sensitive to the glycopeptides, i.e. vancomycin and teicoplanin, and may in addition be sensitive to fusidic acid, rifampicin and co-trimaxozole. These are usually effective as treatment when the patient's underlying state does not herald a poor prognosis, but none of these agents is very effective in eradicating skin carriage.

Brian is started on intravenous vancomycin, administered via a long line, and oral fusidic acid, to which the isolate is sensitive. Assays of serum taken after 2 days indicate sub-therapeutic levels of vancomycin and the dose is therefore increased. Swabs of his nose, axilla and perineum grow MRSA. One week later he returns to theatre for further removal of infected bone tissue, from which MRSA is again isolated.

Q What measures, if any, need to be taken to prevent the spread of MRSA?

A Brian is heavily colonized, as indicated by the positive screening specimens, and requires isolation, preferably in a single room with the door closed to prevent transmission to other patients. This is particularly important on an orthopaedic ward, where there may be other vulnerable patients with open wounds or with orthopaedic screws and nails. Whenever he goes to theatre, personnel there need to be informed so that he can preferably be placed last on the list. Effective and thorough hand-washing, however, remains the single most effective measure in preventing spread.

Q Is it necessary for staff to wear face masks when entering Brian's room?

A No. Protective clothing such as disposable plastic aprons and gloves will reduce the likelihood of transmission via hands or clothing. As this bacterium does not pose a threat to the health of staff or visitors, and as it is furthermore highly unlikely to be acquired by inhalation, masks are unnecessary.

Q Does the isolation of MRSA from a repeat specimen indicate antibiotic failure?

A No. Although it is advisable that the sensitivity tests be repeated on the latest isolate, it would be surprising if it were vancomycin resistant. The presence of necrotic tissue with microabscesses may indicate poor antibiotic penetration to the infected site, hence the necessity of removing dead bone. It is possible, but less likely, that persistent or extensive skin carriage may lead to repeat inoculation of the operative site with MRSA.

Q What measures should be taken to eradicate skin carriage?

A Mupirocin, a topical anti-staphylococcal antibiotic, may be applied to the nose, and chlorhexidine baths are also effective in reducing or eliminating skin carriage. Alternative topical agents include povidone–iodine and triclosan.

Brian receives a total of 2 months antibiotic treatment with vancomycin and fusidic acid. Clinical evaluation, laboratory indices (e.g. C-reactive protein and ESR) and X-rays of his femur indicate resolution of his osteomyelitis. A 5-day course of mupirocin applied to the nose, together with daily chlorhexidine baths, eradicates MRSA from carriage sites and later screening samples are negative. He is subsequently discharged, to be followed up at the orthopaedic outpatients.

Q Do the negative screening samples indicate that Brian no longer poses a risk of spreading MRSA?

A Unfortunately no. Our current understanding of MRSA suggests that we cannot be sure that patients, once colonized or infected but subsequently clear following treatment, will remain free of MRSA indefinitely. Patients such as Brian remain a potential risk and should be isolated and screened when subsequently admitted to hospital. It is therefore important that the patient's case notes indicate clearly that he is an MRSA carrier, and that other hospitals are informed before transfer or referral.

Q Should other patients or staff in contact with Brian be screened for MRSA?

A Large-scale screening is disruptive, expensive and often induces a state of near panic, especially among staff. Decisions on screening should be made by those responsible for infection control (microbiologists or infection control doctors and infection control nurses) and will be influenced by the strain of MRSA, clinical area, extent of carriage and likely dissemination, and the type of ward or unit involved. Because the consequences of spread on an intensive care unit or oncology ward are more serious, screening of patients or staff in these areas is more likely to be necessary than, for example, on a care of the elderly ward. Nonetheless, all patients known to be previously MRSA positive in the past, or suspected of having been so, should preferably be screened on admission and isolated in a single cubicle while awaiting the results.

Summary: Osteomyelitis due to MRSA
Presentation
Local bone pain with possible discharge or sinus. Systemic symptoms and signs unusual
Diagnosis
Clinical, radiological and microbiological evaluation. Tissue or deep aspirates rather than superficial swabs for culture essential. MRSA indicated by sensitivity pattern and more common in certain national or international areas
Management
Debridement with prolonged antibiotics, initially administered intravenously. MRSA requires patient isolation and infection control measures, especially hand-washing

CASE 52
Fever, sweating and weight loss in Richard, recently returned from east Africa

Richard is a 64-year-old retired businessman who returned to England 2 months ago from east Africa, where he had been working for the past 5 years. He is referred by his GP to the medical outpatients clinic because he has been unwell for the past month. He complains of intermittent fever, sweating attacks, weight loss of 3 kg and increasing lassitude. His past medical history inclues occcasional episodes of malaria, for which he was treated in Africa, and a myocardial infarction 10 years previously. He is on no medications. On examination he has a temperature of 38°C, appears pale, and his liver and spleen are palpable. Richard is admitted to hospital for observation and investigation. His elevated temperature is characterized by a twice-daily elevation to 38–39°C and his initial investigations reveal an elevated ESR, a haemoglobin of 9.5 g/dl and a white cell count of 2.7×10^9/l.

Q What is the differential diagnosis?

A The combination of weight loss, increasing lassitude, an enlarged liver and spleen and anaemia suggests possible malignancy, such as a lymphoma. Infection, especially one imported from abroad, must also be borne in mind. The possible infective causes include:

- malaria: a possibility no matter how long the interval between presentation and past exposure (infection with *Plasmodium vivax* and *P. ovale* may be recurrent) or history of chemoprophylaxis. In particular, malaria due to *P. falciparum* should be excluded because of its potential seriousness. Repeated blood films for examination of parasites (see Case 47) may confirm the diagnosis
- typhoid or paratyphoid fever: the normal incubation period is up to 3 weeks, and hence the interval between departure from Africa and the onset of the illness makes this diagnosis less likely. Culture of blood and faeces is the diagnostic test of choice (see Case 21)
- typhus: this and many other arthropod-borne illnesses (see Table 52.1), especially those caused by rickettsia, are often accompanied by a skin rash with fever, headache and myalgia. Confirmation of the diagnosis is by serology
- schistosomiasis: hepatosplenomegaly may be seen with infection due to *Schistosoma mansoni* (bilharzia), a blood fluke (see Case 31), but this is often accompanied by abdominal pain or rectal bleeding. Biopsy of infected tissues, e.g. the rectum, or examination of urine for cysts, may confirm the diagnosis
- miliary tuberculosis: disseminated TB is possible here. One should check for the scar of BCG vaccination (usually protects against disseminated disease), do a Heaf test, carry out a chest X-ray and culture sputum, urine and bone marrow for *Mycobacterium tuberculosis* (see Case 49)

- amoebic liver abscess: the absence of a history of diarrhoea does not exclude this infection, but a tender liver without splenomegaly is more common. Diagnosis may be confirmed by ultrasound examination and elevated antibodies to *Entamoeba histolytica* (see Case 23)
- Chagas' disease: also known as American trypanosomiasis (caused by *Trypanosoma cruzi*) and transmitted by a bite from the tsetse fly (see Table 52.1) but unlikely in Richard who has been to Africa not the Americas. Lymphadenopathy is more prominent and cardiac involvement may result in death
- kala azar: visceral leishmaniasis (caused by *Leishmania donovani*) is accompanied by hepatosplenomegaly and anaemia, and has an incubation period of 1–3 months. Patients often have a temperature pattern characterized by twice-daily peaks. The term 'kala azar' derives its name from the discoloration of the skin which is sometimes seen (kala azar = black fever).

After routine investigations fail to lead to a diagnosis, Richard undergoes a liver biopsy which on histological examination reveals amastigotes (non-flagellated forms) of *Leishmania donovani*. An antibody titre of >256 to *L. donovani* is present in a sample of serum (referred to a national reference laboratory) taken in the outpatients, confirming a diagnosis of visceral leishmaniasis.

Q How is visceral leishmaniasis acquired?

A Leishmaniasis may be cutaneous, mucosal (see Box 52.1) or visceral and is contracted through a bite from the sandfly. These conditions are endemic in Africa, the Middle East, parts of the Mediterranean, Asia and South America. Congenital acquisition or transmission by infected blood has been described but is very rare. *L. donovani*, the

B52.1 Leishmaniasis

Cutaneous

- Caused by *Leishmania tropica*, *L. aethiopica* (both found in Africa and Asia) and *L. braziliensis* (found in Latin America). Transmitted by a bite from the sandfly. Dogs and rodents are the reservoir
- Characterized by shallow skin ulcers with circular well-defined edges, nodules and satellite papules
- Differential diagnosis includes leprosy, cutaneous tuberculosis, fungal infection, syphilis or other spirochaete infections such as yaws
- Diagnosis confirmed by amastigotes in Giemsa-stained smears from lesions, culture after prolonged incubation using specialist media, and serology

Mucosal

- Caused by *L. braziliensis*
- Occurs in 2–3% of cutaneous disease with epistaxis due to nasal mucosal involvement and lesions on the lips, tongue and larynx

Table 52.1 Some arthropod-borne infections and their epidemiology (excluding leishmania)

Disease and organism	Vector	Reservoirs	Geographical distribution	Comments
Malaria, *Plasmodium falciparum*, *vivax*, *ovale* and *malariae*	Female mosquito	Humans	Most tropical and sub-tropical areas	Falciparum malaria is life-threatening (see Case 47). Resistance to prophylaxis increasing
Yellow fever, flavivirus	Mosquito	Humans, monkeys	Africa and South America	Effective live vaccine available
Dengue, flavivirus	Mosquito	Humans	Africa and SE Asia	Like yellow fever, a cause of viral haemorrhagic fever (see Case 63)
Filariasis, *Wuchereria bancrofti*, *Brugia malayi*	Mosquito	Humans	Asia and South America	'Respiratory tract infection', lymphoedema, fever
Typhus, *Rickettsia prowazekii*	Louse	Humans	Africa	Increases during war
Lyme disease, *Borrelia burgdorferi*	Ticks	Humans, deer	USA and Europe	Skin rash with multisystem disorder (see Case 42)
Epidemic encephalitis, α-flaviviruses,	Mosquito, ticks	Humans, rodents, sheep, cattle	North and South America	Different types defined geographically and by vector
Trypanosomiasis, *T. gambiense*, *T. rhodesiense*	Tsetse fly	Humans, wild game	Africa, Central and South America	*African trypanosomiasis*, 'chancre', fever, 'sleeping sickness' *American trypanosomiasis* (Chagas' disease) fever, hepatosplenomegaly, lymphadenopathy

cause of visceral leishmaniasis, exists in the flagellated form in the sandfly, and following transmission to the human host reverts to the non-flagellated form when disseminated throughout the reticuloendothelial system. The haematological features (anaemia, neutropenia and thrombocytopenia) are due to hypersplenism.

Q What is the treatment of choice?

A Pentavalent antimony compounds such as sodium stibogluconate are the mainstay of treatment.

Richard is started on sodium stibogluconate. His fever subsides after 10 days, and over the next couple of weeks there is a rise in his haemoglobin and his liver and spleen become smaller as detected clinically and by ultrasound examination.

Q What serious complications may follow visceral leishmaniasis?

A Splenic rupture and haemorrhage, and secondary bacterial or viral infection – which may be overwhelming because of impaired immune responses due to hypersplenism – are major life-threatening complications.

Summary: Leishmaniasis
Presentation
Fever, anaemia, hepatosplenomegaly, lymphadenopathy (visceral) or skin ulcers/nodules (cutaneous). History of sandfly bite not always present
Diagnosis
Tissue biopsy (liver, spleen, lymph node, skin, as appropriate), culture (specialized technique) and serology
Management
Pentavalent antimony compounds and treatment of complications, e.g. plastic surgery for skin deformities, transfusion for severe anaemia

---

CASE 53
Dilip, a 45-year-old motor mechanic, with diabetes and renal failure

Dilip, a 45-year-old motor mechanic, has had insulin-dependent diabetes since the age of 17. Over the past 3 years his renal function has deteriorated. After referral to the renal physicians, appropriate investigations confirm a diagnosis of diabetic nephropathy and that renal dialysis is indicated.

Q What microbiological investigations should the renal physicians perform?

A All patients entering a dialysis unit should be screened for urinary tract infection with an MSU and for bloodborne virus infections. Such patients are likely to undergo extensive invasive procedures over a long period of time, and therefore represent an infection risk to health-care workers performing these manipulations. Furthermore, haemodialysis machines are a potential source of patient-to-patient spread of bloodborne infection, and well-documented outbreaks of hepatitis B and non-A non-B hepatitis (now known as hepatitis C) have occurred on dialysis units, some with alarmingly high mortality rates. Dilip should therefore be tested for evidence of hepatitis B and C and human immunodeficiency virus infections after appropriate explanation and counselling, prior to entry to the dialysis unit.

Dilip's results are: anti-HIV negative; hepatitis B surface antigen negative; anti-HCV negative

Q What prophylactic measure should be offered to Dilip?

A He should be offered a course of hepatitis B vaccine, with the aim of inducing protective levels of anti-HBs (see Case 22). Individuals who are immunosuppressed, or who have chronic underlying disease, are less likely to make an antibody response to this vaccine, so Dilip should be offered vaccine as soon as it is clear that his renal function is deteriorating and that dialysis may eventually be required.

Q What other measures can be taken to reduce the risk of nosocomial transmission of these bloodborne viral infections on a renal unit?

A

- Optimal infection control practice should be rigorously adhered to (e.g. handwashing, careful disposal of sharps)
- Once-only disposable materials should be used wherever possible, including component parts of dialysis machines
- Health-care workers who are HBe antigen-positive carriers of HBV (see Case 22 for explanation of HBeAg, and definition of HBV carriers) should not be allowed to perform invasive procedures on the unit
- All staff on the unit should be protected from HBV infection by vaccination
- All patients entering the unit should be screened for HBV, HCV and HIV infection. Such screening should be repeated at intervals (e.g. every 6 months) to ensure that no new infections are introduced into the unit, and to provide assurance that spread of infection is not occurring
- All patients should be vaccinated against HBV
- The management of a patient discovered to be a carrier of any of these viruses is problematic. Ideally, there should be dedicated dialysis machines on the unit that are used *only* for these patients, and dialysis should be performed in a suitable isolation facility.

Recent reports of the spread of HCV infection within dialysis units, through routes as yet unknown, highlight the need for continued vigilance of infection control procedures.

After 2 years on haemodialysis a donor kidney becomes available for Dilip.

Q What microbiological investigations should be performed on donor and recipient immediately prior to transplantation?

A Donor serum should be tested for evidence of chronic carriage of HBV, HCV and HIV. Donor organs from HBV or HIV carriers are **not** acceptable for use, as the risks associated with transmission of these infections to the recipient outweigh the potential benefits of the transplantation. The situation with HCV is less clear at present. Recipient serum should also be sent for the same tests, unless by chance screening has been performed recently.

Q What other virological screening assays should be considered?

A Cytomegalovirus (CMV) can be transmitted by organ transplantation, and the immune status of both donor and recipient to CMV should be determined. The immune status of the recipient to varicella-zoster virus (VZV) should also be determined.

Q Why is it necessary to know the VZV immune status of the recipient?

A All transplant recipients receive imunosuppressive agents, and are therefore at risk of serious consequences of infection with organisms that are otherwise relatively innocuous in immunocompetent hosts. Thus, if a recipient is known to be susceptible to VZV infection, and is exposed to someone with chicken-pox, passive immunization with varicella-zoster immune globulin is indicated, with the aim of attenuating a possible attack of chicken-pox.

On looking through Dilip's medical records, you note that viral serology was performed 3

months ago when he presented with a febrile illness. Among other results you find the following: CMV CFT (complement fixation test) <16 (i.e. negative), VZV CFT <16.

Q Does this mean that Dilip has never been exposed to either CMV or VZV?

A No. Complement-fixing antibodies (IgM, and certain subclasses of IgG) appear early during acute infection and tend to disappear over the following few months. Thus, detection of such antibodies by means of a CFT is a useful approach to diagnosis of recent infection. However, much more sensitive assays (e.g. ELISA, latex agglutination) should be employed if immune status is being sought.

The following results are received from Dilip and the kidney donor:

> Donor: anti-CMV (by ELISA): Positive
>
> Dilip: anti-CMV (by ELISA): Negative
> anti-VZV (by ELISA): Positive.

Q How should these results be interpreted?

A The donor has had prior exposure to CMV, whereas Dilip has not. Dilip has been infected with VZV in the past. He is therefore not at risk of acquiring primary VZV infection (i.e. chicken-pox), but he may suffer from reactivation of his own latent VZ virus, i.e. shingles or zoster (see Case 38).

Q Is there a risk that the donor kidney may transmit CMV infection to Dilip?

A Yes. CMV, like VZV, belongs to the herpesvirus family and exhibits the phenomenon of latency (see Case 2). The donor has been infected with CMV in the past; CMV will thus be present within the donor in a latent state and may be transmitted in renal tissue.

Q What types of CMV infection may occur in a recipient of a solid organ?

A The possibilities are:
Primary
• seronegative recipient of seropositive organ
Secondary
(a) reinfection
• seropositive recipient of seropositive organ
(b) reactivation
• seropositive recipient of seronegative or seropositive organ.

Primary infection carries the greatest risk of symptomatic disease.

Dilip undergoes a transplant operation, with a standard immunosuppressive regimen of cyclosporin, azathioprine and prednisolone. The transplant is successful, and Dilip is discharged after 2 weeks with a functioning kidney. He returns for regular follow-up. Seven weeks after the operation he presents with general malaise, and is noted to be febrile (38.5°C). There are no localizing signs.

Q What is the differential diagnosis, and what investigations should be initiated?

A Dilip should be admitted to hospital and investigated thoroughly. Although there is a long list of causes of febrile illness without localizing signs, the following must be considered in particular:

• bacterial infection (e.g. urinary or respiratory tract infection, septicaemia)
• a rejection episode
• CMV infection.

Correct diagnosis is crucial. If this is a rejection episode immunosuppression must be increased, whereas if this is acute CMV it should be decreased to allow Dilip's own immune response to overcome the infection. A range of simple investigations should be ordered, such as full blood count, urea and electrolytes, liver function tests, chest X-ray, and septic screen (MSU, sputum, blood cultures).

The following results are received:

Hb 9.7 g/dl
White cell count 3.2 × 10⁹/l
Differential PMNLs 30%, lymphocytes 65%, monocytes 5%
Urea and electrolytes – within normal ranges
ALT 75 IU/l (normal range up to 45)
Bilirubin, alkaline phosphatase, γ-glutamyl transferase – within normal ranges
Chest X-ray – normal
MSU – no growth
Sputum– commensals only
Blood cultures (after 48 hours) – no growth.

Q How are these results interpreted?

A The absence of a neutrophil response, and failure to isolate a pathogen from a patient with no history of recent antibiotics, are evidence against an acute bacterial infection. The normal renal function makes an acute rejection episode unlikely. The marrow suppression, particularly of the white cells, together with the biochemical evidence of hepatitis (raised ALT), is a typical feature of primary CMV infection.

Q How may CMV infection be acquired?

A

- *Mother to baby*, giving rise to congenital CMV infection (see Case 59)
- *Close contact with small children*. CMV-infected infants excrete CMV in saliva and urine for many months, if not years. Spread of infection, e.g. within a daycare centre, can therefore occur through contamination of the environment
- *Sexual transmission*
- *Blood transfusion and transplantation*: the likely route in

Dilip's case, as he has received a seropositive kidney.

Q What are the consequences of CMV infection?

A These depend on the age and immune status of the patient (see Box 53.1).

Q How can it be confirmed that Dilip has a CMV infection?

A Given the potential seriousness of Dilip's illness, the laboratory should be asked to perform a *rapid diagnostic technique* for the diagnosis of CMV infection on a sample of blood. There are a number of such techniques available, and individual laboratories will differ as to which one they can offer:

- Detection of early antigen fluorescent foci (the DEAFF test): although CMV-infected cells may remain morphologically normal for many days, they will nevertheless be expressing viral antigens on the cell surface. Thus, after inoculation of patient material into cell culture the presence of virus may be seen 24–48 hours later by staining the cells with fluorescent-labelled monoclonal antibodies directed against viral antigens expressed early in the replicative cycle of CMV (the so-called early antigens)
- Direct CMV antigen detection: here, peripheral blood cells taken directly from the patient are stained with labelled monoclonal antibodies, to detect CMV antigen expression occurring *in vivo*
- CMV genome detection: the advent of polymerase chain reaction assays (see Case 2) means that the presence of the DNA genome of CMV in peripheral blood can now be demonstrated. Routine tissue culture, which is the standard assay for demonstration of CMV, is inappropriate here, as it may take up to 4 weeks for the virus to produce a cytopathic effect.

B53.1 Consequences of CMV infection

- In fetus and neonate
  Congenital CMV infection – see Case 59
- In immunocompetent individuals
  Asymptomatic – the vast majority
  Infectious mononucleosis syndrome – see Case 9
- In immunosuppressed individuals
  Multisystem disease may arise from primary *or* secondary infection.
  In HIV infection – see Case 48
  In transplant recipients; fever, marrow suppression and hepatitis are common; pneumonitis may be life-threatening.

Q Why is it important to demonstrate CMV in peripheral blood rather than, say, a urine sample?

A Excretion of CMV in urine is a not uncommon finding, especially in immunosuppressed individuals, and may occur in the absence of disease. The presence of replicating CMV in peripheral blood correlates much better with CMV-induced disease.

Q How should Dilip's CMV infection be managed?

A His immunosuppression should be reduced, e.g. by stopping the azathioprine, although this will require careful monitoring of his renal function. He should also be treated with ganciclovir, an antiviral agent with activity against CMV. This drug, however, has toxic side-effects, principally on the bone marrow, causing yet further suppression of white cell production.

After a stormy 3 weeks, Dilip recovers from his CMV infection with his transplanted kidney intact.

Q Could Dilip's severe CMV-induced disease have been prevented?

A Yes, or at least attenuated. As Dilip was known to be a CMV-seronegative recipient of a seropositive kidney, and therefore at increased risk of serious CMV disease, he should have been offered some form of prophylaxis. A number of prophylactic regimens have been shown to reduce the risk of serious CMV infection in recipients of both solid organs and of bone marrow. These include:

- prophylactic acyclovir. Although this drug has very little anti-CMV effect *in vitro*, trials have nevertheless demonstrated its efficacy in the prevention of CMV infection
- administration of CMV hyper-immune globulin, i.e. passive immunization
- pre-emptive therapy with ganciclovir, i.e. surveillance monitoring for the emergence of CMV infection, including routine bronchoalveolar lavage (for BMT recipients), and institution of ganciclovir therapy at the earliest indication of potential trouble.

Summary: CMV infection in a transplant recipient
Presentation
Multisystem disease with fever, leucopenia, hepatitis; pneumonitis is life-threatening
Diagnosis
Rapid diagnostic techniques on clinically relevant samples, i.e. DEAFF test, antigen or genome detection on blood sample
Management
Prophylaxis for high-risk patients; if symptomatic disease arises, reduce immunosuppression if possible and consider ganciclovir therapy

CASE 54
Irritability, feeding difficulties and hypoxia in Sarah just after birth

After a 3-day pyrexial illness in her mother, Sarah is born by vaginal delivery at 30 weeks and weighs 1.8 kg. She is transferred to the special care baby unit (SCBU) for observation, but on day 4 she becomes irritable, difficult to feed and hypoxic, requiring intubation and ventilation. Biochemical investigations exclude a metabolic cause such as hypoglycaemia, and there is no clinical or other evidence of congenital abnormality or intraventricular haemorrhage.

Q What microbiological investigations should be carried out to exclude infection?

A Non-specific signs such as those described are compatible with neonatal infection, and the presence of risk factors such as maternal pyrexia or prolonged rupture of membranes make infection likely. A septic screen, which includes two sets of blood cultures, cerebrospinal fluid (CSF), urine and respiratory secretions for bacterial culture, should therefore be carried out. A throat swab in viral transport medium, faeces and CSF should also be sent for virological studies,

as enteroviral infection can cause severe neonatal infection.

Q How may neonatal bacterial infection be classified?

A Early-onset infection is defined as occurring during the first 3–4 days of life and is usually caused by pathogens acquired during passage down the birth canal, during traumatic delivery, or immediately following a caesarian section. Late-onset infection presents 5 days after delivery or later, and is usually due to pathogens acquired from the mother, staff, or occasionally from inadequately cleaned or decontaminated

Table 54.1 Bacterial pathogens important in the neonate	
Neonatal bacterial pathogen	**Special features**
β-haemolytic streptococci group B (*S. agalactiae*)	Usually acquired from mother's vagina and accounts for 43% of early-onset neonatal sepsis, including bacteraemia, meningitis (see Case 1) and pneumonia (see Case 36)
Coliforms, including *E. coli*	Similar spectrum of disease to group B streptococci. Outbreaks of multiresistant *Klebsiella aerogenes* in neonatal units occasionally occur
Listeria monocytogenes	Recognized cause of serious infection in the neonate and mother
Pseudomonas spp.	*P. aeruginosa* (see Case 16) causes ventilator-associated pneumonia and other species are implicated in the premature neonate
Staphylococcus aureus	May cause localized (skin pustules, conjunctivitis, infected umbilical cord) or systemic (bacteraemia, pneumonia, osteomyelitis) infection and the scalded skin syndrome (see Case 40)
Staphylococcus epidermidis	Intravascular catheter-associated bacteraemia and, occasionally, meningitis if congenital abnormality present
Neisseria gonorrhoeae	Ophthalmia neonatorum (conjunctivitis) from mother (see Case 56)
Chlamydia trachomatis	Inclusion conjunctivitis during first week and pneumonia in 2nd–3rd weeks of life (see Case 56)

equipment. The most frequently implicated bacteria are listed in Table 54.1.

Blood cultures, urine, CSF and respiratory secretions are taken and sent to the microbiology laboratory. Sarah is started on intravenous penicillin and gentamicin to cover streptococcal and Gram-negative infection pending the results of investigations. The following day it is reported that Gram-positive bacilli are to be seen that morning in a Gram film from all of the blood culture bottles.

Q What is the most likely pathogen?

A Significant bacteraemia and not contamination is likely, as all the bottles are positive (see Case 44). The Gram film findings in the setting of a premature neonate with systemic infection is very suggestive of listeriosis (infection caused by *L. monocytogenes*, see Box 54.1). Sometimes the appearance on the Gram film is said to resemble 'Chinese lettering', but the subsequent culture results will exclude infection due to other Gram-positive bacilli such as *Clostridium* spp. or *Bacillus* spp.

Q What are the clinical features of listeriosis associated with pregnancy?

B54.1 *Listeria monocytogenes*

- Short Gram-positive bacilli with tumbling motility at 25°C, slightly haemolytic on blood agar. There are at least six other species, e.g. *L. ivanovii*, but these are rarely implicated in human disease
- Transmission (see Figure 54.1) is by ingestion of contaminated foodstuffs (see Case 17) or contact, for example with resuscitation equipment
- A haemolysin, listeriolysin O, is a potential virulence factor, but in non-pregnant patients impaired cell-mediated immunity (such as occurs in patients with lymphoma or diabetes mellitus) is a more important predisposing factor to infection

---

A Four clinical syndromes are described:

- Abortion: maternal flu-like illness during the last 4–5 months of the pregnancy, with loss of the fetus
- Maternal infection: flu-like illness just before delivery, with rigors, myalgia and pharyngitis. Early-onset infection in the neonate may follow
- Early-onset neonatal infection: intrauterine acquisition of listeria due to haematogenous spread to the placenta. May present acutely with pneumonia, bacteraemia, diarrhoea and meningitis, or occasionally subclinically

- Late-onset neonatal infection: acquired during passage down the birth canal, especially in premature babies, or may be acquired from a nosocomial source. Presents from the 4th–5th day onwards with meningitis and bacteraemia. Mother is usually well.

The intravenous penicillin is changed to ampicillin, the gentamicin continued (believed to act synergistically with the ampicillin) and serum assays of gentamicin are carried out every other day. *L. monocytogenes* is isolated from blood cultures but the CSF is sterile. Sarah gradually improves over the next 3 days, is discharged from the SCBU after a further 4 days and ultimately goes home to be followed up in the community and at the paediatric outpatients.

Q Is *L. monocytogenes* part of the normal flora of the pregnant woman?

A Yes. Listeria may be detected in the faeces of 30–40% of pregnant women (and many non-pregnant individuals), but is often intermittent or transient.

Q Does maternal carriage predict the development of listeriosis?

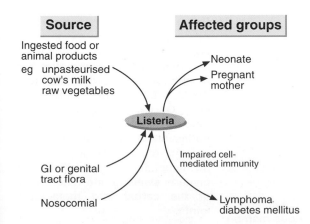

Fig. 54.1 Sources of, and at-risk patients for listeriosis.

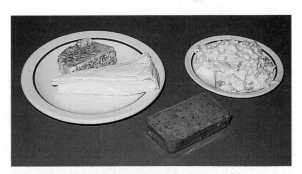

Fig. 54.2 Foods (soft cheese, coleslaw, paté) associated with listeriosis.

A No. Asymptomatic rather than symptomatic carriage is the norm, and systemic maternal infection may not be associated with a positive faeces sample. Isolation from blood cultures or CSF is the only reliable means of diagnosing maternal and neonatal listeriosis, but amniotic fluid or placenta should be cultured when abortions occur, or when listeria infection is suspected at delivery. Reliable serological tests are not available to diagnose listeriosis.

Q Which is more common, sporadic infection due to *L. monocytogenes* or clusters of cases/epidemic infection?

A Most cases are sporadic and no source is usually ever identified. It is true, however, that there was an increase in cases, approaching epidemic proportions, during the late 1980s in the United Kingdom, which may have been related to the increased consumption of contaminated foods such as soft cheeses and paté (see Figure 54.2). Localised outbreaks have also been described associated with animals (eg sheep) and in hospitals where transmission has occurred via hand contact with contaminated equipment (eg thermometers).

Q Is listeriosis associated with recurrent abortions?

A This is a controversial point. A study conducted in the 1960s suggested that listeriosis caused recurrent abortions in some women, but this has not been confirmed in further clinical studies. If listeriosis is a cause, experience suggests that it is quite uncommon and

accounts for a small proportion of recurrent abortions.

Q What advice should be given to pregnant women about avoiding infection due to *L. monocytogenes*?

A Pregnant women and immuno-compromised patients at risk should avoid certain foods, e.g. soft ripened cheeses (brie, camembert), all types of paté, cooked–chilled meals and ready-to-eat poultry unless thoroughly reheated. Patients should also be advised about good hygiene in the storage and preparation of foods, such as keeping food for as short a time as possible, ensuring the refrigerator is working properly, storing cooked foods separately from raw foods, discarding left-over reheated food, and finally, observing the reheating and standing times when using a microwave oven.

Summary: Listeriosis
Presentation
Unexplained fever or meningitis in a pregnant woman, neonate or immunocompromised patient, e.g. lymphoma, diabetes mellitus
Diagnosis
Isolation of *L. monocytogenes* from blood, CSF or birth products
Management
Avoidance of at-risk foods such as soft cheeses. Ampicillin with gentamicin is the treatment of choice

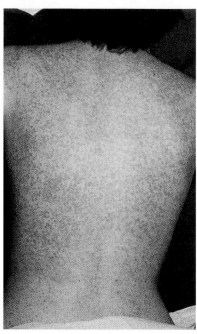

Fig. 55.1 Deborah's rash.

Q Which infectious diseases need to be considered in the differential diagnosis?

A Although there are a number of non-infectious causes of a rash and arthralgia (e.g. a connective tissue disorder such as systemic lupus erythematosus, a drug or other allergy), the important diagnoses to confirm or refute in this case are acute rubella virus and acute parvovirus B19 infections.

Deborah gives a history of rubella vaccination as a teenager. This is her first pregnancy. She remembers looking after her neighbour's son 2–3 weeks ago, the day before he developed a rash. On examination Deborah's rash is maculopapular, most noticeable on the face but also present on the trunk. There is no lymphadenopathy. There is bilateral swelling and tenderness of the carpal and metacarpal joints.

Q What investigations should be carried out?

CASE 55
Deborah, 23 years old and 12 weeks pregnant, develops a rash

Deborah, 23 years old and 12 weeks pregnant, presents to the antenatal clinic with a 1-day history of fever and a diffuse erythematous rash on the face and trunk (see Figure 55.1). She has also noticed some swelling of her wrists.

A Serum should be sent requesting both rubella and parvovirus serology. The history of rubella vaccination is *not* sufficient to rule out a diagnosis of acute primary rubella infection. A percentage of individuals may not respond to the vaccine, or the vaccine may have been incorrectly stored, resulting in failure with the patient remaining susceptible to rubella. Although there may be features in an individual case more suggestive of parvovirus than rubella infection or vice versa (e.g. the parvovirus rash characteristically waxes and wanes; cervical adenopathy is more likely in rubella), a clinical diagnosis cannot be relied upon and thus both serologies should be performed.

Q How should the following rubella serology be interpreted?

Rubella IgG negative, IgM negative?
Rubella IgG negative, IgM positive?
Rubella IgG positive (60 iu/ml), IgM positive?
Rubella IgG positive (60 iu/ml), IgM negative?

A Correct interpretation of these results requires an understanding of the differences between IgG and IgM. Figure 55.2 shows the sequence of events following infection with a virus. As can be seen, the IgM response appears marginally sooner than the IgG, but is only transient whereas the IgG response persists, usually for life. Thus, the laboratory would issue the following reports:

• *Rubella IgG negative, IgM negative*

Laboratory report No evidence of prior infection with rubella. Please send repeat sample in 5 days' time.

Explanation Despite her history of rubella vaccination, Deborah is not immune to rubella and is therefore susceptible to infection. Note that antibody may not appear until a day or two AFTER the rash, so it is still possible that Deborah is suffering an acute rubella infection. To resolve this, a repeat serum sample, taken

5 days or later after appearance of the rash, must be tested. If that serum is also seronegative, then Deborah's current illness is not rubella. She should be advised to have rubella vaccination postpartum.

• *Rubella IgG negative, IgM positive*

Laboratory report Suggests acute rubella. Please send second sample for confirmation.

Explanation The IgM response appears slightly earlier than IgG, although this combination of results is relatively unusual. The implication is that the patient is suffering an attack of acute rubella. However, given the significance of that diagnosis, and the possibility of false positive IgM results, the diagnosis must be confirmed by testing a repeat sample taken a few days later, and demonstrating IgG seroconversion. Indeed, some laboratories may only report the negative IgG result on the first specimen, deferring the IgM testing until a second sample is available.

• *Rubella IgG positive (60 iu/ml), IgM positive*

Laboratory report These results strongly suggest acute rubella infection. Please send second sample for confirmation.

Explanation For reasons given above it is wise to seek a repeat sample, which may enable a rising IgG titre to be demonstrated and will allay any doubts over possible laboratory errors.

• *Rubella IgG positive (60 iu/ml), IgM negative*

Laboratory report No evidence

of primary rubella. Please send second sample for confirmation.

Explanation As there is no IgM present Deborah has not suffered a recent attack of rubella. The presence of IgG indicates that she has been exposed to this virus in the past, either the wild-type or vaccine (or both). This IgG further indicates that she is immune to rubella. Again, it is still wise to ask for a second sample to confirm this.

Q Why is the diagnosis of maternal rubella infection in pregnancy so important?

A Rubella virus may cross the placenta and infect the developing fetus, resulting in the congenital rubella syndrome.

Q What are the main features of the congenital rubella syndrome?

A A wide range of abnormalities have been reported. The common ones include:

• general – growth retardation
• cardiac – patent ductus arteriosus, pulmonary artery stenosis
• eye – cataract, retinopathy, microphthalmia
• ear – sensorineural deafness
• CNS – encephalitis, mental retardation.

Q In a pregnant woman with rubella, what single factor influences the risk of development and the severity of the congenital rubella syndrome?

A The stage in pregnancy at which the rubella infection is acquired. Thus, the risk of congenital rubella syndrome from maternal infection in

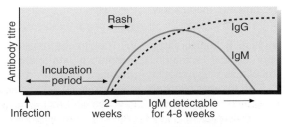

Fig. 55.2 Antibody response in primary rubella.

Table 55.1 Risk of rubella

Gestation	Risk	Clinical features
0–8 weeks	90–100%	Multiple defects, cardiac/eye/CNS
8–12 weeks	80–90%	Multiple defects, cardiac/eye/CNS
12–18 weeks	Declining to 0%	Deafness, mental retardation
>18 weeks	rare (<1%)	Deafness

the first few weeks of pregnancy is almost 100%, whereas maternal rubella in the third trimester carries no risk (see Table 55.1)

Q How may rubella be prevented?

A By the use of a live attenuated vaccine. The UK has recently (1988) changed from a strategy of vaccinating only women of child-bearing age to one of universal vaccination in the second year of life (in combination with measles and mumps – MMR). This has the advantage of interrupting the circulation of rubella virus in the community, rubella being predominantly a disease of childhood, and therefore dramatically reducing the risk of a susceptible pregnant woman coming into contact with rubella.

Q If Deborah's serology had indicated a recent rubella infection, how should she be managed?

A The only alternatives for Deborah are to continue with the pregnancy, with the attendant risk of her baby having the congenital rubella syndrome, or to have a termination.

Q How would your management of Deborah differ if she had presented with only a history of contact with a rash, being herself completely asymptomatic?

A This is, in fact, a considerably more common clinical scenario. Once again, rubella serology should be requested. The interpretation of the results are similar to above, but the timescale of sampling may differ. Possible results would be:

Rubella IgG negative, IgM negative
The patient is seronegative and therefore susceptible. The incubation period between infection and production of antibodies is usually 2–3 weeks (see Figure 55.2), but in rare instances may be delayed as long as 4 weeks. Thus, primary rubella cannot be excluded in this patient until a sample taken 28 days after contact has also been shown to be seronegative.

Rubella IgG negative, IgM positive
This is either early rubella or a false positive IgM. As the IgM response has begun, if this really is rubella the IgG should be detectable very soon, so a repeat sample can be taken in 2–5 days' time.

Rubella IgG positive (60 iu/ml), IgM positive
Strongly suggestive of recent rubella. A second sample for confirmation should be requested.

Rubella IgG positive (60 iu/ml), IgM negative
No evidence of recent (i.e. within the last 6–8 weeks) rubella. A second sample should be requested for confirmation.

In fact, the following results are received on Deborah's serum: rubella IgG positive, IgM negative; parvovirus B19 IgM and DNA positive.

Q How are these results interpreted?

A The rubella results indicate that Deborah is immune to rubella. The presence of IgM directed against parvovirus B19 indicates a recent infection with this virus. This is confirmed by the finding of parvovirus B19 DNA.

Q What effects may parvovirus B19 infection have in pregnancy?

A Although maternal parvovirus infection may be clinically indistinguishable from rubella, and both viruses may cross the placenta and infect the fetus, the consequences to the fetus are very different. Parvovirus B19 infects bone marrow precursor cells (see Case 62), resulting in a temporary cessation of marrow production. The consequences of parvovirus infection in pregnancy are:

- a 10% increased risk of spontaneous termination of the pregnancy
- if the maternal infection occurs in the 2nd or 3rd trimesters, then fetal heart failure secondary to parvovirus-induced fetal anaemia may result in presentation with hydrops fetalis

Note that there are no reports of congenital malformations in babies from those pregnancies that survive.

For those still confused by the various combinations of results given in this case, the essential messages are that it is always advisable to request serology and, if in doubt, discuss the interpretation of results and management with the virologist or microbiologist.

Summary: Rash in pregnancy
Diagnoses to exclude
Rubella, parvovirus infection
Investigations
One or more serum samples for rubella and parvovirus serology
Complications
Congenital rubella syndrome: risk depends on stage of pregnancy; parvovirus – miscarriage or hydrops fetalis in late pregnancy
Prevention
Rubella vaccination; no vaccine for parvovirus

CASE 56
A sticky eye in Daniel, 5 days old

Daniel was born 6 days ago, by vaginal delivery after an uneventful labour, and discharged from hospital 48 hours later. His Apgar scores were 9 at 1 minute and 10 at 5 minutes. His mother, Susan, has brought him back to the postnatal ward as she has noticed swelling and reddening of his left eye, which he is now not opening. He has been breast-feeding without difficulty, and is otherwise well. On examination of his left eye, in addition to the swelling and reddening, there is a mucopurulent discharge (see Fig. 56.1), a thin film of whitish exudate over the cornea, and the conjunctivae are also reddened. The right eye shows similar, but less marked changes. There are no other abnormal physical signs.

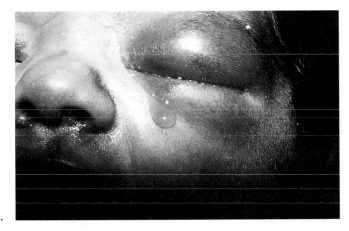

**Fig. 56.1
Daniel's eye.**

> **B56.1 Infectious causes of ophthalmia neonatorum**
>
> *Chlamydia trachomatis*
> * strains D–K (i.e. the same strains responsible for genital infection)
> * onset 5–14 days after birth
> * follicular keratoconjunctivitis
>
> *Neisseria gonorrhoeae*
> * onset on first or second day of life
> * severe purulent conjunctivitis
>
> *Staphylococcus aureus*
> * onset 5–10 days after birth
> * known as 'sticky eye'
> * may be associated with outbreak of staphylococcal sepsis on maternity ward
>
> Other causes include *Streptococcus pneumoniae, Haemophilus influenzae*, herpes simplex virus (HSV)

Q What is the clinical diagnosis?

A The signs are those of acute conjunctivitis. In a young baby this condition is known as **ophthalmia neonatorum.**

Q What are the common causes of ophthalmia neonatorum?

A

* Infection (see Box 56.1)
* Chemical irritation. This was common when it was standard practice to use ocular silver nitrate prophylaxis against *Neisseria gonorrhoeae*, but such prophylaxis is not indicated today. The disease was self-limiting, occurring within the first 24 hours and lasting 1 or 2 days.

Q What investigations should be performed?

A A conjunctival smear should be Gram stained. In acute bacterial conjunctivitis large numbers of neutrophils are seen. Bacteria may be present within or outside leukocytes. Gonococci may be seen as intracellular Gram-negative diplococci. One smear should be stained for chlamydial basophilic intracytoplasmic inclusion bodies in epithelial cells (using Giemsa, or fluorescent antibody stains). Swabs should be taken for culture of *C. trachomatis, N. gonorrhoeae*, other bacteria and HSV. Note that each swab must be sent in appropriate transport medium (e.g. Amies charcoal for *N. gonorrhoeae*, chlamydial and viral transport medium for *C. trachomatis* and HSV respectively) before transport to the laboratory.

Q What is the treatment of choice?

A Definitive treatment will depend on the results of the above investigations, but a likely diagnosis in a 6-day-old baby with conjunctivitis is chlamydia infection, and presumptive therapy with tetracycline ointment should be started after collection of the swab. Systemic erythromycin is also indicated for severe infection, and also to prevent the development of chlamydia pneumonia. Suspected gonococcal conjunctivitis must also be treated promptly with systemic benzylpenicillin (unless there is reason to suspect a penicillin-resistant strain, see Case 28), as corneal ulceration and perforation may occur. Chloramphenicol ointment for the treatment of other bacteria is appropriate only if chlamydia and gonorrhoeal infections have been ruled out.

Q Should any further investigations be performed?

A Yes. The pathogenesis of gonococcal and chlamydial ophthalmia neonatorum involves acquisition of the relevant organism during passage of the baby through the birth canal. If either of these organisms is confirmed in Daniel's eye, then his mother should be counselled and treated appropriately, as should her sexual contacts (see Case 28).

Q What other eye disease is caused by *C. trachomatis*?

A Trachoma is caused by *C. trachomatis* strains A–C. This is endemic in Africa and the Middle East. Organisms are spread between patients by the hands, leading to a chronic follicular keratoconjunctivitis. In overcrowded and unhygienic conditions secondary bacterial infection is a common complication. Scarring of the cornea occurs, leading to blindness, of which trachoma is the most common infectious cause in the world.

Summary: Ophthalmia neonatorum
Presentation
Acute purulent conjunctivitis within 14 days of birth
Pathogenesis
Acquisition of *N. gonorrhoeae*, or *C. trachomatis* infection on passage through birth canal; nosocomial acquisition of *S. aureus* on maternity ward
Management
Identification of causative organism by appropriately stained smears and culture; prompt topical or systemic antibiotics; treatment of mother and her sexual contacts for chlamydial infection and gonorrhoea

CASE 57
A pregnant woman whose son has developed chicken-pox

A 30-year-old mother of two attends the surgery because her 8-year-old son has chicken-pox (see Case 38). She mentions that she is 12 weeks pregnant.

Q Is this situation of concern?

A Yes. Here is a pregnant woman who has been exposed to chicken-pox. If she is susceptible to varicella-zoster virus (VZV) infection then she may herself suffer an attack of chicken-pox during this pregnancy, which may have consequences for both herself and her fetus.

Q What are the complications of chicken-pox in pregnancy?

A There are possible adverse effects for both the mother:

• Chicken-pox pneumonia; this, the commonest life-threatening complication of primary VZV infection, is more likely to occur in an adult than in a child, and is also more likely in a pregnant rather than a non-pregnant woman, with an incidence of 10%

and for her baby:

• Congenital varicella syndrome (see Box 57.1); this rare complication arises in 1–2% of cases of maternal chicken-pox in the first 20 weeks of pregnancy. Virus crosses the placenta and infects the fetus

B57.1 The congenital varicella syndrome
• Skin loss and scarring, usually unilateral, segmented • Hypoplasia of limb bud development, rudimentary digits • CNS – cortical, cerebellar atrophy, microcephaly • Eye – microphthalmia, chorioretinitis, cataracts • General – intrauterine growth retardation, psychomotor retardation

• Herpes zoster in infancy; if the maternal infection is after 20 weeks of pregnancy, then the only potential problem for the offspring is that he or she may develop herpes zoster in early childhood. This proves that virus can indeed cross the placenta

• Neonatal chicken-pox; if the maternal infection occurs at the end of pregnancy, then there is a risk that the baby will be born before the mother has had time to mount an immune response and to transfer immunity, in the form of antibodies, across the placenta. The baby will therefore be at risk of developing neonatal chicken-pox, which carries a high morbidity and mortality.

Q How should this pregnant patient be managed?

A It is necessary to determine whether or not she is at risk of primary VZV infection.

Q How can it be ascertained whether the mother is susceptible to VZV infection?

A The simplest method is to ask the patient – or her parents, if possible – whether she has ever had chicken-pox. The features of chicken-pox are sufficiently distinctive that a clinical diagnosis is usually correct, and therefore a past history of chicken-pox correlates very well with the presence of antibodies to VZV. Thus, if the answer is 'yes' the patient can be reassured that she is immune from an attack of chicken-pox, and no further action need be taken.

Q What if the answer is 'no', or 'don't know'?

A Her immune status should be checked by sending a serum sample to be tested for the presence or absence of anti-VZV antibodies. Eighty per cent of women without a personal history of chicken-pox are nevertheless anti-VZV positive, and therefore immune.

The patient is not aware that she has had chicken-pox in the past. A serum sample is sent for determination of her immune status to VZV, and the result is negative (i.e. no anti-VZV detected).

Q What should be done now?

A The patient should be offered a dose (1000 mg, given intra-muscularly) of varicella-zoster immunoglobulin (VZIg). This is an example of passive immunization: the VZIg will provide her with antibodies to VZV made by someone else. The reason for doing this is that the VZIg will attenuate (but not prevent) the attack of chicken-pox, thereby reducing the risk of maternal chicken-pox pneumonia. There is also evidence that VZIg reduces the risk of transplacental spread of virus, and hence of the congenital varicella syndrome. The sooner after the contact that the VZIg is administered the better, but VZIg is still worth giving up to 10 days after contact.

Q What is the management of a pregnant woman who is exposed to herpes zoster (i.e. shingles)?

A Although a patient with shingles excretes considerably less virus into their surroundings than a patient with chicken-pox, he or she is still infectious – the vesicles contain virus in high titre. Consequently the management is the same as for exposure to chicken-pox, which is summarized in Figure 57.1.

Another antenatal patient gives a history of a recent contact with a child with chicken-pox (chicken-pox is very common). Unfortunately, she did not think to report this at the time, and she now presents with a typical chicken-pox rash. She is 37 weeks pregnant.

Q Is it worth offering her a dose of VZIg?

A No. VZIg given at this stage will have no effect on the course of her illness.

Q How should she be managed?

A The first worry is that she may develop chicken-pox pneumonia. She should therefore be observed carefully over the next few days, and if there is any cause for concern referred to hospital for further investigation and treatment. Although acyclovir is not licensed for use in pregnancy, it is nevertheless a potentially life-saving drug in this situation and thus far it has an excellent safety record.

The patient remains reasonably well, but 3 days after the onset of her rash she goes into labour and delivers a healthy baby girl.

Q What is the optimal management of mother and child?

A This represents the second worry – that she will go into labour before she has had time to pass on any protective antibodies to her fetus. It takes up to 7 days after onset of the maternal rash for the mother to produce antibodies. Thus, all babies born 7 days (or later) after development of the maternal rash will have detectable anti-VZV in their serum. The risk period, therefore, is for babies born within 7 days of onset of the maternal rash, as these babies may be anti-VZV negative. All such babies should be given VZIg (250 mg, i.m.) immediately after birth, once again with the intention of attenuating the severity of the infection. Some authorities also recommend giving prophylactic high-dose acyclovir in addition to VZIg. Separation of mother and baby at birth is not recommended, as there is no evidence that this reduces the risk of neonatal disease.

Note that the same rationale applies to mothers who develop chicken-pox after their baby is born. By definition, they cannot have passed any protective immunity to their offspring, who are therefore at risk of acquiring infection. Babies up to the age of 30 days are at risk of developing chicken-pox with the same high morbidity and mortality as neonatal chicken-pox, and should at least be offered VZIg prophylaxis if exposed to an infectious source.

A third patient gives a history of a painful blistering rash on one side of her trunk for the past 4 days. On examination the rash has the typical appearance of

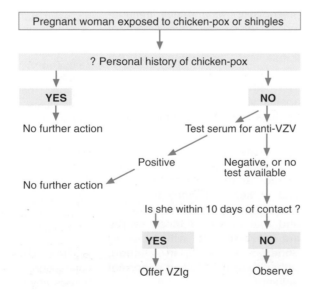

Fig. 57.1 Algorithm for management of exposure to VZV in pregnancy.

CASE 57

herpes zoster. She is 36 weeks pregnant.

Q Is her fetus at any risk?

A No. Herpes zoster is the manifestation of secondary or reactivated VZV infection. This patient will therefore be anti-VZV positive, and antibodies will cross the placenta and protect her fetus.

Summary: Chicken-pox in pregnancy
Risks
Maternal pneumonia; varicella embryopathy; neonatal chicken-pox
Management
• Of pregnant woman in contact with chicken-pox or shingles: check VZV immune status; if negative, offer VZIg • Of pregnant woman with chicken-pox: acyclovir for pneumonia; if at end of pregnancy, VZIg to neonate

CASE 58
Mrs Fisher, 25 years old, pregnant and a history of genital herpes

Mrs Fisher thinks she may be pregnant for the first time. She is 25 years old. Her last menstrual period was 6 weeks ago, and a kit pregnancy test from the pharmacy was positive. She had an attack of genital herpes when she was 17, and she suffers from occasional recurrent attacks about every 6 months. She has heard that this can be very dangerous for her baby, and is therefore worried.

Q What is the serious complication of maternal genital herpes in pregnancy?

A Neonatal herpes simplex infection, arising from passage of the neonate through an infected birth canal.

B58.1 Neonatal herpes simplex infection

- Incidence: UK 10 cases/year, USA 1/10 000 births
- Presents around 8–12 days after delivery, with non-specific signs, e.g. poor feeding, weight loss, fever
- Infection is restricted to skin, mouth or eyes in only 25% of cases
- Spread in the other 75% may involve multiple organs, e.g. liver, adrenals, brain, and may occur in the absence of skin lesions, making diagnosis difficult
- Mortality is 70–90% in disseminated disease
- Long-term morbidity includes severe developmental impairment

---

Q Why is neonatal herpes such a feared disease?

A The clinical features of neonatal herpes simplex infection are shown in Box 58.1. Neonates are unable to control the spread of HSV infection, presumably owing to their immunological immaturity. Involvement of internal organs is common and life threatening, and many of the survivors suffer long-term damage. The advent of potent antiviral agents such as acyclovir has not led to a significant improvement in mortality and morbidity.

Mrs Fisher has heard that she will have to have swabs taken at regular intervals towards the end of her pregnancy to see if she is having a recurrent attack, and that if any of these swabs are positive she will have to undergo a caesarian section, rather than be allowed a normal delivery.

CASE 58

Q Is this statement true?

A No. This strategy was devised to prevent the transmission of HSV from mother to neonate during an asymptomatic recurrent attack of genital herpes (i.e. one of which the mother is unaware), but it is in fact a misconception. Although it is true that asymptomatic recurrences do occur, excretion of virus during such attacks lasts only 24 hours or so. Thus women with a positive culture at, say, 36 weeks, will not necessarily be excreting virus at term. In contrast, the presence of negative swabs up to 40 weeks does not guarantee that the woman will not be excreting virus when she comes in 2 days later in labour. Thus the above policy is likely to result in a large number of unnecessary caesarian sections, while having no effect at all in preventing neonatal HSV. The practice of surveillance cultures should be abandoned.

Q In women with a history of genital herpes, is asymptomatic excretion of virus during delivery always associated with transmission of infection to the neonate?

A No. In fact, the risk of neonatal herpes in a baby born *per vaginam* through a birth canal infected during an asymptomatic recurrence in a woman with a history of genital herpes is very low – much less than 10% – presumably because such women pass on protective immunity to their babies. Thus, even if surveillance cultures succeeded in identifying all asymptomatic excretion during labour in women with a history of genital herpes, caesarian section would not necessarily be the most appropriate management.

Q Is a maternal history of genital herpes common in babies with neonatal HSV infection?

A No. This is another misconception! Most cases of neonatal herpes arise from mothers who are undergoing primary asymptomatic genital herpes infection, and who therefore have no history of recurrent disease. This further illustrates the futility of the surveillance culture strategy referred to above, which concentrates all efforts on those women who have a positive history of genital herpes, as only 10–15% of cases of neonatal herpes arise from such women.

Q Do all individuals who have suffered genital infection with HSV give a history of genital herpes?

A No. The development of serological assays which can distinguish between antibodies to HSV-1 and HSV-2 have demonstrated that many more people are anti-HSV-2 positive than give a history of genital herpes. Thus, the majority of genital HSV infections are asymptomatic, and a negative answer to the question 'have you ever had an attack of genital herpes?' is an unreliable guide to which patients may be excreting virus during their pregnancy.

Q Do all babies with neonatal HSV infection acquire the virus from their mothers?

A No. A small minority (5%) of babies acquire their infection postnatally (rather than perinatally) from a source other than their mother, e.g. a relative or a healthcare worker with a cold sore.

Q Under what circumstances related to the risk of HSV transmission should Mrs Fisher be advised to have a caesarian section?

A If she is suffering a symptomatic attack at the time she presents in labour. Visible lesions contain much higher titres of virus than are shed from the cervix during an asymptomatic attack, and thus the risk of transmission of infection is considerably greater. The only caveat is if the membranes have been ruptured for a considerable time (e.g. more than 6 hours), caesarian

section may not reduce the risk of transmission of infection.

For all of the reasons outlined above it is extremely difficult to devise strategies for reducing the incidence of neonatal herpes, and there are a number of myths surrounding this subject. Such information as is known with certainty is presented in Box 58.2.

The diverse manifestations of HSV infection are presented in Box 58.3.

B58.2 Genital herpes in pregnancy

- A history of genital herpes is an unreliable guide as to which women are genitally infected with HSV
- Surveillance cultures during pregnancy do not predict which women will be excreting virus asymptomatically during delivery
- Asymptomatic excretion of virus during labour in such women poses little risk to their neonates
- Most babies with neonatal herpes do *not* have mothers (or fathers) with a history of genital herpes
- If herpetic lesions are visible when a woman presents in labour, *regardless of her personal history in relation to genital herpes*, she should be delivered by caesarian section

---

B58.3 Manifestations of herpes simplex virus infection

- Asymptomatic seroconversion
- Orolabial herpes (see Case 35)
- Eczema herpeticum (see Case 35)
- Herpetic conjunctivitis (see Case 39)
- Genital herpes (see Case 29)
- Herpetic whitlow (see Case 41)
- Herpes simplex encephalitis (see Case 2)
- Neonatal herpes (this Case)

Summary: Genital herpes in pregnancy

Risk

Neonatal herpes simplex infection, which has high morbidity and mortality

Maternal genital HSV infections

- Primary – high risk of neonatal infection; caesarian section advisable
- Recurrent – low risk; caesarian section only indicated if visible lesions present during labour

---

CASE 59
An unexpected blood count from Mrs Archer, 16 weeks pregnant

Mrs Archer attends for a routine antenatal appointment. By dates she is 16 weeks pregnant. Her history and physical examination are unremarkable, and she is on no regular medication. She is a nurse on one of the paediatric wards at the local hospital. The usual routine antenatal investigations are performed, including a full blood count. Four days later the following report is received from the haematology laboratory:

Full blood count:
Haemoglobin 11.6 g/dl
White cell count 11.0 × 10⁹/l, including 5% large unclassifiable cells (LUC)
Differential white cell count and film:

Neutrophils	**44%**
Lymphocytes	**45%**
Monocytes	**6%**
LUC	**5%**

Atypical mononuclear cells seen. ?recent virus infection

Q How are these results interpreted, and what should be done now?

A These results are something of a surprise. The large unclassifiable cells (LUC) are cells which, on the basis of size and nuclear staining, do not fall into the groups of white blood cells which the automated counter is able to recognize. The high LUC count prompted a film to be made and examined, revealing the atypical mononuclear cells. These cells may appear during many acute viral infections, but are most often seen in cases of infectious mononucleosis (IM) or glandular fever.

The differential diagnosis of acute IM (see Case 9) should therefore be considered:

Epstein–Barr virus (EBV)
Cytomegalovirus (CMV)
Toxoplasma gondii
Acute HIV seroconverting illness.

Mrs Archer is asked to return to the clinic, where it is explained that one of her blood tests is abnormal and some more blood is required for further investigation.

Q What tests should be ordered to determine the cause of Mrs Archer's illness?

A Monospot or Paul Bunnell tests are useful in the diagnosis of EBV infection. Serum should also be sent for CMV and toxoplasma serology. Anti-HIV testing will not be helpful at this point, but Mrs Archer should be asked about possible risk factors for HIV infection (see Case 30).

The following results are received:
Monospot – negative
Toxoplasma latex test <16
CMV titre 256 (by complement fixation test, CFT).

Q How should these be interpreted?

A The negative monospot result decreases the likelihood of this

being EBV infection, although a minority of cases (5–10%) may be negative by both this and the Paul Bunnell test. If no other diagnosis is reached, then EBV-specific serology should be requested (see Case 9).

The toxoplasma latex test is a screening assay for the presence of antibodies to toxoplasma. The titre here is less than 16, which means there is no evidence that Mrs Archer has ever been infected with this agent. Had this result been positive, then a toxoplasma-specific IgM test should be requested to determine whether the infection is recent or not.

The CMV CFT result indicates large amounts of complement-fixing antibody against this virus.

Q Does the CMV result confirm a recent CMV infection?

A No. The serological ways in which recent infection with a given virus can be confirmed are:

- demonstration of the presence of virus-specific IgM
- demonstration of a rise in antibody titre in two separate samples taken a few days apart.

The CFT does not distinguish between IgG and IgM, both of which may fix complement. An assay for the detection of IgM anti-CMV should therefore be performed. It may also be possible to demonstrate a rise in IgG titre, as the laboratory may have received an earlier sample from Mrs Archer for rubella and syphilis serology at around 12 weeks of pregnancy.

On consultation with the laboratory further tests are initiated and the following results received:
Sample 1 (12 weeks)
 CMV CFT <16
Sample 2 (16 weeks)
 CMV CFT 256
 CMV IgM positive (strong reaction)
Indicates recent infection with CMV.

Q What type of CMV infection could this be?

A CMV is one of the herpes viruses. It is therefore possible to undergo both primary and secondary (re-activation or reinfection) infections with CMV (see Case 2). As Mrs Archer has progressed from being antibody negative to antibody positive, i.e. she has seroconverted to CMV, in addition to which she has generated a strong IgM response, it is highly likely that she has undergone a primary infection.

Q What are the risks to Mrs Archer and her fetus of a CMV infection during pregnancy?

A The virus may cross the placenta and infect the fetus. The baby will then be born congenitally infected with CMV (see Box 59.1). The chances of this happening during a primary CMV infection are around 40–50%.

Q What are the possible consequences to the fetus of congenital CMV infection?

A Of all babies congenitally infected with CMV:

- 80–90% are normal at birth, and develop normally
- 5–10% are symptomatic at birth, with cytomegalic inclusion disease (see Box 59.2)

B59.1 Congenital CMV infection

- The most common congenital infection: 1 in 300 births in the UK, i.e. considerably more common than congenital rubella
- May arise as a result of maternal primary or secondary CMV infection, both of which are usually asymptomatic
- Damage to the fetus may arise during any trimester of pregnancy (unlike congenital rubella infection)
- Diagnosis is by detection of IgM anti-CMV in cord blood, or by isolation of CMV from a neonatal throat swab or urine sample in the first 3 weeks of life

B59.2 Clinical features of cytomegalic inclusion disease

In utero
- Intrauterine growth retardation

At birth
- CNS – microcephaly, encephalitis, seizures, apnoea, focal neurological signs
- Outside the CNS – hepatitis, hepatosplenomegaly, thrombocytopaenia, pneumonitis, myocarditis

On follow-up
- 20% mortality during infancy
- Survivors have significant morbidity, which may be severe, e.g. mental retardation, blindness, deafness, or mild, e.g. defects in perceptual skills, learning disability

- 5–10% have no abnormalities at birth but develop defects on follow-up, e.g. hearing defects (uni- or bilateral), impaired intellectual performance, poor motor skills

Q How should Mrs Archer be counselled?

A She has suffered an asymptomatic primary CMV infection in pregnancy. The risks of congenital infection are outlined above. There is no evidence that treatment of the mother with anti-CMV drugs (ganciclovir, foscarnet) has any effect on the outcome – both drugs are toxic, and are not indicated in pregnancy. Mrs Archer may continue with the pregnancy, or opt for a termination. This decision is one that can only be taken by the patient, following consultation with her GP and her obstetrician.

Q How could a strategy for the prevention of congenital CMV infection be devised?

A This is difficult. There is currently no vaccine available to prevent CMV infection. Both primary and secondary CMV infections are almost invariably asymptomatic. Thus diagnosis of maternal infection would necessitate diagnostic screening during pregnancy. In the UK, screening all antenatal sera for the

presence of anti-CMV is not indicated because:

- serious congenital infection may arise from both maternal primary and secondary CMV infections (i.e. in women initially seronegative or seropositive)
- avoidance of sources of CMV infection (small children, sexual partners) by seronegative women is not practicable.

However, contrary views have been expressed in the USA, where maternal secondary CMV infection is believed to pose very little risk to the fetus. Thus, efforts are made to identify seronegative women and counsel them about avoidance of CMV infection.

Q Should Mrs Archer's baby receive antiviral treatment if it is shown to be congenitally infected with CMV?

A There is some logic to this suggestion, in order to prevent the late complications of congenital CMV. However, there is no way of distinguishing the small proportion of those babies who will develop CMV-related problems from the vast majority who will not, and the currently available anti-CMV agents are too toxic to be administered to all CMV-infected babies.

Q Mrs Archer was working on a paediatric ward. Do you think that a nurse on such a ward, who becomes pregnant, should be moved to a different working environment?

A This is another controversial topic. Certain groups of workers are more likely to be exposed to CMV at work, including health-care workers looking after children and immunosuppressed patients, as both of these patient groups are significant excretors of CMV. Nursery and child daycare workers are similarly at risk. However, the significance of such occupational exposure is unclear, as women may be exposed to CMV during pregnancy from their (and other) children, and their sexual partners. Congenital CMV infection

is no more common in the occupational groups mentioned above. Thus, a nurse in this setting does not need to be moved. She should, however, be reminded to be scrupulous about handwashing, which is the key to the prevention of hospital-acquired infection.

Q What other infections in pregnancy may give rise to congenital abnormalities?

A

- Rubella (see Case 55)
- Cytomegalovirus
- Toxoplasmosis
- Varicella-zoster virus (see Case 57)
- Syphilis (see Case 28).

In addition, a number of virus infections can be transmitted vertically (i.e. from mother to baby), e.g. hepatitis B virus (Case 22), HIV (Case 30), HTLV-1 (Case 61). Although these infections are clinically important to the baby, they do not give rise to congenital abnormalities.

Q What is toxoplasmosis, and how may it be acquired?

A Infection with the protozoon parasite *Toxoplasma gondii*. The definitive host of this organism is any member of the cat family, which becomes infected by eating tissues of infected prey and sheds oocysts in the faeces. Oocysts may infect intermediate hosts, e.g. sheep, pigs, cattle and humans, within whom a parasitaemia is followed by invasion of organs and tissues, and the formation of tissue cysts. Humans may become infected by four routes:

- ingestion of oocysts from soil or water contaminated with cat faeces
- ingestion of viable tissue cysts in raw or undercooked meat, or in milk from infected intermediate hosts
- transplantation of organs containing tissue cysts
- transplacental transmission from a mother who is acutely infected.

B59.3 Clinical features of toxoplasmosis

Presentation

Acute infection, acquired postnatally
- may be asymptomatic
- fever, malaise, myalgia
- lymphadenopathy – usually cervical; may be one isolated enlarged node which may persist for months
- glandular fever-like illness (see Case 9)

In the immunosuppressed
- reactivation of latent tissue cysts may occur, with manifestations dependent on the site of reactivation
- encephalitis
- myocarditis

Congenital infection – varied manifestations
- asymptomatic (the majority)
- non-specific symptoms, e.g. intrauterine growth retardation, hepatosplenomegaly
- severe disease with hydrocephalus, intracranial calcification, retinochoroiditis (the 'classic triad'); extensive internal organ involvement (liver, heart, lungs)
- ocular complications – retinochoroiditis; may not present until many years after birth; due to reactivation of retinal cysts

Diagnosis

- Serology – a rise in antibody titre and the presence of specific IgM.
- Antigen or genome detection techniques are available in reference laboratories

Treatment

- Immunocompetent hosts – therapy usually not indicated
- Immunosuppressed hosts – sulphadiazine and pyrimethamine, with folinic acid replacement; clindamycin is an alternative
- In pregnancy – spiramycin, a macrolide similar to erythromycin
- Congenital infection – specific therapy should be given during the first year of life in order to reduce the incidence of late ocular sequelae

Q What are the clinical features of toxoplasmosis?

A These vary with the age and immune status of the host (see Box 59.3). There is some controversy as to whether acute infection may be associated with retinochoroiditis, or whether the latter is always due to the reactivation of retinal cysts acquired *in utero*.

Q How may congenital toxoplasmosis be prevented?

A Pregnant women should be educated as to the routes of transmission of the organism, and given clear advice as to how to reduce the risk of infection:

- Avoid cleaning out cat litter trays. Otherwise, use gloves and wash hands afterwards
- Wear gloves when gardening, and wash hands afterwards
- Do not eat raw/undercooked meat, or drink unpasteurized milk. Wash hands after handling raw meat

There is currently no antenatal screening programme in the UK to identify toxoplasma-seronegative pregnant women. Retesting such women at intervals during pregnancy would allow the identification of cases of acute infection, which could then be managed appropriately. Such programmes do exist in other countries.

Summary: Congenital CMV infection

Incidence

The most common congenital infection; 1 in 300 babies affected

Clinical features

Cytomegalic inclusion disease (5–10%); normal at birth, defects evident later (5–10%); normal at birth, normal development (80–85%)

Pathogenesis

From maternal primary or secondary CMV infections, which are usually asymptomatic

Diagnosis

IgM in cord blood; culture of CMV from throat or urine within 3 weeks of birth

CASE 60
David, a 22-year-old student with a swollen testis

David, a 22-year-old medical student, limps gingerly into the surgery. His main complaint is that of a painful, swollen left testis. He was well until 2 days ago, when he felt unable to attend lectures, with non-specific aches and pains, a headache, and a temperature of 37.8°C. He first noticed his testicular swelling this morning, when he woke up feeling sick. He is an active sportsman, but can recall no recent injury or trauma which might account for the swelling. He has no history of sexually transmitted diseases, and has no dysuria or urethral discharge. He has a steady girlfriend, who is well. He has had no serious illnesses in the past. On examination he has a low-grade fever, but no other abnormal physical signs apart from his left testis, which is about double the size of his right testis, and tender (see Figure 60.1).

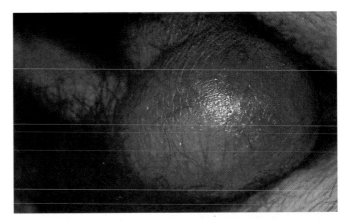

Fig. 60.1
David's swollen testis.

Q What is the diagnosis? Name one infectious cause of this condition.

A David has symptoms and signs of orchitis. The most likely cause, in someone of this age, is mumps virus infection.

On checking David's history it transpires that he has never received mumps vaccine. Re-examination pays particular attention to his face and neck, but there is no evidence of salivary gland enlargement and the orifices of his parotid ducts are not inflamed.

Q Is mumps virus infection still likely?

A Yes. Although parotitis is usually the dominant clinical feature of mumps, any of the associated manifestations of mumps can occur

before, simultaneously with or after the parotitis, or even in its complete absence. The pathogenesis of mumps infection includes a viraemic phase, where virus spreads in the bloodstream and can infect many end-organs, giving rise to a number of clinical manifestations (see Table 60.1). Most of the complications are more common in postpubertal patients than in children.

A clinical diagnosis of mumps is made.

Q Are there any investigations that will confirm the diagnosis?

A Mumps virus can be grown in tissue culture in the laboratory, from saliva, urine or CSF. The easiest sample to send to the laboratory is urine. Sending an acute serum sample is also good practice.

During the next few days the parotid gland swelling becomes evident, confirming the clinical diagnosis. A laboratory report a week later states that mumps virus was isolated from the urine sample.

Q What type of vaccine is available for the prevention of mumps?

A Mumps vaccines contain live attenuated strains of virus (see Appendix 2). One potential drawback of the use of such vaccines is that failure to achieve sufficient attenuation may result in the vaccine causing clinical disease. One of the mumps vaccines used in the UK (the Urabe strain), which gave rise to an unacceptably high incidence of vaccine-induced mumps meningitis (about 1/10 000 doses of vaccine), has now been withdrawn.

Q Why is mumps now included in the recommended list of childhood vaccinations?

A Mumps virus infection may result in a range of clinical syndromes (see Table 60.1). The principal reason for including mumps in the measles/mumps/rubella vaccine was to reduce the incidence of the central nervous system complications of mumps infection. Even though the prognosis of these complications is good, cost–benefit analysis demonstrated that the cost of universal vaccination would be more than offset by the savings to be made from reducing hospitalizations due to these particular manifestations of mumps virus infection.

However, there is one cautionary note to be struck when considering mumps vaccination. All of the non-parotitic manifestations of mumps are more common in older patients. Vaccination of a proportion of children may reduce circulating wild-type virus, and therefore more non-immunized children will evade natural infection during their childhood. However, these individuals remain susceptible to mumps infection as they become older, and so overall, suboptimal vaccination may paradoxically generate an increase in the incidence of mumps complications as the average age of infection increases.

Table 60.1 Mumps virus infection

Asymptomatic seroconversion (i.e. subclinical infection)
Approximately 30% of infections

Prodromal illness
Malaise, myalgia, low-grade fever, for 1–2 days

Parotitis
Occurs in 95% of cases of symptomatic disease
Is bilateral in 75% cases
Glands are swollen and tender, duct orifices red and oedematous
Swelling lasts 4–7 days
Submandibular and sublingual glands occasionally involved

Central nervous system
Meningitis (see Case 1)
Aseptic meningitis in 5–10% of mumps patients (males >females)
Encephalitis (see Case 2)
About 1 in 6000 cases
May cause convulsions, focal neurological signs, motor or sensory disorders
Other
Hearing loss may occur in absence of meningitis or encephalitis
Guillain–Barré syndrome (rare)

Orchitis, epididymitis and oophoritis
20–40% postpubertal males, 5% postpubertal females
Bilateral orchitis in one-third of cases
Risk of sterility due to testicular atrophy is, however, very small
Oophoritis, presenting with lower abdominal pain and pelvic tenderness, may cause diagnostic difficulties

Pancreatitis
? around 5% incidence

Other manifestations
Myocarditis (rare)
Arthritis (rare)
Renal dysfunction (rare)
In a pregnant female, increased risk of abortion
The role of mumps infection as a trigger for juvenile-onset insulin dependent diabetes mellitus is controversial

Summary: Mumps

Clinical features

Parotitis, meningitis, meningoencephalitis, orchitis, oophoritis, pancreatitis

Diagnosis

Clinical; virus isolation from urine, CSF, saliva; serology

Management

Symptomatic

Prevention

Live attenuated vaccine; given to prevent CNS complications

CASE 61
Lenny, a 38-year-old Jamaican with a palpable skin rash

Lenny, a 38-year-old Jamaican man who has lived in the UK for 30 years, is referred to the dermatology clinic because of a skin rash. He first noticed slightly raised patches of itchy skin some months ago. The skin in those patches has recently become further thickened, and in the past 2 months discrete nodules have appeared. There is nothing else of note in his history, except that his mother died of 'a blood disorder'. The only abnormal signs on examination are moderately enlarged axillary lymph nodes and several nodules in the skin. Routine investigations reveal a normal haemoglobin and white cell count, but a decreased platelet count of $70 \times 10^9/l$. A biopsy of a skin nodule is reported as showing a T-cell lymphoma.

B61.1 Adult T-cell leukaemia lymphoma

Epidemiology – common in Japan, the Caribbean, Central and South America, equatorial Africa, but rare elsewhere

Clinical presentation – variable. Acute or chronic leukaemia, or cutaneous lymphoma

Malignant cell – T cell, CD4+ (i.e. helper subset), expresses high levels of the receptor for interleukin-2. Unlike HIV, HTLV-1 does not bind to CD4. The nature of the viral receptor on the cell has not yet been identified

Prognosis – usually culminates as a highly malignant monoclonal proliferation of T cells

Q Is there any further diagnostic test which should be performed?

A There is a distinct possibility that this patient may be suffering from adult T-cell leukaemia lymphoma (ATLL, see Box 61.1), which is known to arise from infection with human T-cell lymphotropic virus type 1 (HTLV-1). HTLV-1 serology should therefore be requested plus a careful review of the blood film.

Lenny is shown to be anti-HTLV-1 positive. Abnormal white cells with the characteristic morphology shown in Figure 61.1 are seen in his blood film, which confirms the diagnosis of ATLL.

Q What type of virus is HTLV-1?

A A retrovirus, i.e. it possesses a reverse transcriptase enzyme which enables it to copy its RNA genome into DNA (see Case 30). Retroviruses are widespread in nature, but HTLV-1 was the first human retrovirus to be discovered. Other human retroviruses include HTLV-2 and the human immunodeficiency viruses HIV-1 and HIV-2.

Q What is the treatment of ATLL?

A First-line therapy is aggressive chemotherapy using standard lymphoma treatment regimens. Azidothymidine (AZT), a reverse transcriptase inhibitor, has not been shown to be of any clinical benefit in this disease.

Lenny is admitted to hospital and a regimen of four chemotherapeutic agents is instituted. While in hospital, he complains of constipation, frequency in passing urine, and an intense thirst. He also becomes noticeably depressed.

Q What complication of ATLL is he suffering from now?

A Constipation, polyuria, polydypsia and depression are all features of hypercalcaemia, which is frequently present in ATLL. The mechanism of this is unclear, but may be due to the release of cytokines, such as interleukin-1 and T-cell growth factor β, from the malignant cells, which have osteoclast-activating properties.

Q What is the evidence implicating HTLV-1 as the causative agent of ATLL?

A

- The epidemiology of HTLV-1 infection exactly parallels that of ATLL (i.e. common in Japan, the Caribbean, South America).
- Patients with ATLL are invariably HTLV-1 seropositive.
- Virus can be isolated from malignant ATLL cells. The viral genome is integrated into the chromosomal DNA of the cell.

Q How could Lenny have acquired his infection with HTLV-1?

A The routes of spread of HTLV-1 are:

- vertical (i.e. mother to baby)
- sexual
- blood-borne (e.g. transfusion, intravenous drug abuse).

Lenny's mother who died of a 'blood disease' may have had leukaemia, which suggests that he may have acquired his infection from her. This would be entirely compatible with his presentation 38 years later. As with other virus-associated malignancies, ATLL has a long latent period, i.e. 30–40 years.

The exact mode of vertical transmission of HTLV-1 is believed to be postnatally via breast milk, rather than in utero or perinatally. Advice to anti-HTLV-1-positive mothers not to breast-feed their babies, plus exclusion of anti-HTLV-1-positive blood from the blood supply, has resulted in a dramatic fall in the rate of seropositivity in Japan. HTLV-1 is highly cell associated and thus administration of acellular blood products, such as factor VIII, does not transmit infection.

Q Is HTLV-1 infection associated with any other clinical conditions?

A Yes. Tropical spastic paraparesis (TSP), the features of which are outlined in Box 61.2. This syndrome is known in Japan as HTLV-1-associated myelopathy (HAM). TSP

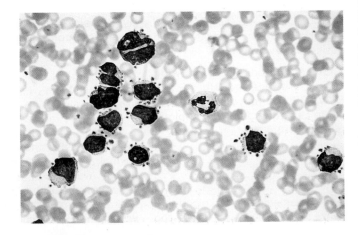

Fig. 61.1 Malignant HTLV-1 infected cells in peripheral blood.

B61.2 Tropical spastic paraparesis

Epidemiology – mean age of onset 40 years. Female: male = 2:1. Geographic distribution parallels HTLV-1 seroprevalence

Clinical features – insidious presentation, stiffness/weakness in one or both legs, resulting in spastic paraparesis. Sphincter disturbance and penile impotence are common. Cranial nerve and upper limb involvement rare. Only minor objective sensory impairment

Diagnosis – anti-HTLV-1 found in serum and CSF, often in very high titre

Treatment – steroids of short-term benefit only

Prognosis – 30% of patients are bedridden after 10 years; 45% cannot walk unaided by crutches

debilitating lymphocytic infiltration of the skin, have all been described in HTLV-II-infected individuals. However, the vast majority of sero-positive individuals (mostly intra-venous drug abusers) do not have any of these manifestations of disease.

Summary: HTLV-1 Infection	
Routes of spread	
Vertical (breast milk); sexual; blood transfusion	
Geographic distribution	
High prevalence in Japan, Caribbean, South America	
Disease associations	
Adult T-cell leukaemic lymphoma; tropical spastic paraparesis	
Prevention	
Avoid breastfeeding; screen blood donors in endemic areas	

has been recognized as a distinct syndrome in the Caribbean for many years, where it is the most common cause of demyelinating disease, i.e. it occurs more frequently than multiple sclerosis. The pathogenesis of TSP is unclear. To date, no major differences between 'leukaemogenic' and 'neurogenic' strains of HTLV-1 have been reported.

Q What is the likelihood of an HTLV-1-infected individual developing ATLL or TSP?

A Only a small minority of HTLV-1-infected individuals will present with ATLL or TSP. The lifetime risk of the former is of the order of 3% in individuals infected in the first year of life, and of the latter is 0.25%. TSP has been documented in individuals who acquired their HTLV-1 infection from blood transfusion, but ATLL has not.

Q What diseases are associated with HTLV-II infection?

A The data implicating HTLV-II as a cause of disease are much less clearcut. Neurological disease similar to TSP, large granulocytic-cell leukaemia, and cutaneous diseases ranging from eczema to

CASE 62
Richard, a young man with lethargy and breathlessness

Richard, an 18-year-old student, complains of lethargy and weakness which have become more prominent since he first became ill 3 days ago, with general malaise, a fever, a runny nose and an irritating cough. Today he has also noticed some shortness of breath after climbing the stairs in his home. He has had no serious illness in the past, and is on no regular medication. His mother and sister both suffer from an uncharacterized chronic haemolytic anaemia. On examination Richard is pale and his resting pulse is 90/min. He has a palpable spleen.

Q What initial investigations should be performed?

A A full blood count and film should be done as this patient has symptoms (lethargy, shortness of breath) and signs (pale, resting tachycardia) of anaemia, with a background of a positive family history.

That afternoon the following results are received: Hb 5.0 g/dl MCV 86 fl. No reticulocytes seen; white cell count 2.2 × 10⁹/l; platelets 80 × 10⁹/l.

Q How are these results interpreted, and what should the next investigation be?

A All elements of the blood are below normal values, suggesting

bone marrow failure. Examination of a bone marrow aspirate is therefore indicated.

The bone marrow report shows marked erythroid hypoplasia. Granulopoiesis and megakaryopoiesis are active but mildly reduced.

Q Is Richard's family history likely to be relevant to his presentation with acute bone marrow failure?

A Richard was in fact investigated as a child, but his haemoglobin was normal at that time and nothing further was done. However, the history of a 'flu-like illness' followed by bone marrow failure in a patient with a family history of chronic haemolytic anaemia is highly suggestive of acute infection with parvovirus B19, resulting in an aplastic crisis.

Q How might the diagnosis be confirmed?

A At this stage of infection patients are viraemic, i.e. virus particles are present in their peripheral blood. Electron microscopy of a serum sample may thus reveal such particles. Alternatively, parvovirus DNA can be identified in peripheral blood by hybridization techniques, or by using the polymerase chain reaction assay.

Richard is observed carefully over the next few days. His haemoglobin, white cell and platelet counts gradually begin to rise. However, 9 days after his initial presentation an erythematous maculopapular rash develops on his face, trunk and limbs, and the next day he complains of pain in the small joints of his hands.

Q Do these new symptoms and signs indicate that the patient has acquired a new infection?

A No. Rash and arthralgia/arthritis are well recognized complications of parvovirus infection, arising typically 7–10 days after the viraemic febrile stage of the illness. Clinical manifestations of acute parvovirus B19 infection are listed in Box 62.1.

Richard's rash lasts 4 days and his joint symptoms, initially relieved by paracetamol, also disappear. On follow-up in outpatients, his full blood count shows an Hb of 11.3 g/dl, a white cell count of 5.4 × 10⁹/l and a platelet count of 180 × 10⁹/l. Subsequent investigations confirm a diagnosis of chronic haemolytic anaemia due to pyruvate kinase deficiency.

Q What are the pathogenetic mechanisms underlying the various

manifestations of parvovirus infection seen in this patient?

A The pathogenesis of parvovirus B19 infection has been studied in healthy adult volunteers intranasally inoculated with virus. The salient features, illustrated in Figure 62.1 are:

- a viraemic phase (1 week postinoculation), associated with a non-specific febrile illness
- infection of bone marrow progenitor cells leading to transient bone marrow arrest
- immune complex manifestations (i.e. rash and joint involvement) evident at 18–21 days, as the IgG antibody response to infection becomes detectable.

The effects of the bone marrow arrest are not clinically evident in otherwise healthy individuals. However, in patients with chronic haemolytic anaemia, in whom erythrocytes have a shortened life-span, the profound reticulocytopenia may result in the depression of haemoglobin concentrations to critical levels – a so-called aplastic crisis.

Treatment of an aplastic crisis involves blood transfusion until the bone marrow recovers. Family members with chronic haemolytic anaemia who are seronegative for parvovirus antibody will also be at risk, especially as the index patient

will be excreting virus at this stage of the illness. Normal human

---

B62.1 Clinical manifestations of parvovirus B19 infection

Prodromal illness

- Fever, malaise 1 week before other manifestations (except aplastic crisis)

Rash

- Known as erythema infectiosum, 5th disease, or 'slapped-cheek' syndrome, due to the most prominent site of the rash

Arthralgia/arthritis

- Usually in adult females
- Self-limiting, although may take months to resolve

Aplastic crisis

- In individuals with underlying chronic haemolytic anaemia
- Can become chronic in immunocompromised patients

In pregnancy

- Rash ± arthritis may mimic rubella (see Case 55)
- Increased risk of spontaneous miscarriage
- Cause of fetal hydrops late in pregnancy
- No congenital malformations described

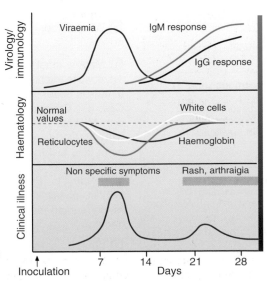

Fig. 62.1 Pathogenesis of parvovirus infection.

immunoglobulin contains anti-parvovirus antibody and may protect those susceptible individuals.

Immunosuppressed patients (e.g. due to HIV infection, leukaemia, or bone marrow transplant recipients) may fail to eliminate the virus, resulting in chronic infection with consequent chronic anaemia and transfusion dependence. Treatment with intravenous normal human immunoglobulin may be succesful in eliminating infection.

Q Could Richard's aplastic crisis have been diagnosed by detection of parvovirus-specific IgM in his serum?

A No. The reason for this is evident in Figure 62.1 – the aplastic crisis occurs during the viraemic phase of the illness, before the patient has mounted a detectable immune response. However, specific IgM detection is the mainstay of diagnosis in patients presenting with rash and/or joint manifestations.

Q What diseases are caused by parvovirus B5?

A There is no such virus. The rather clumsy nomenclature of parvovirus B19 arose from the code number of the original serum sample in which it was discovered. Thus there are no parvovirus A or parvovirus B 1–18 viruses.

Summary: Parvovirus B19 infection
Disease associations
Erythema infectiosum; arthritis; aplastic crisis; in pregnancy: miscarriage; hydrops fetalis
Pathogenesis
Manifestations arise from virus infection of rapidly dividing cells in bone marrow, and immune complex formation
Diagnosis
Serology; detection of viral DNA

CASE 63
Michael, a medical student recently returned from Africa with a fever

Michael, a 19-year-old medical student, presents in A and E complaining of feverishness, shivering, headache and generalized aches and pains. He first felt ill 2 days ago, and feels he is getting worse. On direct questioning he also reports that his throat has become painful since yesterday. He has no relevant past medical history. He has just returned to the UK from abroad, and although on no regular medication he has been taking malaria prophylaxis. On examination he is febrile (39°C), his pharynx is inflamed, but there are no other physical signs.

Q What further history is relevant?

A The information provided thus far is non-specific, and there is a long list of possible differential diagnoses. The first point to clarify is exactly where and when Michael has been on his travels.

Michael took a year out between leaving school and starting medical school. For the past 6 months he has been backpacking around west Africa, returning to England 7 days ago. Apart from some moderate diarrhoea 4 weeks after his arrival in Africa, he was well during the trip and is adamant that he complied with his prescribed malaria prophylaxis throughout. For the last month of his travels he stayed in a rural hospital in Nigeria, where he was able to sit in on the various clinics and participate on ward rounds.

Q What is your differential diagnosis now?

A Malaria must remain high on the list, despite the history of prophylaxis, as this is never 100% effective (see Case 47). Other infections compatible with Michael's presentation include typhoid, typhus and influenza. However, the history of time spent in rural west Africa immediately before his return to England raises the distinct possibility of lassa fever, which should set the alarm bells ringing!

Q What is lassa fever, and why is the diagnosis of such major importance?

A Lassa is one of a group of diseases known collectively as the viral haemorrhagic fevers (VHF). The key features of lassa fever are listed in Box 63.1. Apart from the associated high mortality, its formidable reputation for person-to-person spread has major management implications.

B63.1 Lassa fever
Aetiology: infection with lassa fever virus (an arena virus) **Natural reservoir of infection:** rodents **Geographic distribution:** West Africa, e.g. Nigeria, Sierra Leone **Incubation period:** 3–21 days **Presentation:** insidious onset, fever, malaise, flu-like illness **Complications:** hypotension, oliguria, haemorrhage **Mortality:** 5–40% in different outbreaks

Q What are the principles of management of a case of VHF such as lassa fever?

A There are strict guidelines issued by the UK Department of Health, which are designed to achieve optimal patient care and minimize the risks of spread of infection. As with any serious medical problem, the most important point to remember is 'if in doubt, ask for help'. The local infectious diseases physician/medical microbiologist should have access to the national guidelines, and will know how to trigger the correct chain of response. The broad principles of management are:

- no laboratory work must be carried out on specimens from

these patients until a blood film has been examined for the presence of malarial parasites. Malaria is itself a medical emergency (see Case 47), and statistically is more likely than any viral haemorrhagic fever

- the blood film and any other patient samples must be taken with extreme care and rendered safe where possible by immersion in 10% formalin. Strict attention must be paid to the safe disposal of all instruments used in specimen taking and preparation
- laboratories undertaking work on any samples from these patients must be notified in advance, and must have suitable containment facilities
- the patient must be transferred to an isolation facility. If there is a strong likelihood of VHF, the patient must be admitted directly to a designated high-security isolation unit
- the local Consultant for Communicable Disease Control or equivalent must be informed, and through him or her the appropriate surveillance unit (e.g. in the UK, the Communicable Disease Surveillance Centre, CDSC), which holds national responsibility on behalf of the Department of Health
- if the diagnosis is strongly suspected or confirmed, then close contacts of the patient must be identified and placed under surveillance.

CDSC confirms that the area in Nigeria in which Michael was staying is endemic for lassa fever. Repeat blood films are sent to the laboratory and no malarial parasites are seen. Lassa fever is therefore strongly suspected, and Michael is transferred to the nearest high-security isolation unit. The diagnosis is confirmed by identification of the virus in clinical material in a laboratory with Category 4 isolation facilities.

Q Is there any antiviral agent available for the treatment of lassa fever?

A Yes. Ribavirin, a nucleoside analogue with a broad antiviral spectrum, is active against the lassa fever virus. It can also be used prophylactically for individuals visiting endemic areas.

Intravenous ribavirin therapy is started. Over the next few days Michael becomes prostrate, with a high fever, and shows evidence of plasma leakage (facial oedema, pleural effusion, ascites) and bleeding (petechiae on the skin and mucous membranes). However, his fever subsides after 7 days and he makes a rapid recovery, although his tiredness persists for many weeks. Happily, no family member, close friend or health-care worker develops symptoms.

Q What are the other viral haemorrhagic fevers?

A There are a number of virus infections which can produce severe haemorrhagic disease in humans. These belong to a number of different virus families, have distinct geographic distributions, and utilize different modes of spread. The salient features of some of them are listed in Table 63.1.

Summary: Viral haemorrhagic fevers

Presentation

Febrile illness followed by hypovolaemic shock and haemorrhage, in a patient with a history of recent travel

Diagnosis

Clinical suspicion; laboratory diagnosis in specialized centres

Management

Exclude malaria; isolation and referral to tropical disease specialist; notify authorities

Table 63.1 Viral haemorrhagic fever syndromes

Yellow fever

Causative agent: Yellow fever virus (flavivirus family)
Clinical features: Multisystem disease with jaundice and haemorrhagic manifestations
Geographic distribution: Central and South America, Africa
Transmission: Mosquito
Comment: Preventable by vaccination

Dengue haemorrhagic fever

Causative agent: Dengue virus (flavivirus family)
Clinical features: Uncomplicated dengue – adults, older children, fever, muscle and joint pain, rash. Dengue haemorrhagic fever (DHF) – young children, hypovolaemic shock, bleeding, 5% mortality
Geographic distribution: Pacific Islands, Asia, Caribbean
Transmission: Mosquito
Comment: Pathogenesis unknown

Haemorrhagic disease with renal syndrome

Causative agent: Hantaviruses (bunyavirus family)
Clinical features: Vary – asymptomatic disease; mild (nephropathica endemica, N. Europe); severe (Korean haemorrhagic fever)
Geographic distribution: China, Southeast Asia, Europe
Transmission: Rodents
Comment: Hantavirus pulmonary syndrome recently described in USA

Ebola and Marburg diseases

Causative agent: Ebola and Marburg viruses
Clinical features: Outbreaks associated with very high mortality rates (50–90%)
Geographic distribution: Sub-Saharan, central and East Africa
Transmission: From monkeys, human to human spread
Comment: Natural reservoir of infection unknown

CASE 64
Polyarthralgia in Susan, a 25-year-old

Susan, a 25-year-old woman, has a 5-day history of polyarthralgia involving the toes, fingers and wrists. Two weeks earlier she had a bout of acute diarrhoea, vomiting and abdominal pain lasting 6 days for which no microbiological cause was found. There is no history of a skin rash, eye symptoms or urethral discharge.

Q What are the likely causes of her polyarthralgia?

A The following should be considered:

- Connective tissue diseases, such as rheumatoid arthritis, may present as described above. Subsequent episodes and a positive rheumatoid factor will confirm the diagnosis.
- Viral arthritis, due to rubella (see Case 55) or parvovirus (see Case 62) should be considered. A history of exposure, the presence of a characteristic rash or vaccination history (rubella) may help in diagnosis. Other viruses less commonly implicated in arthralgia include Epstein–Barr virus, mumps, enteroviruses, e.g. echoviruses, adenoviruses and hepatitis B.
- Enteropathic arthropathies, associated with Crohn's disease and ulcerative colitis in 20% of cases. This usually involves the larger joints of the lower limbs and recurrent gastrointestinal symptoms are likely.
- Psoriasis-associated joint disease, which characteristically affects the sacroiliac joint. The presence of characteristic skin lesions suggests the diagnosis.
- Septic arthritis, due to *Staphylococcus aureus*, streptococci etc. is often accompanied by risk factors such as trauma, previous joint disease or immunosuppression, and affects one or at most two joints. The absence of systemic symptoms such as fever and arthritis makes the diagnosis less likely here.
- Reactive arthropathies, which may follow gastroenteritis due to *Salmonella*, *Shigella*, *Campy-*

lobacter and *Yersinia*. The history of a diarrhoeal illness makes this possible here. This condition is analogous to Reiter's disease, in which skin lesions occur in 50% of cases and in which urethritis and conjunctivitis are also present.

Q Which gastrointestinal pathogen is likely to have been responsible here?

A *Campylobacter*, *Salmonella* and *Shigella* are isolated from stool samples by most microbiology laboratories using selective (e.g. desoxycholate-citrate agar for *Shigella*) and enrichment (e.g. selenite broth for *Salmonella*) techniques. *Yersinia* species (see Box 64.1) cause gastroenteritis less commonly and are not routinely sought in clinical specimens.

Q How may yersiniosis be diagnosed?

A Attempts to isolate these bacteria from faeces are hampered by slow growth, and cold enrichment or selective agar media are required. *Yersinia* spp. may occasionally be recovered from lymph nodes taken at laparotomy when associated with intra-abdominal pathology. Synovial effusions are usually sterile in the presence of polymorphonuclear cells. Paired sera, 10–14 days apart, may confirm a diagnosis by showing a rise in antibodies, but sera should be appropriately absorbed to prevent cross-reaction with other bacteria, including *Salmonella*, and yersinia serology is usually confined to regional or reference laboratories. A reactive polyarthralgia is seen in 10–30% of adults following infection with *Y. enterocolitica* and is related to the presence of HLA-B27.

Susan's faeces are negative on culture for *Campylobacter*, *Shigella*, *Salmonella* and *Yersinia*, and blood cultures are sterile. Serum taken from her confirms that she has been vaccinated against or been infected with rubella in the past, and she has no markers for a connective tissue disorder. A repeat serum sample taken 2 weeks later shows a rise in antibody titre to *Y. enterocolitica* from 1 in 32 in the first specimen to 1 in 512, confirming a diagnosis of reactive arthritis due to yersiniosis.

B64.1 *Yersinia* species

- *Y. enterocolitica* and *Y. pseudotuberculosis* are Gram-negative motile non-lactose-fermenting rods
- May survive and replicate at 4°C
- Reservoirs include domestic, agricultural and wild animals and aquatic environments
- *Y. pestis*, the aetiological cause of human plague, is a worldwide zoonotic infection transmitted by flea bites

---

Q What other clinical conditions are associated with *Yersinia*?

A A number of conditions of unconfirmed aetiology have been associated with *Yersinia* but the most widely recognized of these are:

- gastroenteritis, clinically indistinguishable from many other causes but often accompanied by blood and mucus
- mesenteric adenitis/terminal ileitis, often indistinguishable from appendicitis. Usually due to *Y. pseudotuberculosis*
- bacteraemia, especially in immuno-compromised patients or those with liver disease, including those with iron overload, e.g. thalassaemia requiring frequent transfusions
- erythema nodosum.
- Plague (*Y. Pestis*)

Q How is yersiniosis treated?

A Many of the various forms of yersiniosis are self-limiting and it is not clear whether antimicrobial chemotherapy significantly alters the natural history. Exceptions to this include systemic infection such as bacteraemia or deep-seated infection such as liver abscesses or osteomyelitis. *Y. enterocolitica* is usually resistant to penicillin, ampicillin and many of the cephalosporins. Trimethoprim, a tetracycline, or more recently, a fluoroquinolone such as ciprofloxacin, are preferred. Bacteraemic infection is probably best treated with a combination of one of the above plus an aminoglycoside such as gentamicin.

Summary: Yersiniosis
Presentation
Variable, but includes gastroenteritis, arthralgia, abdominal pain
Diagnosis
Culture of faeces, joint fluid etc. Rise in antibodies
Management
Often self-limiting. Antibiotics such as tetracyclines, trimethoprim or a quinolone

CASE 65
Problems on a Friday afternoon for a junior house officer

Virginia, a recently appointed Junior House Officer in health care of the elderly is called to see an 84-year-old man with vomiting and diarrhoea at 3 p.m. on Friday 13th August! Cedric has been an inpatient for 2 weeks for assessment of increasing immobility and treatment of a mild chest infection. He has been vomiting since earlier that day, and in the last 3 hours has passed two watery stools. He appears mildly dehydrated; Virginia takes blood to check his urea and electrolytes and he is started on intravenous normal saline. One of the nurses remarks that Cedric is the fourth patient on the ward with diarrhoea and vomiting occurring over the last 48 hours.

Q What should Virginia do first?

A She should ascertain the nature of the symptoms of the other patients to determine whether they are similar to Cedric's, and again treat dehydration if present. If they appear similar and there are no identifiable reasons why these patients should have gastrointestinal symptoms, e.g. laxative use, diverticular disease, recent antibiotics, it seems very likely that there is an outbreak of gastroenteritis on the ward.

Q Who should she contact now?

A After informing and discussing the problem with a senior colleague, preferably the consultant in health care of the elderly, she should inform the hospital infection control team, i.e. the infection control doctor (most likely a consultant microbiologist) and infection control nurses to ensure that early control measures may be implemented.

The infection control team visit the ward that afternoon and investigate the outbreak in conjunction with the medical and nursing staff. It transpires that over the previous 5 days, seven patients have developed gastrointestinal symptoms and two staff nurses and a physiotherapist have gone off work with similar symptoms (see Figure 65.1). Vomiting, sometimes projectile in character, has almost always been the initial symptom and this has usually been followed by moderate to severe diarrhoea for 2–3 days. Abdominal pain has not been a prominent symptom. Only two patients are or have recently been on antibiotics in the preceding couple of weeks, and no obvious food source is implicated. Sadly, no specimens from patients or staff have been sent to microbiology to confirm a diagnosis.

Q What is the likely aetiological cause of the outbreak?

A The occurrence of this outbreak on a health care of the elderly ward, the short and generally mild nature of the symptoms, and the absence of an obvious food source all point to a viral aetiology. Other causes such as *Salmonella*, *Shigella* and *Campylobacter* must be excluded by stool culture and because antibiotic-associated diarrhoea caused by *Clostridium difficile* (see Case 17) is more common in the elderly (Cedric had a recent respiratory infection for which he most likely received antibiotics), cytotoxin analysis (indicating *C. difficile* disease) should also be requested when faeces samples are submitted to the microbiology laboratory.

Q How may a viral aetiology be confirmed?

A Elecron microscopy of a fresh sample of faeces taken early in the course of the illness (i.e. in the first 24 hours) may confirm the presence of small round structured viruses (SRSV) such as Norwalk virus (see Case 18). In the elderly this is the most likely viral aetiology, as rotavirus, astrovirus, calicivirus and adenovirus (types 40 and 41, see Case 18) are less common in this setting and are more commonly implicated in childhood diarrhoea. Enzyme immunoassay or immuno-

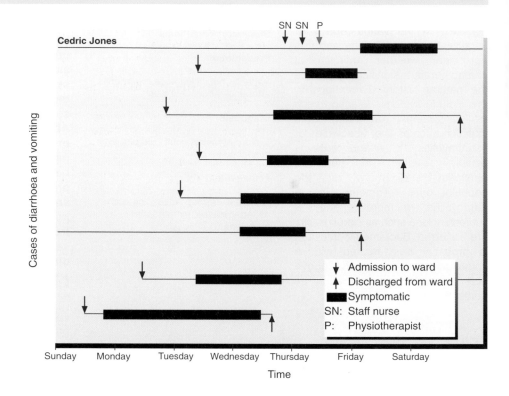

**Fig. 65.1 Time course
of the outbreak.**

electron microscopy are other less commonly used techniques. Tissue culture isolation of SRSVs from stools is very difficult and is therefore not routinely carried out. In the future, the polymerase chain reaction (PCR, for the detection of viral genome) may provide a rapid and more sensitive means of diagnosis.

Q What measures should be taken to control spread?

A Symptomatic patients should be nursed in isolation cubicles with their own toilet facilities. As ever, hand-washing is the single most important infection control measure. Staff movement to other wards should be restricted and those who have symptoms must not work, as they are a potential source of further spread. Symptomatic patients should not be transferred to other wards or institutions because of the risk of spreading the outbreak to these areas. Affected patients or staff are considered non-infectious when they have been asymptomatic for 48–72 hours. Asymptomatic patients should

also not be transferred to other institutions until 48 hours or more after the last symptomatic case has elapsed, because they might be incubating the infection.

Electron microscopy of faeces is carried out on Saturday morning and reveals SRSVs in two of five stool specimens. There are only two isolation cubicles on the ward, however, and by Monday eight patients are symptomatic and a further two members of staff have gone off ill; another ward is by now also affected. One of the patients, Doris, is visited by her son who is the local MP and in passing, he remarks that he is surprised that in this day and age the ward is tiled rather than carpeted.

Q What alternative is there to nursing patients in isolation cubicles?

A During outbreaks there may be insufficient isolation cubicles in which to care for all affected patients. If

this is the case, cohort nursing – that is, nursing affected patients in the same part of the ward together, using the same nursing staff – is recommended. Thus, physical separation of patients with symptoms from those without, together with restriction of the movements of nursing and other staff contacts, will help reduce the chances of spread.

Q Why do you think the ward has tiled floors instead of carpets?

A Tiled floors are in general easy to clean and in particular are not damaged by commonly used surface disinfectants. Carpets, however, are difficult to keep clean, do not withstand the use of surface disinfectants such as hypochlorite and, if stained, are unsightly. Furthermore, dust accumulating in carpets may be a potential source of spread of some hospital pathogens, such as methicillin-resistant *Staphylococcus aureus* (MRSA, see Case 51). Therefore, carpets should not be fitted in clinical areas.

Q How long is the outbreak likely to continue for?

A Nosocomial outbreaks of gastro-enteritis due to SRSVs can 'rumble' on for some weeks, and may spread to involve further wards and clinical areas. This is because these agents are very infectious and aerosol spread derived from projectile vomiting results in secondary cases. Attempts to limit spread may be hampered by inadequate isolation facilities, poor communications and a failure to close wards to admissions and discharges early on.

Cedric makes a speedy recovery from his illness but the outbreak spreads to involve a further three general medical and health care of the elderly wards, resulting in considerable disruption of clinical services and additional expense. Doris's son, the local MP, however, writes to the hospital's chief executive to compliment staff on their professionalism and the high standard of care received by his mother!

Summary: Nosocomial diarrhoea
Presentation
A cluster of patients with diarrhoea and vomiting, acquired in hospital, with evidence of spread (viral gastroenteritis) or a point source (food-borne *Salmonella*)
Diagnosis
Clinical presentation, culture for conventional bacterial pathogens, electron microscopy of stools for viruses, and toxin detection for *C. difficile*
Management
Fluid replacement and isolation or cohort nursing of symptomatic patients, with scrupulous hand-washing to prevent spread. Staff with symptoms should not continue to work

APPENDIX 1
Rational Use of the Microbiology Laboratory

General

- Specimens should be taken BEFORE the start of antimicrobial chemotherapy, especially if the infection is life-threatening, e.g. bacteraemia.
- Specimens and accompanying request forms should include name, age, full clinical details and whether the patient is on antibiotics.
- If there is likely to be a delay, specimens should be refrigerated. Blood cultures, however, should be placed in an incubator.
- The laboratory should be contacted in advance for vital or difficult to repeat specimens, e.g. joint aspirates, CSF especially if taken out of hours.
- The results from bacteriological investigations are usually available within 24–48 hours and positive blood or CSF results will usually be 'phoned.
- If in doubt about diagnosis, treatment, prevention or control of infection, RING UP AND ASK!

Genitourinary Tract Investigation

Urine
- Urine culture, i.e. a mid-stream urine (MSU) is not always essential in the management of uncomplicated urinary infection/cystitis except in children and pregnant women.
- An early morning large volume specimen is required for the investigation of tuberculosis.

Genital
- Cervical and urethral rather than vaginal swabs are required to confirm infection with *Neisseria gonorrhoeae* or *Chlamydia trachomatis*.
- Candidosis, trichomonas and anaerobic vaginosis are diagnosed with a vaginal swab.
- Vesicle fluid or a swab in viral transport medium is needed to diagnose genital herpes; serology is not helpful here.
- A serum sample is appropriate to exclude syphilis, hepatitis B and HIV disease when assessing a patient for sexually transmitted disease.

Gastrointestinal and Abdominal Investigations

Faeces
- 2–3 consecutive daily specimens are required to exclude salmonella, shigella, campylobacter and especially protozoan (e.g. giardia) infections.
- Details of travel abroad should be supplied to ensure appropriate investigations, and of recent antibiotics to exclude *Clostridium difficile* disease.
- In the investigation of possible viral gastroenteritis, it is essential that a faecal sample is sent for electron miscroscopy *as early as possible* in the course of the illness.

Intra-abdominal
- Pus or tissue is preferable to a swab in diagnosing infection, especially that due to anaerobes.
- Fresh fluid from external drains rather than fluid in drainage bags, which may be contaminated or stale, should be sent for culture.

Skin Investigations

- Wound swabs are only indicated if there is clinical evidence of local (e.g. erythema) or systemic (e.g. pyrexia) infection and should not be taken routinely post-operatively.
- Pus, if present, is superior to a swab in isolating the cause of wound infection.
- Blood cultures should always be taken in patients with cellulitis or erysipelas as β haemolytic streptococci may not be recovered from superficial swabs and the presence of bacteraemia has

therapeutic and prognostic implications.

- Skin scrapings from the edge, not the centre, of lesions placed in a sterile container or between two glass slides, nails or hairs should be taken to isolate the aetiological agent of dermatophyte infections.
- Skin rashes due to viral illnesses, may require laboratory investigation e.g. serology.
- In vesicular disease, vesicle fluid should be sent for viral culture, or dried onto a glass slide for subsequent electron microscopy.

Respiratory Tract Investigations

Upper
- Most 'viral-type illnesses' do not require laboratory confirmation.
- A throat swab may be indicated to confirm or exclude streptococcal tonsillitis but if diphtheria is suspected (e.g. recently returned from eastern Europe), *the laboratory must be informed* to ensure appropriate culture methods are used.
- A pernasal rather than a nasopharyngeal swab is required to confirm a diagnosis of whooping cough (pertussis).

Lower
- Mucoid sputum (i.e. saliva) rarely if ever reflects pathology in the lung parenchyma.
- Bronchoscopy specimens, e.g. bronchoalveolar lavage are preferable when microbiologically confirming the aetiology of pneumonia, especially if atypical or occurring in the immunocompromised patient where opportunist pathogens such as *Pneumocystis carinii* are important.
- Three consecutive early morning sputa should be taken when investigating possible tuberculosis. Phone to request an urgent Ziehl-Neelsen stain if patient is gravely ill or 'open' tuberculosis suspected.
- A nasopharyngeal aspirate for antigen detection is the optimal approach for the diagnosis of viral bronchiolitis or pneumonia in infants and small children. In adults, a throat swab in viral transport medium may be useful in the diagnosis of influenza. Paired serum samples to detect a rise in antibodies should also be taken; this approach is also useful in the investigation of atypical pneumonia.

Neurological Investigations

- CSF, a throat swab in viral transport medium, faeces (enteroviruses) and urine (mumps) for viral culture, with paired sera are recommended to confirm viral meningitis.
- The diagnosis of herpes encephalitis is best made by neurological imaging techniques or by brain biopsy. Investigation of CSF using the polymerase chain reaction (PCR) may in the near future become the microbiological test of choice.

Investigations of Systemic Disease

- Two sets of blood cultures (at least three if infective endocarditis suspected) are required in diagnosing bacteraemia. Details of time and site of venepuncture, clinical features and proposed antibiotic treatment should be supplied with the specimens.
- A number of thick and thin blood smears are necessary to diagnose malaria in a pyrexial patient recently returned from an endemic area.
- A single high titre (e.g. >1/256 for legionellosis), demonstration of a fourfold or greater rise in titre (e.g. <1/16 rising to 1/128 for mycoplasma) or a positive IgM (e.g. rubella) are required for serological confirmation of infection.
- Tissue specimens may be required to definitely diagnose certain infections, e.g. invasive pulmonary aspergillosis, cytomegalovirus infection of the intestine, cutaneous leishmaniasis.

APPENDIX 2
Immunisation against infectious diseases (UK recommendations)

Active immunisation (i.e. induction of protective host immune response)

Routine universal vaccines

	Organism	Nature of vaccine	Primary course	Booster
D/T/P	Diphtheria	toxoid	3 doses at 2, 3, 4 months	Pre-school (D and T only) 15–18 years (T only)
	Tetanus	toxoid		
	Pertussis	killed		
Hib	Haemophilus influenzae type b	conjugated capsular antigen	3 doses at 2, 3, 4 months	
Polio	Poliovirus	live attenuated (Sabin)	3 doses at 2, 3, 4 months	Pre-school and 15–18 years
MMR	Measles	live attenuated	12–15 months	
	Mumps	live attenuated		
	Rubella	live attenuated		
BCG	Tuberculosis	live attenuated	10–14 years	

Vaccines for at-risk groups only

Hepatitis B virus

Nature of vaccine:
Hepatitis B surface antigen i.e. subunit vaccine

Course of vaccination:
3 doses; at 0, 1, 6 monthly intervals

Booster:
at 5 years; earlier if anti-HBs response sub-optimal

Target groups:
health-care personnel
sexually promiscuous
sexual and family contacts of known carriers
newborn of carrier mothers (also given HBIg at birth)
recipients of blood/blood products e.g. haemophiliacs, dialysis patients

Note: anti-HBs response should be checked 2 months after last dose. Non-responders are not protected

Influenza

Nature of vaccine:
killed
contents revised yearly to account for changes in circulating virus
currently must contain A/H1N1, A/H3N2 and B strains

Course of vaccination:
one dose in early winter

Booster:
repeat vaccine annually

Target groups:
1. adults and children with:
   chronic respiratory disease, including asthma
   chronic heart disease
   chronic renal failure
   endocrine disease, including diabetes mellitus
   immunosuppression due to disease or treatment
2. residents of facilities where rapid spread may follow introduction of infection:
   nursing homes
   old people's homes

Pneumococcal vaccine

Nature of vaccine:
capsular polysaccharide from 23 serotypes

Course of vaccination:
one dose

Booster:
repeat after 5–10 years

Target groups: patients with:
1. splenic dysfunction e.g. splenectomy, sickle cell disease
2. chronic disease e.g. diabetes mellitus, lung, heart, renal disease
3. immunosuppression e.g. HIV infection

Varicella vaccine

Nature of vaccine:
live attenuated

Course of vaccination:
single dose

Booster:
not indicated at present

Target groups:
immunosuppressed children

Note: not licensed in UK at present; available on named-patient basis

Rabies vaccine

Nature of vaccine:
whole virus grown in human diploid cells and killed

Course of vaccination:
3 doses at 0, 7, 28 days

Booster:
every 2–3 years if still at risk

Target groups:
occupationally exposed individuals

Note: this is pre-exposure prophylaxis; for post-exposure use see Case 5.

Vaccines primarily for foreign travel
• Vaccines include hepatitis A, rabies, yellow fever, Japanese encephalitis, tick-borne encephalitis, cholera, typhoid, meningococcal meningitis.
• Exact requirements depend on destination, planned activities, level of sanitation.
• Seek expert advice on current indications and administration protocols.

Passive immunisation (i.e. administration of pre-formed antibodies)

Human normal immunoglobulin (HNIg)
derived from normal blood donors, contains antibodies to viruses currently prevalent in the general population
prophylaxis against hepatitis A (decreasing as vaccine is now available)
protection of immunosuppressed children exposed to measles

Hepatitis B immunoglobulin (HBIg)
derived from blood donors with high titres of anti-HBs; provides immediate protection against HBV infection; can be administered simultaneously with vaccine; should be given as soon as possible after exposure to HBV, including (i) infants of carrier mothers, and (ii) individuals with needle-stick injury (post-exposure prophylaxis)

Human rabies immunoglobulin (HRIg)
derived from vaccinees with high titre anti-rabies antibodies
given as post-exposure prophylaxis if high-risk exposure

Varicella-zoster immune globulin (VZIg)
derived from individuals recently recovered from zoster
given to seronegative individuals, at high risk of severe disease after exposure to VZV i.e.
pregnant women; neonates of non-immune mothers, or whose mother develops chicken-pox within the period 7 days prior to birth to 30 days thereafter; immunosuppressed patients

Tetanus immunoglobulin
given within 24 hours to unvaccinated individuals or those whose immune status is unknown following a wound:
with a significant degree of devitalised tissue
puncture-type with contact with soil or manure
with clinical evidence of sepsis

APPENDIX 3
Some of the more commonly used antimicrobial agents

Anti-bacterial agents			
Antimicrobial agent	**Spectrum of activity**	**Side-effects/comment**	**Main therapeutic uses**
Penicillins			
benzylpenicillin	Gram positive bacteria	parenteral administration only	streptococcal infections, syphilis, endocarditis, meningitis
ampicillin	Gram positive bacteria & some GNB	most hospital GNBs resistant	respiratory (RTI) & urinary infections (UTI)
flucloxacillin	staphylococci (most strains of *S. aureus* are pen. amp. resistant)		wound, skin infections etc,
piperacillin/azlocillin	GNB including *Pseudomonas*	parenteral administration only	bacteraemia, pneumonia
Cephalosporins			
cephradine & cephalexin	Gram positive bacteria & GNB	parenteral & oral administration	UTI, soft tissue infections
cefuroxime	better Gram negative activity	parenteral & oral administration	as above plus surg. prophylaxis
cefotaxime	Gram positive bacteria & GNB but not *Pseudomonas*	parenteral only	pneumonia, abdominal sepsis
ceftazidime	Gram positive bacteria & GNB including *Pseudomonas*	parenteral only; reserved for *Pseudomonas*	pneumonia, bacteraemia
cefixime	Gram positive bacteria & GNB but not *Pseudomonas*	oral administration (use in community)	UTI, RTI, soft tissue infections
Other β-lactam agents			
co-amoxyclav (amoxycillin + clavulanic acid)	Gram positive bacteria & GNB (stable to many bacterial β lactamases)	oral & parenteral administration, used in hospital & community	UTI, soft tissue & RTI, surgical prophylaxis
imipenem	Gram positive bacteria & GNB including *Pseudomonas* & some enterococci	2nd or 3rd line agent, e.g. in ITU	polymicrobial/intra-abdominal infection
aztreonam	GNB only	alternative to aminoglycosides	bacteraemia & RTI
Aminoglycosides			
e.g. gentamicin, tobramycin	GNB, staphylococci, inactive against anaerobes, streptococci (when used alone)	renal and VIII cranial nerve toxicity: regular serum levels essential	bacteraemia, complicated UTI, hospital-acquired pneumonia, neutropenic fever, endocarditis (with a penicillin)
Macrolides			
erythromycin	staphylococci, streptococci, *Mycoplasma*, *Chlamydia*, *Legionella*	poor activity against *Haemophilus*, GI side-effects impair compliance	alternative to penicillin if allergic, soft tissue, RTI & genital infections
clarithromycin & azithromycin	above plus some GNB including *Haemophilus influenzae*	new agents; still under clinical evaluation	pneumonia, acute exacerbations of chronic bronchitis (COAD)

Table continued overleaf

Anti-bacterial agents (cont'd)			
Antimicrobial agent	**Spectrum of activity**	**Side-effects/comment**	**Main therapeutic uses**
Quinolones			
nalidixic acid	GNB except *Pseudomonas*	less frequently used now	UTI (urinary antiseptic)
norfloxacin,	GNB including *Pseudomonas*,		UTI,
ciprofloxacin, ofloxacin	variable activity against Gram positive bacteria	affects growing cartilage; use with caution in children	gastroenteritis, traveller's diarrhoea, bacteraemia, hospital-acquired RTI, genital infections
Miscellaneous agents			
trimethoprim	GNB, some activity against Gram positive bacteria, *Pneumocystis carinii**	oral administration; used in hospital & community	UTI, pneumocystis pneumonia
tetracyclines	Gram positive bacteria & GNB, rickettsia (e.g. Q fever), *Chlamydia*	less frequently used now; contra-indicated in childhood	non-gonococcal urethritis, plague, atypical pneumonia
clindamycin	Gram positive bacteria, anaerobes	antibiotic-associated diarrhoea due to *Clostridium difficile*	soft tissue infections, gangrene
rifampicin	mycobacteria, meningococci, staphylococci	rarely used alone; induces liver enzymes	tuberculosis, staphylococcal CNS infections, meningitis prophylaxis
fusidic acid	staphylococci	rarely used alone; cholestatic jaundice with parenteral administration	bone & joint infections
fosfomycin	GNB	widely used in Europe for years	single dose for uncomplicated UTI
metronidazole	anaerobes, protozoa (see below)	oral, parenteral & rectal administration; antabuse reaction with alcohol	surgical infections, antibiotic prophylaxis

*with sulphamethoxazole as co-trimoxazole

Antiviral Agents			
Antimicrobial agent	**Spectrum of activity**	**Side-effects/comment**	**Main therapeutic uses**
Nucleoside analogues			
acyclovir (now available as valacyclovir, a valyl ester with better oral absorption)	herpes simplex (HSV), varicella zoster (VZV). Epstein-Barr & CMV less susceptible	renal dysfunction occasionally, resistance possible	primary HSV – mucosal, keratitis recurrent HSV – prophylaxis other – encephalitis, disseminated primary & recurrent VZV
famciclovir	as for acyclovir	similiar to acyclovir, less frequent doses required	
ganciclovir	herpes viruses, more active against CMV	quite toxic; renal failure, convulsions & bone marrow suppression (e.g. neutropenia)	prophylaxis & treatment of CMV infections in immunocompromised patients
idoxuridine	herpes viruses, less active against CMV	too toxic for systemic use	eye infections; largely superceded by acyclovir
tribavirin (ribavrin)	broad-spectrum i.e. DNA (e.g. herpes) & RNA (e.g. RSV, influenza) viruses	administered by nebuliser for RSV	severe RSV infections rarely, Lassa fever
Reverse transcriptase inhibitors			
zidovudine (AZT)	HIV	bone marrow toxicity, myopathy	prophylaxis & treatment of HIV disease
zalcitabine (DDC)	HIV	neuropathy, pancreatitis	used with AZT
didanosine (DDI)	HIV	neuropathy, pancreatitis	used with AZT
lamivudine (3Tc)	HIV	New drugs currently under trial	
stavudine (d4t)	HIV		
HIV protease inhibitors			
ritonavir	HIV	New drugs currently under trial	
saquinavir	HIV		
indinavir			
Amantanes			
amantadine, rimantadine	influenza A	confusion & CNS stimulation in the elderly	treatment & prevention of influenza
Others			
foscarnet (sodium phosphonoformate)	herpes viruses (DNA polymerase inhibitor)	nephrotoxic	prophylaxis & treatment of CMV infections acyclovir-resistant HSV
Immunomodulators			
interferon (α)	most viruses, modulates inflammatory response	'flu-like' illness, bone marrow suppression	topical (warts), intramuscular (hepatitis B & C)

APPENDIX 3

Antifungal Agents			
Antimicrobial agent	**Spectrum of activity**	**Side-effects/comment**	**Main therapeutic uses**
Polyenes			
nystatin	most fungi		treatment of oral & genital candidiasis
amphotericin B	most fungi, dermatophytes less sensitive	highly protein bound, poor CSF penetration, renal failure, electrolyte disturbances. New preparations less toxic	local administration for UTI & CAPD peritonitis. Intravenous for most systemic fungal infections (1st line agent for aspergillosis)
Imidazoles			
miconazole/clotinagole	most fungi	poor absorption from gut	mucosal and superficial mycoses
ketoconazole	most fungi except aspergillus & mucor	hepatitis (1:10,000), gynaecomastia	chronic mucocutaneous candidiasis, dermatophytosis
itraconazole	most fungi	oral administration only; variable absorption	superficial mycoses, 2nd line agent for systemic fungal infection such as aspergillosis
fluconazole	most fungi except aspergillus	very good tissue penetration; non-albicans candida species may be resistant, few side-effects	superficial candidiasis, 2nd line agent for systemic candida infections, treatment & prevention of cryptococcal disease
Griseofulvin	dermatophytes	oral treatment for at least 3 weeks; concentrates in keratin	hair & nail dermatophyte infections
Flucytosine (5-FC)	yeasts only	bone marrow suppression, liver toxicity, serum levels recommended, penetrates well into CSF	UTI (used alone), with amphotericin B to treat systemic candida & cryptococcal infections
Terbinafine	dermatophytes	good penetration to skin & nails	dermatophytosis

Antiprotozoal & Antihelminth Agents			
Antimicrobial agent	**Spectrum of activity**	**Side-effects/comments**	**Main therapeutic uses**
Antimalarials			
quinine	all 4 plasmodium species	cardiac arrhythmias, especially if used with mefloquine	treatment of complicated or resistant falciparum malaria
chloroquine	hepatic phases	retinopathy; resistance increasing	treatment & prophylaxis of falciparum malaria
pyrimethamine	folate antagonist; active against plasmodia & toxoplasma	marrow depression (e.g. neutropenia)	treatment & prophylaxis of malaria & toxoplasmosis
primaquine	all 4 plasmodium species	marrow depression if G-6-PD deficient	treatment & prophylaxis of malaria
Metronidazole	anti-bacterial (anaerobes) some flagellates, amoebae	antabuse reaction with alcohol; neuropathy following prolonged use	giardiasis, amoebiasis (colitis & hepatic abscesses), trichomonas vaginitis
Sodium stibogluconate	*Leishmania* spp.	anaphylaxis; renal & hepatic toxicity	viscereal, cutaneous, mucosal leishmaniasis; Kala-azar
Praziquantal	trematodes & cestodes	diarrhoea	schistosomiasis, liver & lung fluke, tapeworm infestations (eg cysticercosis)
Mebendazole	broad-spectrum anti-helminth agent	teratogenic	hookworm, roundworm, threadworm & whipworm infestations
GNB: Gram negative bacilli, RTI: respiratory tract infection, G-6-PD: glucose-6-phosphate dehydrogenase			

APPENDIX 4
AIDS defining illnesses (modified from CDC Surveillance Case Definition for AIDS)

Patients with no other cause of immunodeficiency, but without confirmation of HIV infection
- Systemic candidiasis
- Extrapulmonary cryptococcosis
- Cryptosporidiosis > 1 month
- CMV infection of any organ other than liver, spleen, or lymph nodes- in patients > 1 month old
- Prolonged mucocutaneous HSV infection, or HSV pneumonitis or oesophagitis
- Kaposi sarcoma in patients <60 years old
- Primary CNS lymphoma in patients <60 years old
- Lymphoid interstitial pneumonitis in patients <13 years old
- *Mycobacterium avium* complex or disseminated *M. kansasii*
- *Pneumocystis carinii* pneumonia
- Progressive multifocal leukoencephalopathy
- Cerebral toxoplasmosis in patients >1 month old

Known HIV-infected patients
- Recurrent pyogenic bacterial infections in patients >13 years old
- Disseminated coccidioidomycosis
- Disseminated histoplasmosis
- Isosporiasis >1 month duration
- Kaposi sarcoma, any age
- Primary CNS lymphoma, any age
- Non-Hodgkin's lymphoma

- Invasive cancer of the cervix
- Disseminated mycobacterial disease, other than *M. tuberculosis*
- Extrapulmonary or pulmonary *M. tuberculosis*
- Recurrent bacterial pneumonia
- Recurrent *Salmonella septicaemia*
- Oesophageal candidiasis*
- CMV retinitis*
- Lymphoid interstitial pneumonitis in patients <13 years old*
- *Pneumocystis carinii* pneumonia*
- Cerebral toxoplasmosis in patients >1 month old*
- HIV encephalopathy*
- HIV wasting syndrome*
- Multiple pyogenic bacterial infections in patients <13 years old

*Diseases which may be diagnosed presumptively

Note: This case definition may well be altered as the list of diseases recognised as complications of HIV infection increases. Indeed a recent modification to include the presence of a CD4 cell count of less than 200 as an AIDS-defining illness has recently been adopted in the USA. This modification has not, for various reasons, found acceptance in Europe.

Abdomen, specimens, 152, *see also* Hepatic mass
Abendazole, 56
Abortion, *Listeria monocytogenes*, 129, 130
Abscesses
  brain, 7–8
  liver, amoebiasis, 57, 123
  lung, 37
Acanthamoeba, eye, 90
Acid-fast bacilli, 114
Acquired immunodeficiency syndrome, 110–112
  defining illnesses, 160
Acute laryngotracheobronchitis, 18
Acyclovir, 5, 157
  CMV chemoprophylaxis, 127
  derivatives, 88
  herpes simplex virus
    genital infection, 68, 69
    oral infection, 79
  varicella-zoster virus, 88
    pregnancy, 135
Adenoviruses, 90–91, 91
  conjunctivitis, 89, 90–91
  cystitis, 72
  enteric, 41
Adult T-cell leukaemia lymphoma, 142–144
Aerophobia, 11
AIDS, *see* Acquired immunodeficiency syndrome
Airway obstruction, exudative pharyngotonsillitis, 20
Alcohol, metronidazole, 44
α-interferon therapy, 54, 157
α-streptococci, *see* Viridans streptococci
Alzheimer's disease *vs* Creutzfeldt-Jakob disease, 13
Amantadine, 23, 157
  chemoprophylaxis, 26
American trypanosomiasis, 123
Amikacin, serum assays, 46
Aminoglycosides, 155
  and blood-brain barrier, 8
  and renal function, 46–47
Amoebiasis, 44
  liver abscess, 57, 123
Amoxycillin
  central nervous system infections, 8
  chronic bronchitis, 32
  infective endocarditis prophylaxis, 107
  and leg ulcers, 78–79
  otitis media, 16
Amphotericin B, 102, 158
Ampicillin, 155
  chronic bronchitis, 32
  enteric fever, 49
  otitis media, 16
  urinary tract infections, 61
Anaemia, 144–146
  malaria, 108
Anaerobic bacteria, perianal ulcers, 78
Anergy, 117
Anthrax, 78, 94
Anthropophilic dermatophytosis, 75
Antiarrhythmic agents, in tetanus, 9
Antibiotic-associated diarrhoea, 40, 47, 149
Antibiotic resistance, *Haemophilus influenzae*, 16
Antibiotics, 155–156, *see also* Chemoprophylaxis
  bacteraemia, 100
  brain abscess, 7–8

cholera, 58
common cold, 17
cystic fibrosis, 36
food poisoning, 40
infective endocarditis, 105
meningococcal meningitis, 2–3
in MMR vaccine, 86
osteomyelitis, 120
peritonitis, 46
pneumonia, 27
post-surgical infection, 101
toxic shock syndrome, 92
Antibodies
  toxic shock syndrome, 93
  viral hepatitis, 52
  VZV, placental transfer, 135
Antidiarrhoeal agents, 40
Antifungal agents, 158
Antigenic drift and shift, 24–25
Antihelminthics, 159
Anti-HIV testing, 70
Antihyaluronidase titre, 84
Antimalarials, 108, 159
Antimony compounds (sodium stibogluconate), 124, 159
Antiprotozoal agents, 159
Antistreptolysin O titre, 84
Antiviral agents, 157
Aortic valve, endocarditis, 105
Aplastic crisis, 145–146
Apnoeic attacks, 33
Arterial disease, ulcers, 78
Arthralgia, 148
  parvovirus B19, 145
Arthropathies, enteropathic, 148
Arthropod-borne infections, 122, 123
  viruses, encephalitis, 4
Ascaris lumbricoides, 59
Aseptic meningitis, 2
Aspergillosis, 103
Aspirin, 24
Asthma
  colds, 17–18
  vs respiratory syncytial virus, 34
Astroviruses, 41
Ataxia, dementia, 13–14
Athlete's foot, 75–76
Atypical mycobacteria, 115
Atypical pneumonia, 28–30
Auroscopy, otitis media, 15 (Fig.)
Autoimmune diseases, FUO, 117
Azidothymidine, 71, 157
  and HTLV-1, 143
Azithromycin, 155
  chronic bronchitis, 32
Azlocillin, 155
Azoles, 76
Aztreonam, 155

Bacille Calmette-Guérin vaccine, 115, 153
Bacillus cereus, food poisoning, 38, 39
Bacteraemia, 91
  Escherichia coli, 59
  vs septicaemia, 99
Bacterial meningitis, 1–3
Bacterial vaginosis, 67
Bacteriophages, 92
BCG vaccine, 115, 153
Behavioural changes
  herpes simplex encephalitis, 4
  rabies, 11

Benzodiazepines, 9
Benzylpenicillin, 155
    for ophthalmia neonatorum, 133
    streptococci, 82
β-lactams, 16, 155
Bilharzia, 59, 72–73, 122
Biliary tract infections, bacteraemia from, 99
Biofilms, 63
Bismuth compounds, traveller's diarrhoea,
    44
Bites, animals, 10–11
Bladder carcinoma, 72
Blind antibiotic therapy
    meningitis, 3
    otitis media, 16
Blindness, see also Ocular infections
    leprosy, 97
Blisters, 93–94
    genital herpes, 67
Blood-brain barrier, function testing, 5
Blood cultures, 152–153
    candidiasis, 102
    FUO, 117
    infective endocarditis, 104, 153
    pneumonia, 27
    pyelonephritis, 98–99
Blood films, see also Anaemia malaria, 107–108
Bone marrow failure, 144–146
Bone tuberculosis, 115, 120
Bordetella pertussis, 21
Bornholm disease (pleurodynia), 81
Borrelia burgdorferi, 95, see also Lyme
    disease
Botulism, 9
Bovine spongiform encephalopathy, 13, 14
Brain, see also Central nervous system
    abscess, 7–8
    biopsy, herpes simplex encephalitis, 4
Breastfeeding
    HIV infection, 72
    HTLV-1, 143
    protective effects, 42
Bronchiectasis, 35, 36, 37
Bronchiolitis, 32–35
Bronchopneumonia, 26
Bronchoscopy, 153
    Pneumocystis carinii pneumonia, 111
Brucellosis, 118–119
Brugia malayi, 123
Bulbar motor system, 9–10
Burkholderia cepacia
    cystic fibrosis, 36
Burkitt's lymphoma, 20–21

Caesarean section
    genital herpes, 136, 137
    HIV transmission, 71
Caliciviruses, 41
Campylobacter jejuni, food poisoning, 39, 40
Candidiasis, 47, 76
    genital swabs, 152
    systemic, 101–102
    vaginal, 67
Capnocytophaga canimorsus, 83
Caramel-like aroma, Streptococcus milleri,
    7
Carcinoma
    bladder, 72
    cervix, 74
    nasopharyngeal, Epstein-Barr virus, 20
    skin, squamous-cell, 74
Carpets, 150
Carriage
    hepatitis B virus, 53
    latent viruses, 4
    Staphylococcus aureus, 64
        methicillin-resistant, 121
Caseating granulomata, tuberculosis, 114
Casoni test, 56

Catheters, intravascular, 64
CD4-positive lymphocytes, HIV infection, 71,
    112, 160
Cefixime, 155
Cefotaxime, 155
Ceftazidime, 155
Ceftriaxone, Lyme disease, 95
Cefuroxime, 155
Cell cultures, Chlamydia trachomatis, 65
Cellulitis, 81–84
Centers for Disease Control
    AIDS definition, 110, 160
    HIV infection classification, 71
Central lines, see Intravascular line infections
Central nervous system, 1–14
    diseases in AIDS, 112
    infectious mononucleosis, 20
    investigations, 153
    malaria, 108
    mumps virus, 142
    toxoplasmosis, 111
Cephalexin, 155
Cephalosporins, 155
    central nervous system infections, 8
    chronic bronchitis, 32
    peritonitis, 46
    urinary tract infections, 61
Cephradine, 155
Cerebral abscess, 7–8
Cerebral malaria, 108
Cerebral toxoplasmosis, 111
Cerebrospinal fluid
    bacterial meningitis, 2
    herpes simplex encephalitis, 5
    intracranial haemorrhage, 6
Cervical smears, bacteriology, 65
Cervicitis, mucopurulent, 65–67
Cervix
    carcinoma, 74
    herpes simplex virus, 67
Cestodes, 59
Chagas' disease, 123
Chancroid, 69
Chemicals, food poisoning, 39, 43
Chemoprophylaxis
    AIDS patients, 112
    amantadine, 26
    cytomegalovirus, 126–127
    infective endocarditis, 107
    malaria, 109–110
    meningitis, 3
    surgery, 46
    systemic fungal infections, 103
    traveller's diarrhoea, 44
    tuberculosis, 115
Chest X-ray, fine opacities, 113
Chicken-pox, 86-87
    pregnancy, 134–136
Children
    cytomegalovirus, 126
    FUO, 117
    and tetracyclines, 16
Chlamydia spp., pneumonia, 29
Chlamydia trachomatis, 65, 66
    eye, 89, 134
    genital swabs, 152
    neonates, 128, 129, 133
Chloramphenicol
    central nervous system infections, 8
    enteric fever, 49
    for ophthalmia neonatorum, 133
Chloroquine, 108, 109–110, 159
Cholera, 57–58
    prevention, 44
Chronic active hepatitis, 54
Chronic bronchitis, 30–32
    colds, 17–18
Chronic obstructive airways disease, 31
Chronic suppurative otitis media, 16
Ciliation, 24

Ciprofloxacin, 156
    chronic bronchitis, 32
    enteric fever, 49
    Pseudomonas aeruginosa, 37
    traveller's diarrhoea, 45
    urinary tract infections, 61
Clarithromycin, 155
    chronic bronchitis, 32
Clavulanic acid, 16, see also Co-amoxyclav
Clindamycin, 156
    infective endocarditis prophylaxis, 107
    malaria, 108
Clofazimine, 97
Close contacts, meningitis, 3
Clostridium difficile, antibiotic-associated
    diarrhoea, 40, 47, 149
Clostridium perfringens, food poisoning, 39
Clostridium tetani, see Tetanus
'Clue' cells, 67
Coagulase negative staphylococci, 64
Co-amoxyclav, 155
    chronic bronchitis, 32
    leg ulcers, 79
    urinary tract infections, 61
Coccidioidomycosis, 103
Cold sores, 4, 79
    and genital herpes, 68
Coliforms, neonates, 128
Colistin, nebulized, 37
Colloidal amphotericin B, 102
Colorado tick fever, 95
Combination antimicrobial chemotherapy,
    cystic fibrosis, 36
Common cold, 17–18
Communicable Disease Surveillance Centre,
    147
Community-acquired pneumonia, organisms,
    27
Complement fixation tests
    cytomegalovirus, 138
    varicella-zoster virus, 125
Computed tomography
    brain abscess, 7
    cerebral toxoplasmosis, 111
    encephalitis, 5
Condylomata acuminata, 74
Congenital cytomegalovirus infection,
    138–139
Congenital heart disease, brain abscess
    organisms from, 8
Congenital rubella syndrome, 131–132
Congenital toxoplasmosis, 140
Congenital varicella syndrome, 134
Conjugated polysaccharide vaccine,
    Haemophilus influenzae type b, 3, 153
Conjunctivitis, 89–90
    enteroviruses, 81, 89
Connective tissue diseases, FUO, 117
Consciousness, disturbance, 1–6
Consultants for Communicable Disease
    Control, 147
Contact lenses, 90
Contacts
    hepatitis B, 53
    Lyme disease, 95–96
    meningitis, 3
    rubella, 132
    sexually transmitted diseases, 66
Continuous ambulatory peritoneal dialysis,
    62–64
Core antigen, hepatitis B, 53
Corneal impressions, rabies, 12
Corneal lesions, 89–90
Coronaviruses, 17
Cor pulmonale, schistosomiasis, 73
Coryza, 17–18
Co-trimoxazole, 156
    brucellosis, 119
    methicillin-resistant S. aureus, 121
    Pneumocystis carinii pneumonia, 111

Co-trimoxazole (contd)
traveller's diarrhoea, 44, 45
Cough
croup, 18
paroxysmal, 21–22
Coxiella burnettii, pneumonia, 29
Coxsackieviruses, 80
C-reactive protein, infective endocarditis, 105
Creutzfeldt-Jakob disease, 13–14
Crohn's disease, arthropathy, 148
Cross-allergy, cephalosporins, 46
Cross-infection
group A streptococci, 83
methicillin-resistant S. aureus, 121
Salmonella spp., 49
Croup, 18
Cryotherapy, warts, 74
Cryptococcus spp., 103
meningitis, 111
Cryptosporidium spp., 43 (Fig.), 44, 111
Culture-negative endocarditis, 106
Cyclophosphamide, 72
Cycloplegic agents, 89
Cystic fibrosis, 35–37
Cystitis, 60
haemorrhagic, 72–73
Cystoscopy, 62
Cysts, liver, 56
Cytokines, malaria, 108
Cytomegalovirus, 111, 126–127
donor organs, 125
pregnancy, 138–139
Cytopathic effect, respiratory syncytial virus, 33
Cytotoxin-producing Escherichia coli, 44

Dapsone, 97
Dementia, and myoclonic jerks, 12–14
Dengue haemorrhagic fever, 147
Dental care, chemoprophylaxis, 107
Dental sepsis, brain abscess organisms from, 8
Dental workers, herpetic whitlow, 94
Deoxyribonucleases, streptococci, 82
Dermatophytosis, 75–76
specimens, 76, 153
Desquamation, skin, 92
Detection of early antigen fluorescent foci (DEAFF), cytomegalovirus, 126
Developing countries
enteric fever, 49
immigrants from, 47
measles, 85–86
rotaviruses, 42
schistosomiasis prevention, 73
Diabetes mellitus
and mumps virus, 142
ulcers, 78
Dialysis, 124–125
Diarrhoea, see also Food poisoning; Traveller's diarrhoea
legionnaire's disease, 29
management, 40
rotaviruses, 42
Diazepam, 9
Didanosine, 157
Diphtheria, 19
Direct immunofluorescence, herpes simplex virus, 69
Disinfection, adenoviruses, 90
Disulfiram-like reaction, metronidazole, 44
Dog bites, 10–11, 83
Donor organs, infections, 125
Doxycycline, traveller's diarrhoea, 44
Drug abuse, endocarditis, 106
D/T/P vaccine (triple vaccine), 10, 153
Dumb rabies, 11
Duncan's syndrome, 20
Dysentery, 40

E antigen, hepatitis B, 53–54
Eardrum, otitis media, 15 (Fig.)
Early-onset neonatal infection, Listeria monocytogenes, 129
Ebola disease, 147
Echinococcus granulosus, 56, 59
Echocardiography, vegetations, 104
Echoviruses, 80
Ecthyma gangrenosum, 78
Eczema herpeticum, 79
Eggs
allergy, 86
Salmonella spp., 39
Electrolytes, gastroenteritis, 41
Electron microscopy, gastroenteritis, 41, 149, 152
Elephantiasis, 59
ELISA, viral gastroenteritis, 41
Emboli, infective endocarditis, 106
Emphysema, exacerbations, 31
Empirical antibiotic therapy, see Blind antibiotic therapy
Encephalitis, 3–6
chicken-pox, 86, 87
enteroviruses, 4, 81
measles, 4, 85
mumps virus, 142
pertussis vaccine, 22
postinfectious, 24, 85, 87
rabies vaccine, 12
Endocarditis
Candida spp., 103
coagulase negative staphylococci, 64
Endotoxic shock, 91
Entamoeba histolytica, 43 (Fig.), 44
liver abscess, 57, 123
Enteric fever, 48–50, 122
Enteric spread, viral hepatitis, 51
Enterobacteria, chronic bronchitis, 31
Enterobius vermicularis, 59
Enterococci, 46, 78, 82
urinary tract infections, 47
Enteropathic arthropathies, 148
Enterotoxins, 93
cholera, 57–58
Enteroviruses, 80–81, 91
conjunctivitis, 81, 89
encephalitis, 4, 81
meningitis, 1–2, 81
neonates, 81, 128
Epidemic MRSA (methicillin-resistant S. aureus), 120–122
Epidemic myalgia (pleurodynia), 81
Epidemics, influenza, 24
Epidermodysplasia verruciformis, 74
Epididymitis, mumps, 142
Epithelial cells, urine, 61
Epstein-Barr virus, 19
Erysipelas, 82
Erythema chronicum migrans, 95
Erythema infectiosum, 145
Erythema multiforme, 69
Erythema nodosum leprosum, 96–97
Erythrogenic toxins, group A streptococci, 82
Erythromycin, 46, 155
atypical pneumonia, 29
chronic bronchitis, 32
for ophthalmia neonatorum, 133
whooping cough, 21–22
Escherichia coli, 44, 99
bacteraemia, 59
enterotoxigenic, 39, 44
neonates, 128
meningitis, 1
urinary tract infections, 61
wound infections, 83
Exanthem subitum (roseola infantum), 84
Exudative pharyngotonsillitis, 20
Eye clinics, infection control, 90
Eye infections, see Ocular infections

Face-masks, see Masks
Factitious temperature, 117
Faecal specimens, 152
electron microscopy, 149
encephalitis, 5
food poisoning, 39
Famciclovir, 157
Fasciola hepatica, 59
Female patients, genitourinary medicine clinics, 65–66
Fever
transplant patients, 125–126
of unknown origin, 116–118
5th disease (erythema infectiosum), 145
Filariasis, 123
Fishtank granuloma, 115
FitzHugh—Curtis syndrome, 66
Flaviviruses, 123
Floors, infection control, 150
Flucloxacillin, 155
Fluconazole, 102, 103, 158
Flucytosine, 102, 158
Fluid replacement, 40, 58
Flukes, 59
Focal lesions, herpes simplex encephalitis, 4
Follicle stimulating hormone, prions in, 14
Food-handlers, Salmonella spp., 50
Food hygiene, Listeria monocytogenes, 130
Food poisoning, 38–40, see also Traveller's diarrhoea
Salmonella spp., 39, 40, 49–50
Staphylococcus spp., 39, 93
Foreign bodies, 64
Foreign travel, vaccines, 154
Foscarnet, 157
cytomegalovirus, 111
Fosfomycin, 156
urinary tract infections, 61
Frontal lobe abscess, 8
Fulminant hepatitis, 53
Fundoscopy, FUO, 117
Fungal infections, see also Dermatophytosis
brain abscesses, 8
chemoprophylaxis, 103
liver, 57
FUO, 116–118
Furious rabies, 11
Fusidic acid, 156
methicillin-resistant S. aureus, 121

Gamma streptococci, 82
Ganciclovir, 157
CMV chemoprophylaxis, 127
cytomegalovirus, 111, 126
Gastroenteritis, 38–40, see also Food poisoning
adenoviruses, 90
arthropathy, 148
infants, 41–42
nosocomial infection, 149–151
Gastrointestinal system, 38–59
bacteraemia from infections, 99
normal flora, 45
specimens, 152, see also Faecal specimens
surgical chemoprophylaxis, 46
Genes, isoforms, 14
Genital herpes, 67–69
and encephalitis, 4
pregnancy, 136–137
Genitalia, specimens, 152
Genital warts, 73–74
Genitourinary medicine clinics, 65–66
Genitourinary system, 60–74
laboratory investigations, 152
tuberculosis, 115
Gentamicin
infective endocarditis prophylaxis, 107
with penicillin, 106

Gentamicin (contd)
  peritonitis, 46
  and renal function, 46–47
  serum assays, 46
Geophilic dermatophytosis, 75
Gerstmann-Straussler-Sheinker syndrome, 13
Giant-cell pneumonia, 85
Giardia lamblia, 43 (Fig.), 44
Glandular fever, 18–21, 138
Glomerulonephritis, post-streptococcal, 83
Glue ear, 16
Gonorrhoea, 65, 66
Granuloma inguinale, 69
Granulomata, tuberculosis, 114
Griseofulvin, 76, 158
Growth hormone, prions in, 14

Haemagglutinins, influenza viruses, 24
Haematuria, 104, see also Haemorrhagic
      cystitis
Haemodialysis, 124–125
Haemolysis, Streptococcus spp., 81
Haemolytic anaemia, chronic, 145
Haemolytic-uraemic syndrome, 39
Haemophilus influenzae, 3, 16
  chronic bronchitis, 31
  cystic fibrosis, 36
  eye, 89
  type b, 1
    conjugated polysaccharide vaccine, 3, 153
Haemorrhage, intracranial, 6
Haemorrhagic cystitis, 72–73
Haemorrhagic disease with renal syndrome,
      147
Haemorrhagic necrosis, herpes simplex
      encephalitis, 5
Haemorrhagic varicella, 86
Hairy leukoplakia, oral, 110
Halofantrine, 108
Hand, foot and mouth disease, 80, 81, 94
Hantavirus infections, 147
Headache, progressive, 6–8
Head-boxes, 35
Heaf test, 114
Health-care workers
  Creutzfeldt-Jakob disease, 14
  cytomegalovirus, 139
Helminths, 59
Hepatic failure, schistosomiasis, 73
Hepatic mass, 55–57
Hepatitis
  acute infective, 50–55
  infectious mononucleosis, 20
Hepatitis B immunoglobulin, 154
Hepatitis B vaccine, 54–55, 124, 154
Hepatitis B virus, 51, 52–55
Hepatitis viruses, 51–55
  donor organs, 125
  renal dialysis units, 124–125
  tumours from, 21
Hepatosplenic candidiasis, 103
Herpangina, 81
Herpes simplex virus
  encephalitis, 4, 153
  genital herpes, 67–69
  meningitis, 2
  neonates, 136–137
  ocular infection, 88, 89
  oral infection, 79
  typing, 69
  whitlow, 94
Herpes simplex virus type 2, epidemiology,
      68
Herpesviruses, 4, see also Cytomegalovirus;
      Epstein-Barr virus
Herpes zoster, 87–88
  infants, 134
  pregnancy, 135–136
Heterophile antibodies, 20

Histoplasmosis, 103
HIV infection, 70–73, 110–112, see also
      Acquired immunodeficiency syndrome
  Centers for Disease Control classification,
      71
  donor organs, 125
  seroconverting illness, 19, 70
Hodgkin's disease, 20
Hospital-acquired infections, see Nosocomial
      infections
Human normal immunoglobulin, 154
Human papillomaviruses, 74
  tumour from, 21
Human pituitary-derived growth hormone,
      prions in, 14
Human rabies immunoglobulin, 154
Human T-cell lymphotropic viruses
  type 1, 143–144
    tumour from, 21
  type 2, 144
Hyaluronidase, streptococci, 82
Hydatid disease, 56–57
Hydrophobia, 11
Hypercalcaemia, ATLL, 143
Hypersensitivity reactions, leprosy, 96
Hypoglycaemia, malaria, 108
Hypotension, and rash, 91–93

Iatrogenic transmission, Creutzfeldt-Jakob
      disease, 14
Idoxuridine, 157
IgG antibodies
  vs IgM, rubella, 131, 132
  viral hepatitis, 52
IgM antibodies
  infectious mononucleosis, 20
  viral hepatitis, 52, 53
Imidazoles, 158
Imipenem, 155
Immigrants from developing countries, 47
Immunization, 153–154, see also Vaccines
  and chronic bronchitis, 32
  and cystic fibrosis, 37
  hepatitis B, 54–55
  influenza, 25–26
  rabies, 12
Immunocompromised patient, 58–59
  atypical mycobacteria, 115
  Epstein-Barr virus, 20
  genital herpes, 69
  hepatitis B virus, 53
  herpes simplex virus, 79
  herpes zoster, 88
  parvovirus B19, 146
  pneumonia, 27
  respiratory syncytial virus, 34
  rotaviruses, 42
  superinfections, 47
Immunofluorescence, 33
  direct, herpes simplex virus, 69
  influenza, 23
  Legionella, 29
Immunoglobulins, 154
  rabies, 12
  tetanus, 9, 10
Immunosuppression by measles, 85
Immunotherapy, bacteraemia, 100
Impetigo, 82
Inclusion conjunctivitis (trachoma), 66, 134
Incubation period, rabies, 11
Induced sputum specimens, 111
Infants
  chicken-pox, 135
  cytomegalovirus, 126
  gastroenteritis, 41–42
  herpes zoster, 134
  pneumonia, 32–35
Infection control teams, 149
Infectious mononucleosis, 18–21, 138

Infective endocarditis, 104–107
  blood cultures, 104, 153
  brain abscess organisms from, 8
Infective hepatitis, acute, 50–55
Influenza, 22–26
  vs common cold, 17
  encephalitis, 4
  investigations, 153
  pneumonia, 23, 29
  vaccine, 25, 154
  viruses, 24
Interferon therapy, 54, 157
  warts, 74
Interpandemic epidemic influenza, 24
Intracranial haemorrhage, 6
Intrathecal antibody synthesis, herpes simplex
      encephalitis, 4–5
Intravascular line infections, 64
  bacteraemia from, 99
  candidiasis, 101–102
Intravenous drug abuse, endocarditis, 106
Intravenous urography, 62
Iron overload, yersiniosis, 148
Isoforms, genes, 14
Isolation of patients
  chicken-pox, 87
  lassa fever, 147
  methicillin-resistant S. aureus, 121
  SRSV gastroenteritis, 150
  tuberculosis, 115
Itraconazole, 102, 103, 158

Jaundice, 50–55
Joint implants, chemoprophylaxis, 46
Joints, tuberculosis, 115

Kala azar, 123
Kanamycin, allergy, 86
Katayama fever, 73
Kawasaki syndrome, 91–92
Keratoconjunctivitis, 89–90
Ketoconazole, 76, 158
Klebsiella spp.
  bacteraemia, 99
  urinary tract infections, 61
  wound infections, 83

Laboratory investigations, 152–153
Laboratory technicians, Creutzfeldt-Jakob
      disease, 14
Lag time, AIDS, 70
Lancefield groups, streptococci, 82
Large unclassifiable cells, pregnancy,
      137–138
Laryngotracheobronchitis, acute, 18
Lassa fever, 146–147
Latency
  cytomegalovirus, 125
  herpesviruses, 4, 68
  varicella-zoster virus, 87
Late-onset neonatal infection, Listeria
      monocytogenes, 129
Legionnaire's disease, 29–30
Leg ulcers, 77–79
Leishmaniasis, 123–124
Leprosy, 96–97
Leptospirosis, 91, 118
Leukaemias
  adult T-cell leukaemia lymphoma, 142–144
  chronic, 58–59
Lice, 77
Liposomal amphotericin B, 102
Listeria monocytogenes
  meningitis, 2
  neonates, 128
  pregnancy, 129–130

Liver, see also Hepatitis
    function tests
        chronic active hepatitis, 54
        infectious mononucleosis, 19
    mass, 55–57
Lobar pneumonia, 26–28
Louping ill, 95
Lucio's phenomenon, 97
Lumbar puncture, 1
    for progressive headache, 6
Lung abscess, 37
    brain abscess organisms from, 8
Lyme disease, 95–96, 123
Lymphadenopathy, 18–21
    mycobacteria, 115
Lymphocytosis, infectious mononucleosis, 19
Lymphogranuloma venereum, 69
Lymphomas
    adult T-cell leukaemia lymphoma, 142–144
    Epstein-Barr virus, 20–21
    non-Hodgkin's lymphoma, 118
Lysis centrifugation, 102

Macrolides, 155
Mad cow disease (BSE), 13, 14
Magnetic resonance imaging, cerebral
        toxoplasmosis, 111
Malaria, 48, 107–110, 122, 123, 147
    and Burkitt's lymphoma, 21
    investigations, 153
Male patients, genitourinary medicine clinics,
        65–66
Malignant disease (neoplasms), see also
        Carcinoma; Leukaemias; Lymphomas
    AIDS, 112
    FUO, 117
Malignant otitis externa, 15
Malignant pustule, 78
Marburg disease, 147
Markers, hepatitis B, 53–54
Masks
    methicillin-resistant S. aureus, 121
    TB nursing, 115
Mass, hepatic, 55–57
Mastoiditis, 16
    brain abscess organisms from, 8
Measles, 84–85
    conjunctivitis, 89
    encephalitis, 4, 85
Mebendazole, 159
Mediterranean spotted fever, 95
Mefloquine, 108, 110
Meningitis bacterial, 1–3
    Cryptococcus spp., 111
    enteroviruses, 1–2, 81
    investigations, 153
    mumps, 2, 142
    tuberculosis, 2, 115
Menstruation, toxic shock syndrome, 92–93
Mesenteric adenitis, 148
Metastatic infection, infective endocarditis,
        106
Methicillin-resistant Staphylococcus aureus,
        120–122
Metronidazole, 44, 156, 159
    central nervous system infections, 8
    peritonitis, 46
Miconazole, 158
Microbiology laboratory, rational use, 152–153
Microsporum infection, 76
Micturating cystourethrography, 62
Miliary tuberculosis, 113, 122
MMR vaccine, 85–86, 131, 132, 142, 153
Monoclonal antibodies, virus
        immunofluorescence, 33
Monospot test, 19–20, 138
Moraxella catarrhalis, 32
    chronic bronchitis, 31
Mortality, pneumococcal pneumonia, 27

Mosquitoes, 109
Motor system, 9–10
    herpes zoster, 88
Mucopurulent cervicitis, 65–67
Multi-dose vials, 90
Multiorgan failure, 46
Multiresistant Staphylococcus aureus, 120–122
Mumps, 141–142
    encephalitis, 4
    meningitis, 2, 142
Mupirocin, 64, 121
Murmurs, 104
Muscle weakness, 9
Mycobacterium avium complex disease, 111
Mycobacterium leprae, 96–97
Mycobacterium spp., 114, 115, see also
        Tuberculosis
Mycoplasma pneumoniae, 27, 29
    chronic bronchitis, 31
    infants, 33
Myocarditis
    enteroviruses, 81
    influenza, 24
Myoclonic jerks, and dementia, 12–14

Nailbiting, 94
Nalidixic acid, 61, 156
NANB hepatitis, 51
Nasopharyngeal aspirates, 33, 153
Nasopharyngeal carcinoma, Epstein-Barr
        virus, 20
Nebulized colistin, 37
Necrotizing fasciitis, 83
Needlestick incidents
    herpetic whitlow, 94
    HIV, 70
Negri bodies, 12
Neisseria gonorrhoeae, 65, 66
    eye, 90
    genital swabs, 152
    neonates, 128, 133
Neisseria meningitidis, 1, 2
    rash, 91
Neisseria spp., vs Moraxella catarrhalis, 32
Nematodes, 59
Neomycin, allergy, 86
Neonates, 128–130, see also Ophthalmia
        neonatorum
    anti-HIV, 72
    bacterial meningitis, 1
        Salmonella spp., 39
    chicken-pox, 134
        pneumonia, 87
    enteroviruses, 81, 128
    hepatitis B prophylaxis, 55
    herpes simplex virus, 136–137
    ophthalmia neonatorum, 133–134
    tetanus, 10
Neoplasms, see Carcinoma; Leukaemias;
        Lymphomas; Malignant disease
Netilmicin, serum assays, 46
Neuraminidase, influenza viruses, 24
Nitrofurantoin, 61
Non-Hodgkin's lymphoma, 118
Non-specific urethritis, 66
Non-specific vaginitis, 67
Norfloxacin, 156
    urinary tract infections, 61
Norwalk viruses (small round structured
        viruses), 41, 149–151
    food poisoning, 38–39
Nosocomial infections
    adenoviral conjunctivitis, 90
    gastroenteritis, 42, 149–151
    Legionella, 30
    methicillin-resistant S. aureus, 121
    pneumonia, organisms, 27
    respiratory syncytial virus, 34
    tuberculosis, 115

viral hepatitis, 124–125
Nystatin, 158

Ocular infections, 89–91
    herpes simplex virus, 88, 89
Ofloxacin, 156
    chronic bronchitis, 32
Oka strain, varicella-zoster vaccine, 88
Old people's homes, influenza immunization,
        25–26
Omsk haemorrhagic fever, 95
Onchocerciasis, 59, 90
Oncogenic viruses, Epstein-Barr virus, 20–21
Onychomycosis, 76
Oophoritis, mumps, 142
Open tuberculosis, 114–115
Ophthalmia neonatorum, 133–134
Ophthalmic infections, see Fundoscopy;
        Ocular infections
Opportunistic infections, see also
        Immunocompromised patient
    AIDS, 111–112
    Mycobacterium spp., 115
Oral hairy leukoplakia, 110
Oral ulcers, 79–81
Orchitis, mumps, 141–142
Orf, 93–94
Organ transplantation, 125–127
Osteomyelitis, 119–120
Otitis externa, 15
Otitis media, 15–16
    brain abscess organisms from, 8
    colds, 17
    meningitis, 2 (Fig.)
    respiratory syncytial virus, 34
Otoscopy, otitis media, 15 (Fig.)

P24 antigen, 71
Pancreatitis, mumps virus, 142
Pandemic influenza, 24
Papillomas, 74
Papovaviruses, 74
Paraesthesia, rabies, 10
Parainfluenza virus, 33
Paralysis
    Clostridium spp., 9
    rabies, 11
Parapox viruses, 94
Paratyphoid fever, 48, 122
Parenteral spread, viral hepatitis, 51
Parotitis, mumps virus, 142
Parvovirus B19, 130–131, 132, 145–146
Passive immunization, 154
Pasteurella multocida, 83
Paul Bunnell test, 19–20, 138
Pelvic inflammatory disease, 66
    herpes simplex virus, 68
Penicillin, see also Benzylpenicillin
    central nervous system infections, 8
    with gentamicin, 106
    meningococcal meningitis, 2–3
    after splenectomy, 119
    streptococcal sore throat, 19
    tetanus, 10
Penicillin allergy, 46
Penicillins, 155
Penicillin V, and otitis media, 16
Pentavalent antimony compounds (sodium
        stibogluconate), 124, 159
Perianal ulcers, anaerobic bacteria, 78
Pericarditis, enteroviruses, 81
Peritonitis, 45–47
    Candida spp., 103
    continuous ambulatory peritoneal dialysis,
        62–64
Permethrin, 76
Pernasal swabs, whooping cough, 153
Persistent generalized lymphadenopathy, 110

Pertussis, 21–22, 153
Peru, cholera, 57
Petechiae, meningococcal meningitis, 1
Phage typing, 92
Pharyngitis, 18
Pharyngoconjunctival fever, 90
Pharyngotonsillitis, exudative, 20
Piperacillin, 155
Pituitary-derived growth hormone, prions in, 14
Pityriasis versicolor, 76
Placental transfer
    hepatitis antigens, 52
    VZV antibodies, 135
Plasmodium spp., 107–109
Pleurodynia, 81
Pneumococcal vaccine, 154
    and cystic fibrosis, 37
Pneumocystis carinii pneumonia, 111
    chemoprophylaxis, 112
Pneumonia
    adenoviruses, 90
    atypical, 28–30
    chicken-pox, 86, 87, 134
    infants, 32–35
    from influenza, 23, 29
    lobar, 26–28
    measles, 85
Podophyllin, 74
Poliomyelitis, 81
Poliovirus vaccines, 80–81, 153
Polyarthralgia, 148
Polymerase chain reaction
    candidiasis, 102
    herpes simplex virus, 6
    human papillomavirus, 74
Polymyxin E, 37
Polyomaviruses, cystitis, 72
Pontiac fever, 30
Postherpetic neuralgia, 88
Postinfectious encephalitis, 24, 85, 87
Postpartum period
    hepatitis B prophylaxis, 55
    meningitis, 2
Post-primary tuberculosis, 113
Post-streptococcal glomerulonephritis, 83
Post-surgical infections, 101–103
    wound infections, 83
Poultry, *Salmonella* spp., 39
Pox viruses, orf, 94
Praziquantel, 56, 73, 159
Pre-emptive therapy, cytomegalovirus, 127
Pregnancy
    chicken-pox, 134–136
        pneumonia, 87
    cytomegalovirus, 138–139
    genital herpes, 136–137
    halofantrine, 108
    herpes zoster, 135–136
    HIV transmission, 71–72
    large unclassifiable cells, 137–138
    Listeria monocytogenes, 129–130
    meningitis, 2
    parvovirus B19, 145
    rashes, 130–132
Pressure sores, 78
Primaquine, 108, 159
Primary tuberculosis, 113
Prions, prion diseases, 13–14
Progressive multifocal leukoencephalopathy, 111
Prophylaxis, *see* Chemoprophylaxis;
    Immunization; Vaccines
Prostheses, coagulase negative
    staphylococci, 64
Prosthetic valve endocarditis, 106
Prostitutes, sexually transmitted diseases, 64–67
Proteus spp.
    skin, 78
    urinary tract infections, 61

PrP gene, Creutzfeldt-Jakob disease, 14
Pseudomonas aeruginosa, 36, 37
    bacteraemia, 99
    ecthyma gangrenosum, 78
    eye, 90
    otitis externa, 15
    urinary tract infections, 61
    wound infections, 83
Pseudomonas cepacia, cystic fibrosis, 36
Pseudomonas spp., neonates, 128
Psoriasis-associated joint disease, 148
Pulmonary function tests, bronchiectasis, 35
PUO (FUO), 116–118
Purpuric rash, meningococcal meningitis, 1, 3
Pus specimens, 45
Pyaemia, 99
Pyelonephritis, 60, 98–99
Pyrimethamine, 159
Pyrimethamine-sulfadoxine, 108

Q fever, 118
Quartan malaria, 109
Quinine, 108, 159
Quinolones, 156
    CAPD peritonitis, 63
    traveller's diarrhoea, 44
Quinsy, 82

Rabies, 10–12
    human immunoglobulin, 154
    vaccine, 12, 154
    virus particle, 12
Rapid diagnostic techniques, cytomegalovirus, 126
Rashes, 84–88
    and hypotension, 91–93
    meningitis, 1–3
    non-bacterial skin infections, 76–77
    parvovirus B19, 145
    pregnancy, 130–132
    schistosomiasis, 73
Reactive arthropathies, 148
Recurrence, genital herpes, 68–69
Red blood cells, malaria, 108
Reiter's disease, 66, 72, 148
Rejection episodes, transplant patients, 125–126
Relapsing fever, 95
Renal dialysis, 124–125
Renal failure, *see also* Haemorrhagic disease
    with renal syndrome
    malaria, 108
Renal function, aminoglycosides, 46–47
Respiratory syncytial virus, 33–35
Respiratory tract infections, 15–37
    adenoviruses, 90
    AIDS, 110–111
    atypical mycobacteria, 115
    bacteraemia from, 99
    classification, 17
    enteroviruses, 81
    investigations, 153
Retinochoroiditis, and toxoplasmosis, 140
Retroviruses, 71, 103, *see also* HIV infection
Reverse transcriptase, 71
Rheumatic fever, 83
Rhinoviruses, 17
Ribavirin, 23, 157
    adenovirus infections, 91
    lassa fever, 147
    respiratory syncytial virus, 35
Rickettsiae, 123
    fevers, 92, 122
    pneumonia, 29
Rifampicin, 156
    leprosy, 97
    methicillin-resistant *S. aureus*, 121

Rimantadine, 23, 157
Ringworm, 76
River blindness, 90
Rocky Mountain spotted fever, 92
Roseola infantum, 84
Rose spots, 48
Rotaviruses, 42
Roundworms, 59
Rubella, 130–132
    arthralgia, 148
    encephalitis, 4
    vs measles, 84

Sabin vaccine, 80
Sacral nerve roots, herpes simplex virus, 68
Salk vaccine, 80
Salmonella spp., 49–50
    food poisoning, 39, 40
Scabies, 76
Scalded skin syndrome, 93
Scars, tingling, 10–11
Schistosomiasis, 59, 72–73, 122
Scintigraphy, urinary tract infections, 62
Scrapie, 13
Scrapings, skin infections, 153
Screening
    cytomegalovirus, 139
    human papillomavirus, 74
    methicillin-resistant *S. aureus*, 122
    renal dialysis patients, 124
    toxoplasmosis, 140
Seizures, brain abscess, 8
Sepsis syndrome, 99
Septicaemia
    vs bacteraemia, 99
    meningococcal, 1, 3
    Salmonella spp., 39
Septic arthritis, 120, 148
Septic screen, 101, 128
Septic shock, 99–100
Seroconverting illness, HIV infection, 19, 70
Serology, 153
Serum bactericidal test, 105
Sexual abuse, herpes simplex virus typing, 69
Sexual intercourse
    cystitis, 72
    HIV transmission risk, 71
Sexually transmitted diseases, 60, 64–67
    serum samples, 152
Sheep, 56, 93–94
Shigellosis, 40
Shingles, *see* Herpes zoster
Silver nitrate, ophthalmia neonatorum, 133
Sinusitis
    acute, 17
    brain abscess, 7
        organisms from, 8
    6th disease (roseola infantum), 84
Skin, 75–97
    atypical mycobacteria, 115
    bacteria, 64, 77–78
    biopsy, rabies, 12
    desquamation, 92
    investigations, 152–153
    methicillin-resistant *S. aureus*, 121
    squamous-cell carcinoma, 74
Skin tests, FUO, 117
Slapped-cheek syndrome (erythema infectiosum), 145
Slow infections, 13–14
Small round (featureless) viruses, 41
Small round structured viruses, *see* Norwalk viruses
Smoking, chronic bronchitis, 31
Sodium stibogluconate, 124, 159
Solitary ulcers, genitalia, 69
Sore throat, 17
    pharyngitis, 18

Specimens, 152–153
  CAPD, 63
  dermatophytosis, 76, 153
  HIV infection, 70
  peritonitis, 45
  viral hepatitis, 52
Spleen
  infectious mononucleosis, 20
  leishmaniasis, 124
Splenectomy, 119
  Streptococcus pneumoniae vaccination, 28
Spongiform encephalopathies, 13–14
Sputum specimens, 31, 153
  induced, 111
Squamous-cell carcinoma, skin, 74
Staphylococcus aureus
  bacteraemia, 99
  carriage, 64
  chronic bronchitis, 31
  cystic fibrosis, 36
  methicillin-resistant, 120–122
  neonates, 128
  otitis media, 16
  sticky eye, 89, 133
  toxic shock syndrome, 92, 93
  wound infections, 83, 119–122
Staphylococcus epidermidis, 64
  CAPD peritonitis, 63
  neonates, 128
  wound infections, 83
Staphylococcus saprophyticus, urinary tract
    infections, 61
Staphylococcus spp.
  bacteraemia, 91
  coagulase-negative, bacteraemia, 99
  endocarditis, 105, 106
  food poisoning, 39, 93
  urinary tract infections, 61
Stevens-Johnson syndrome, 91
Stool, *see* Faecal specimens
Streptococcus agalactiae, 82
Streptococcus milleri (*S. anginosus*), 82
  brain abscess, 7
Streptococcus mitis, 105
Streptococcus pneumoniae, see also
    Pneumococcal vaccine
  bacteraemia, 99
  chronic bronchitis, 31
  eye, 89
  meningitis, 1, 2
  pneumonia, 27
Streptococcus pyogenes, 82
Streptococcus spp., 81–84, *see also*
    Enterococci
  bacteraemia, 91
  endocarditis, 105, 106
    β-haemolytic, 82
    group A, 82, 83–84
    group B, 1, 92, 93, 128
  otitis media, 16
  sore throat, 19
Streptokinase, 82
Streptolysins, 82
Streptomycin, and brucellosis, 119
Stridor, 18
Strongyloides stercoralis, 59
Subacute bacterial endocarditis, 105
Subacute sclerosing panencephalitis, 85
Sudden infant death syndrome, 33
Superantigens, 93
Superinfections, 47
Suppurative otitis media, chronic, 16
Surgical debridement, 120
Surgical wounds, 83
Surrogate markers
  HBsAg carriers, 54
  HIV infection, 71
Surveillance cultures, neonatal HSV,
    136–137
Swimmer's itch, 73

Sylvatic rabies, 12
Syphilis, 65
  skin, 78
Systemic infections, 98–127
  investigations, 153

Taenia solium, 59
Tampons, 92, 93
Tapeworms, 59
Target lesions, orf, 94
Teicoplanin, methicillin-resistant *S. aureus*,
    121
Temporal lobe
  abscess, 8
  herpes simplex encephalitis, 4, 5
Tenckhoff catheter, 62–63
Terbinafine, 76, 158
Terminal ileitis, 148
Tertian malaria, 109
Testis, mumps, 141–142
Tetanospasmin, 9–10
Tetanus, 9–10
  immunoglobulin, 154
Tetracycline, 75, 156
  atypical pneumonia, 29
  and children, 16
  brucellosis, 118–119
  chronic bronchitis, 32
  malaria, 108
  non-gonococcal urethritis, 66
  Q fever, 118
Thick and thin blood films, 107–108
Throat swabs, 153
  encephalitis, 5
Thrush, 47
Tick-borne diseases, 95–96
Tick-borne encephalitis, 95
Tinea (dermatophytosis), 75–76
  specimens, 153
Tine test, 114
Tingling of wound, 10
Tissue biopsy, 153
  candidiasis, 102
Tissue invasion, food poisoning, 38–39
Tobramycin, serum assays, 46
Tonsillitis, 82
Toxic shock syndrome, 92–93
Toxins, food poisoning, 38–39
Toxocara canis, 59
Toxoid, tetanus, 10
Toxoplasma latex test, 138
Toxoplasmosis, 139–140
  cerebral, 111
Trachoma, 66, 134
Transient flora, skin, 77–78
Transmissible dementias, 13–14
Transplants, 125–127
Transport media, 133
Trauma, *see also* Wound infections
  brain abscess organisms from, 8
  herpes zoster, 88
Traveller's diarrhoea, 43–45, *see also* Food
    poisoning
Trematodes, 59
Triazoles, 102
Tribavirin, *see* Ribavirin
Trichomoniasis, 67
  genital swabs, 152
Trimethoprim, 156
  chronic bronchitis, 32
  urinary tract infections, 61
Triple vaccine, 10, 153
Tropical spastic paraparesis, 143–144
Trypanosomiasis, 123
  American, 123
Tuberculin skin test, 114
Tuberculoid leprosy, 97
Tuberculosis, 113–115, 118, 122
  meningitis, 2, 115

osteomyelitis, 120
  skin, 78
  sputum specimens, 153
  urine specimens, 152
Tumorigenic viruses, Epstein-Barr virus,
    20–21
Tumour necrosis factor-α, malaria, 108
Tympanic membrane, otitis media, 15 (Fig.)
Typhoid fever, 48–50, 122
Typhus, 122, 123

Ulcerative colitis, arthropathy, 148
Ulcers
  leg, 77–79
  oral, 79–81
  solitary, genitalia, 69
Ultrasound
  liver mass, 56
  urinary tract infections, 62
Upper respiratory tract infections, 17
  adenoviruses, 90
Urabe strain, mumps vaccine, 142
Urban rabies, 12
Urethral syndrome, 62
Urinary tract infections, 60-62, 72–73, 98–100
  Candida spp., 103
  enterococci, 47
Urine
  FUO, 117
  laboratory investigations, 152
  microscopy, 60–61
Urinogenital system, *see* Genitourinary
    system

Vaccines
  BCG, 115
  cholera, 58
  enteric fever, 49
  Haemophilus influenzae type b, 16
  hepatitis B, 54-55, 124, 154
  influenza, 25, 154
  for meningitis, 3
  MMR (measles, mumps, rubella), 85–86,
      131, 132, 142
  pertussis, 22
  polioviruses, 80–81, 153
  rabies, 12, 154
  splenectomy, 119
  Streptococcus pneumoniae, 27–28, 154
  tetanus, 10
  triple, 10, 153
  varicella-zoster virus, 88, 154
Vagina
  infections, 67
  swabs, 152
Vancomycin, methicillin-resistant *S. aureus*,
    121
Varicella-zoster immunoglobulin, 135, 154
Varicella-zoster virus, 86–88
  encephalitis, 4
  organ transplantation, 125
  pregnancy, 134–136
  vaccines, 88, 154
Varicose ulcers, 77–78
Vascular grafts, coagulase negative
    staphylococci, 64
Vasculitis, leprosy, 97
Vegetations, echocardiography, 104
Venous ulcers, 77–78
Ventricular shunts, coagulase negative
    staphylococci, 64
Verrucas, 74
Vertical transmission of viruses, 139
  HIV, 71–72
  HTLV-1, 143
Vesicles, 93–94
  fluid virology, 68
  genital herpes, 67

Vibrio cholerae, 57–58
Viral haemorrhagic fevers, 146
Viral hepatitis, 50–55
  renal dialysis units, 124
Viral pneumonia, 23
Viridans streptococci, 82
  bacteraemia, 99
Viruses
  chronic bronchitis, 31
  conjunctivitis, 89
  encephalitis, 4
  gastroenteritis, 41, 149–150
  meningitis, 1–2
  rashes, 77
  vertical transmission, 139
Visceral leishmaniasis, 123

Warts, 73–74
Water-borne pathogens, 40, *see also*
    Legionnaire's disease; Schistosomiasis
  Vibrio cholerae, 58
Water systems, *Legionella*, 30
Weil's disease, 118
West Africa, 47, 146
Whitfield's ointment, 76
Whitlow, herpes simplex virus, 94
Whooping cough, 21–22, 153
Widal test, 48
Window period, AIDS, 70
Wood's light, ringworm, 76
World Health Organization, rabies
    immunization, 12
Wound debridement, 10

Wound infections, 83, 119–122
Wound swabs, 152
Wuchereria *bancrofti*, 59, 123

X-linked lymphoproliferative syndrome, 20

Yellow fever, 51, 123, 147
Yersinia spp., 148–149

Zalcitabine, 157
Zidovudine, *see* Azidothymidine
Zoonoses, 116
Zoophilic dermatophytosis, 75